Procedures for

Primary Care Pediatricians

Procedures for

Primary Care Pediatricians

Julius G. Goepp, M.D.

Associate Professor of Emergency Medicine and Pediatrics
Director, Pediatric Emergency Medicine
University of Rochester School of Medicine and Dentistry
Rochester, New York

Mark A. Hostetler, M.D., M.P.H.

Instructor, Department of Pediatrics
Division of Emergency Medicine
Instructor, Division of Emergency Medicine
Washington University School of Medicine
St. Louis Children's Hospital
St. Louis, Missouri;
Former Assistant Professor of Emergency Medicine and Pediatrics
Associate Director, Pediatric Emergency Medicine
Vanderbilt University School of Medicine
Nashville, Tennessee

Mosby

A Harcourt Health Sciences Company

St. Louis London Philadelphia Sydney Toronto

Mosby
A Harcourt Health Sciences Company

Publisher: Richard Zorab
Editor: Elizabeth M. Fathman
Developmental Editor: Ellen Baker Geisel
Project Manager: Carol Sullivan Weis
Production Editor: Karen M. Rehwinkel
Designer: Mark A. Oberkrom

NOTICE

Pharmacology is an ever-changing field. Standard safety precautions must be followed, but as new research and clinical experience broaden our knowledge, changes in treatment and drug therapy may become necessary or appropriate. Readers are advised to check the most current product information provided by the manufacturer of each drug to be administered to verify the recommended dose, the method and duration of administration, and contraindications. It is the responsibility of the licensed prescriber, relying on experience and knowledge of the patient, to determine dosages and the best treatment for each individual patient. Neither the publisher nor the editor assumes any liability for any injury and/or damage to persons or property arising from this publication.

Mosby Inc.
A Harcourt Health Sciences Company
11830 Westline Industrial Drive
St. Louis, Missouri 63146

Printed in the United States of America

Library of Congress Cataloging-in-Publication Data

Procedures for primary care pediatricians / [edited by] Julius G. Goepp, Mark A. Hostetler.
p. ; cm.
Includes bibliographical references and index.
ISBN 0-323-00908-5
1. Pediatrics. 2. Primary care (Medicine) 3. Pediatric emergencies. I. Goepp, Julius G. II. Hostetler, Mark A.
[DNLM: 1. Pediatrics—methods. 2. Emergencies—Child. 3. Primary Health Care—methods—Child. WS 200 P9628 2001]
RJ47.P76 2001
618.92—dc21 00-052526

01 02 03 04 05 GW/FF 9 8 7 6 5 4 3 2 1

Contributors

Terry A. Adirim, M.D., M.P.H.
Assistant Professor of Pediatrics and Emergency Medicine
George Washington University School of Medicine and Health Sciences
Attending Physician
Department of Emergency Medicine
Children's National Medical Center
Washington, D.C.

Mohamed Badawy, M.D.
Fellow, Pediatric Emergency Medicine
Department of Emergency Medicine
University of Rochester Medical Center
Rochester, New York

Sam Bartle, M.D.
Fellow of Pediatric Emergency Medicine
Department of Pediatrics, Division of Emergency Medicine
University of Alabama at Birmingham
Fellow of Pediatric Emergency Medicine
Department of Emergency Medicine
Children's Hospital of Alabama
Birmingham, Alabama

John T. Benjamin, M.D.
Professor of Pediatrics
Medical College of Georgia
Chief of Medicine
Department of Pediatrics
Children's Medical Center
Augusta, Georgia

Robert J. Berkowitz, D.D.S.
Professor and Chief, Division of Pediatric Dentistry
Eastman Department of Dentistry
University of Rochester School of Medicine and Dentistry
Clinical Service Chief, Pediatric Dentistry
Department of Dentistry
Strong Memorial Hospital
Rochester, New York

David W. Bernard, M.D.
Assistant Professor of Pediatrics
Department of Emergency Medicine
University of Alabama at Birmingham
Attending Physician, Pediatric Emergency Department
Children's Hospital of Alabama
Birmingham, Alabama

Anne F. Brayer, M.D.
Assistant Professor of Emergency Medicine and Pediatrics
Department of Emergency Medicine
University of Rochester School of Medicine and Dentistry
Attending Physician
Department of Pediatric Emergency Medicine
Strong Memorial Hospital
Rochester, New York

Bernard A. Cohen, M.D.
Associate Professor of Pediatrics and Dermatology
Division of Pediatric Dermatology
The Johns Hopkins University School of Medicine
Director of Pediatric Dermatology
The Johns Hopkins Children's Center
Baltimore, Maryland

Colleen O. Davis, M.D.
Associate Professor
Departments of Emergency Medicine and Pediatrics
University of Rochester School of Medicine and Dentistry
Associate Professor
Departments of Emergency Medicine and Pediatrics
Strong Memorial Hospital
Rochester, New York

Ann-Christine Duhaime, M.D.
Associate Professor, Department of Neurosurgery
University of Pennsylvania School of Medicine
Associate Neurosurgeon
Division of Neurosurgery
The Children's Hospital of Philadelphia
Philadelphia, Pennsylvania

Alison Ensor Dunn, M.D.
Resident, Department of Pediatrics
The Johns Hopkins Hospital
Baltimore, Maryland

Robert J. Freishtat, M.D.
Fellow, Pediatric Emergency Medicine
Department of Pediatric Emergency Medicine
Children's Hospital
Washington, D.C.

Julius G. Goepp, M.D.
Associate Professor of Emergency Medicine and Pediatrics
Director, Pediatric Emergency Medicine
University of Rochester School of Medicine and Dentistry
Rochester, New York

Robin R. Hemphill, M.D.
Assistant Professor
Department of Emergency Medicine
Vanderbilt University Medical Center
Nashville, Tennessee

Mark A. Hostetler, M.D., M.P.H.
Instructor, Department of Pediatrics
Division of Emergency Medicine
Instructor, Division of Emergency Medicine
Washington University School of Medicine
St. Louis Children's Hospital
St. Louis, Missouri;
Former Assistant Professor of Emergency Medicine and Pediatrics
Associate Director, Pediatric Emergency Medicine
Vanderbilt University School of Medicine
Nashville, Tennessee

Christina M.S. Johns, M.D.
Assistant Professor of Pediatrics
The George Washington University School of Medicine and Health Sciences
Assistant Professor and Attending Physician
Department of Emergency Medicine and Trauma Center
Children's National Medical Center
Washington, D.C.

Sean P. Kelly, M.D.
Department of Emergency Medicine
Vanderbilt University Medical Center
Nashville, Tennessee

Ann M. Lenane, M.D.
Clinical Associate Professor of Emergency Pediatrics
Departments of Emergency Medicine and Pediatrics
University of Rochester
Rochester, New York

James G. Linakis, Ph.D., M.D.
Associate Professor of Pediatrics
Brown University School of Medicine
Associate Director
Department of Pediatric Emergency Medicine
Hasbro Children's Hospital
Rhode Island Hospital
Providence, Rhode Island

Frank A. Maffei, M.D.
Assistant Professor
Departments of Pediatric Critical Care and Emergency Medicine
University of Rochester School of Medicine and Dentistry
Strong Memorial Hospital
Rochester, New York

Andrew K. McVie, M.D.
Department of Emergency Medicine
Vanderbilt University
Nashville, Tennessee

C. Jean Ogborn, M.D.
Assistant Professor of Pediatrics
Division of Pediatric Emergency Medicine
The Johns Hopkins University School of Medicine
Assistant Director of the Pediatric Emergency Department
The Johns Hopkins Children's Center
Baltimore, Maryland

Lynne M. Palmisciano, M.D.
Clinical Teaching Fellow
Department of Pediatrics
Brown University School of Medicine
Fellow, Department of Pediatric Emergency Medicine
Rhode Island Hospital
Hasbro Children's Hospital
Providence, Rhode Island

Sally A. Santen, M.D.
Assistant Professor
Department of Emergency Medicine
Vanderbilt University Medical Center
Nashville, Tennessee

Robert Shapiro, D.D.S.
Associate Professor and Chief
Division of Oral and Maxillofacial Surgery
Eastman Department of Dentistry
University of Rochester School of Medicine and Dentistry
Clinical Service Chief, Oral and Maxillofacial Surgery
Department of Dentistry
Strong Memorial Hospital
Rochester, New York

John C.H. Steele, Jr., M.D., Ph.D.
Professor and Vice Chairman for Academic Affairs
Department of Pathology
Medical College of Georgia
Medical Director of Clinical Microbiology Laboratory
Deputy Director, Clinical Pathology Laboratories
MCG Health, Inc.
Augusta, Georgia

Tamara Thomas, M.D.
Associate Professor
Department of Emergency Medicine
Loma Linda University School of Medicine
Director, International Emergency Medicine
Loma Linda University Medical Center
Loma Linda, California

Gretchen R. Volk, M.D.
Instructor, Emergency Medicine and Pediatrics
Department of Emergency Medicine
Division of Pediatric Medicine
University of Rochester Medical Center
Strong Memorial Hospital
Rochester, New York

Allen Walker, M.D.
Director of Pediatric Emergency Medicine
Assistant Professor of Pediatrics
The Johns Hopkins University School of Medicine
Director of the Pediatric Emergency Department
The Johns Hopkins Children's Center
Baltimore, Maryland

David S. Weisman, M.D.
Assistant Professor
Division of Pediatric Orthopaedics
Department of Orthopaedics
University of Rochester Medical Center
Rochester, New York

Steven J. White, M.D.
Assistant Professor of Emergency Medicine
Vanderbilt University School of Medicine
Nashville, Tennessee

James A. Wilde, M.D.
Assistant Professor of Emergency Medicine and Pediatrics
Medical College of Georgia
Children's Medical Center
Augusta, Georgia

Joseph J. Zorc, M.D.
Assistant Professor of Pediatrics
Department of Pediatrics
University of Pennsylvania School of Medicine
Attending Physician
Department of Emergency Medicine
The Children's Hospital of Philadelphia
Philadelphia, Pennsylvania

To my wife Judy in recognition of her support and encouragement.
JGG

To Garth and Moose for their continued support and dedication.
MAH

Preface

When a physician must perform a medical procedure, even a trivial one, for a young child, there is generally more than enough anxiety to go around. For the child, there is the fear of the unknown, the inevitable loss of control, and the reality of a certain amount of discomfort and even pain. For the parent, there is the tension between wanting to do what is best for the child and wanting to avoid further pain and fear, and the sometimes heartbreaking necessity to collaborate with someone whom the child feels is trying to hurt her. Any decent and sensitive physician feels the anxiety of both the parent and the child. The physician must integrate that feeling with the stresses brought on by the need to do the procedure itself, the desire to do the procedure properly, and the need to help reduce the apprehension of parent and child by providing adequate explanation and comfort throughout.

Although no single book can promise to alleviate all of the anxiety associated with performing procedures in children, we hope in this work to offer the assurance that comes with knowledge and the comfort of familiarity. Procedures in children are generally not technically more difficult than they are in adults, but because of the high emotional stakes they often seem more intimidating. Our goal here is to provide clear and simple instructions to any health care provider who cares for children. For those whose practice is exclusively pediatric, these pages will offer quick refreshers for most procedures and step-by-step guidance for the less common ones. For those who care for children as part of a broader practice (family and emergency medicine physicians, for instance), this book can serve as a convenient reference, offering guidance for procedures with which they are familiar in adults but perform infrequently in children.

The book is designed not only to offer details about *how* to do procedures, but also to offer guidelines about *when* and *why* to do procedures (and occasionally, *when* and *why not* to do them). We believe that this kind of information will go a long way toward making a bearable necessity of medical procedures among children. We have tried to provide concrete instructions where called for, while at the same time offering a variety of options and alternatives to allow each practitioner to customize an approach for each individual child. We have included some information about doing procedures under circumstances in which resources and equipment might be limited. We thought this might be helpful for the large numbers of physicians who do relief work in the developing world or those who practice in underserved areas in the United States. Along those lines, we have included an entire section on travel medicine, to provide information to those who might be planning a trip and anticipate functioning as a physician during the journey. Finally, we have asked all of our authors to provide material for aftercare instructions that may be copied and used as office handouts to help physicians provide accurate and consistent instructions to parents (Appendix B).

Many people have helped in the preparation of this work—our colleagues who have chosen to contribute chapters; our residents and fellows, who helped us to see which kinds of information needed to be included; and our long-suffering secretarial staffs, who managed to keep the production process more or less on schedule. We especially wish to thank Mohani Ramphal, who has been intimately involved in every detail of this project and has suffered through it from its inception to this final stage with grace, good humor, and skill.

Julius G. Goepp
Mark A. Hostetler

Contents

Procedures for

Primary Care Pediatricians

CHAPTER 1

General Approach to Pediatric Office Procedures

Julius G. Goepp

This book is intended for anyone who provides medical care to children. It is meant to be particularly useful for practitioners in a primary care setting, and thus might be considered especially appropriate for pediatricians, family practitioners, and nurse practitioners in such environments. It should be equally helpful, however, for practitioners of general emergency medicine who are responsible for the care of young patients in a community hospital emergency department. Many of the procedures we describe herein might be considered fairly advanced and would not be attempted in many practitioners' offices. We include such procedures because most practitioners find themselves, at some point, caring for an acutely ill or injured child in a hospital or clinic setting where a good outcome may hinge on their ability to perform a procedure that they have not done in quite some time. Finally, we expect that this book may help primary care practitioners who wish to educate parents about procedures that may be done for their children on referral to a tertiary care medical center.

My co-editor and I have had experience providing medical care in the developing world and in remote and rural settings in the United States. Therefore we have chosen to include lists of equipment that might be considered "bare minimums" for performing each procedure. We have also asked each author to specify modifications to the technique that might be required under circumstances in which resources (physical and educational) might be limited. Because practitioners are often asked to be official or unofficial medical officers for traveling groups, we have also included an appendix devoted exclusively to the construction of "medical travel kits," with special emphasis on travel to the developing world and remote settings.

We have organized each chapter in a similar format, wherever possible, to create the greatest consistency among chapters on different subjects. Although not every chapter contains every section, we have attempted to include as many of the following sections as possible.

Each chapter begins with a section on *Background and Introduction*. In this section a brief outline of basic concepts and principles is presented, along with any relevant pathophysiology and diagnostic or therapeutic considerations.

The *Relevant Anatomy* section provides a review of the anatomical considerations that are important to the successful performance of each procedure and includes, where necessary, alternative landmarks.

The *Indications* for each procedure are given in the next section. Here practitioners may double-check that they are choosing the appropriate procedure for each given situation. This section may also prove helpful in explaining the rationale for a procedure to parents or guardians.

The next section, *Contraindications and Reasons for Referral to a Specialist,* describes absolute and relative contraindications for each procedure and includes warnings about possible untoward results. Although this book is intended to be comprehensive, situations will inevitably arise in which the complexity of a procedure is too great or multiple attempts will fail, in which case referral to a specialist or a higher-level facility is appropriate. Criteria for making such a decision are offered in this section as well.

For procedures of greater than minimal complexity, a brief description of *Required/Recommended Nursing Skills* is offered. Although seemingly obvious, we believe this section is critical in determining whether a given setting is appropriate for performing each procedure. Practitioners often believe themselves to be adequately trained and qualified to perform a procedure, only to find that the nursing staff has inadequate training or experience to provide much-needed assistance. Nursing skills include not only practical skills but also levels of sophistication sufficient to allow interpretation of monitoring devices, when used.

The section on *Supplies and Equipment* provides an exhaustive listing of those items required to perform each procedure. Each listing is divided into those items that are absolutely necessary to perform the procedure and those that are "nice to have" to make the procedure go more smoothly and comfortably for all concerned. We hope this approach is helpful for practitioners who find themselves needing to perform a procedure in less than ideal circumstances.

The next section describes the actual performance of the *Procedure,* with step-by-step instructions. Where relevant, alternative approaches are listed, along with potential risks for each alternative. This section is generally the most thoroughly illustrated.

Because many procedures are performed at least in part for diagnostic purposes, we include a section where appropriate on the *Interpretation of Results*. This section should also be helpful in determining whether the procedure has been performed in a technically correct fashion and can assist in the decision whether to attempt to repeat the procedure or to refer the patient to a higher level of care.

We include the section *What the Patient and Family Should Know* to help with teaching before and after the procedure. We have found that children naturally are better able to cooperate when they have a clear idea of what will be done, and parents are equally sensitive to the need to be informed.

The section on *Possible Complications* should also help practitioners in educating families; it may also be useful in the decision-making process about whether to perform a procedure in the primary care setting. For more complicated procedures, we recommend that practitioners familiarize themselves with the likely complications through direct training and experience. This section is included to provide a quick overview, not a comprehensive listing.

Aftercare Instructions are listed in the text of each chapter to help the provider with teaching and anticipatory guidance. Detailed instructions for the family, suitable for photocopying, are included in a separate section in Appendix B.

Finally, a brief section on *Modifications for Situations of Limited Resources* is provided. As noted previously, many practitioners find themselves in situations, either in the United States or abroad, in which they must perform procedures with fewer resources and under more trying circumstances than they are used to. Although more complex procedures should generally be deferred in such circumstances until the patient can be transferred to a more acute care facility, many simpler procedures can be performed using only basic medical equipment.

No book or set of written instructions can replace proper clinical experience. This book is intended as a review and reference for practitioners who have performed these procedures previously. It should also provide a useful memory aid for practitioners who have not performed the procedures recently. We hope and expect that this book will be helpful to health care providers who care for children in a broad variety of circumstances.

CHAPTER 2

Venous Sampling

David W. Bernard
Sam Bartle

PERIPHERAL VENOUS SAMPLING

Background and Introduction

Peripheral venous sampling is one of the most frequently performed procedures in pediatrics. It is the preferred method for phlebotomy and for obtaining intravenous access for the delivery of fluids and medications. Although many practitioners are intimidated by venipuncture in children, success can be readily achieved by carefully selecting appropriate landmarks, providing gentle patient restraint, and utilizing available pain-relief techniques. Although more invasive means of access, such as central or intraosseous lines, are occasionally indicated, peripheral venous access is preferred in most cases.

Relevant Anatomy

The veins of the upper and lower extremities are located in a predictable distribution. Although sites for cannulation are often easily visible, a "blind stick" is sometimes necessary when the amount of subcutaneous fat and/or clinical status makes visualization of the vessel difficult. Important anatomical sites in the upper extremity are the cephalic, basilic, and median cubital veins. The saphenous vein is the primary vein in the lower extremity (Figs. 2-1 and 2-2). Because the tributaries of the arm and leg venous systems form arches in the dorsum of the foot and hand, these are good places for finding acceptable veins. The saphenous vein just above the medial malleolus and the cephalic vein proximal to the thumb on the radial border of the forearm are good choices for "blind sticks" when other vessels cannot be seen or palpated. The locations of the two veins are predictable, and they are solidly anchored in the surrounding subcutaneous tissues.

Indications

Peripheral venous sampling is indicated whenever blood is needed for laboratory analysis or when intravenous access is required. Venipuncture is the preferred

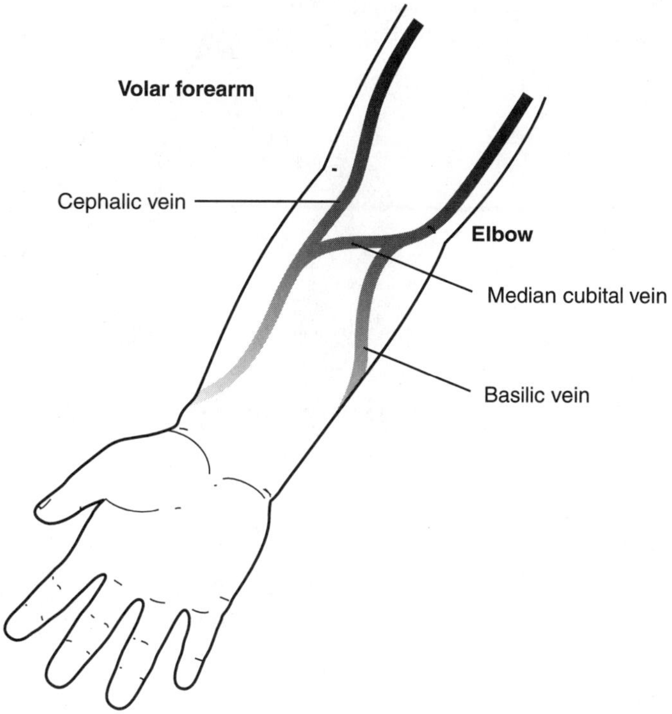

FIG. 2-1. Anatomy of the cephalic and basilic veins in the forearm.

method for blood sampling when intravenous access is not necessary. When an intravenous line is needed, blood specimens can normally be drawn through the intravenous catheter immediately after it is placed. Heel sticks are an alternative method for blood sampling in the newborn. Specimens obtained by heel stick are more likely to be hemolyzed and cannot be used for blood cultures. Arterial puncture is an alternative for blood sampling when venous samples are unobtainable. Because arterial puncture is more painful and is associated with more risks, it should be used only when absolutely necessary.

Contraindications and Reasons for Referral to a Specialist

There are no absolute contraindications to peripheral venous sampling. Children with coagulopathies are at risk for continued bleeding after skin puncture. Intravenous catheters should not be placed in areas with soft tissue infections, in burns, or in fractured extremities.

Recommended Nursing Skills and Procedures

Appropriate restraint techniques are essential. The uncooperative younger child can be immobilized in an appropriately sized papoose board or may be wrapped

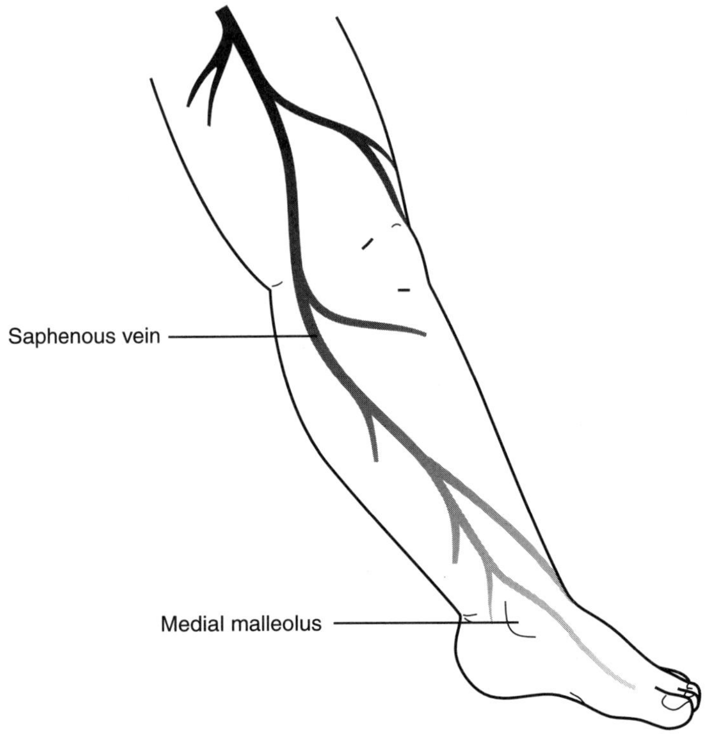

FIG. 2-2. Anatomy of the saphenous vein in the lower leg.

snugly in a sheet. The extremity in which the procedure is being performed must be immobilized, preferably by an assistant whose only role is to help restrain the child. Taping the extremity to a prepadded board before the procedure further secures the site. When the child is properly restrained, the person performing the procedure can focus exclusively on successful completion of the task. The parents should not be asked to assist in restraining the child. Many venous sampling efforts fail because of inappropriate immobilization. Older children often cooperate with the procedure by holding still when time is taken to explain the procedure before beginning, especially when appropriate analgesia is used. Restraint of the fully cooperative child is unnecessary.

In many practices, nurses or assistants perform most venous sampling. Special training or pediatric-specific experience is essential for support staff given the additional difficulty associated with venipuncture of small veins in uncooperative patients.

Supplies and Equipment

Need to have

If possible, arrange all necessary supplies in a self-contained storage box so they are readily available at the beginning of the procedure. Venipuncture is performed with butterfly needles. Over-the-needle catheters are preferred for intravenous cannulas. Suggested supplies for peripheral venous sampling include the following:

- Alcohol wipes
- Adhesive tape (multiple sizes)
- Blood tubes for laboratory analysis
- Butterfly needles (23- and 25-gauge)
- Gloves (sterile and nonsterile)
- Lidocaine (1%) without epinephrine
- Needles (27- and 30-gauge)
- Normal saline flush solution
- Over-the-needle catheters (14- through 24-gauge)
- Padded arm boards
- Povidone-iodine solution (Betadine)
- Restraint boards (papoose)
- Sodium bicarbonate (8.4%)
- Sterile gauze
- Syringes (1, 3, 5 ml)
- Tourniquets and rubber bands

Nice to have

- Antibiotic ointment
- Multicolored stickers and adhesive strips
- Primed intravenous tubing
- Razors
- T-connectors
- Transparent adhesive dressings

Procedure

Before beginning venous sampling, a standard skin preparation regimen should be followed. Hands should be washed before gloving. Gloves must be worn for all procedures. The overlying skin should be cleaned with alcohol. Povidone-iodine (Betadine) should be painted three times on the overlying skin and allowed to dry. Some practitioners, however, use alcohol alone for cleansing before peripheral venous sampling. If blood is being obtained for culture specimens, sterile gloves should be worn and the povidone-iodine step must be included.

Many techniques exist for minimizing the pain of venous sampling. Parents or play therapists can use distraction techniques that may decrease the child's perception of pain. Intradermal lidocaine (1%) given before placing intravenous catheters is helpful. Buffering the lidocaine with sodium bicarbonate (8.4%) in a ratio of nine parts lidocaine to one part sodium bicarbonate decreases the pain of injection. Additionally, using smaller-gauge needles such as 27- or 30-gauge and injecting slowly decreases pain. A eutectic mixture of local anesthetics (EMLA cream) may be applied and will induce local anesthesia. Unfortunately, topical anesthesia is not fully achieved for 1 hour. EMLA is therefore less useful for urgent or emergent access.

Several techniques can be utilized to maximize success in venous cannulation. Tourniquets should always be used in extremities. Placing the site in a dependent position relative to the heart increases venous distention. Warming the extremity and the patient can be helpful. Veins often roll out from the overlying skin; this can be minimized by stretching the skin tightly over the vein before puncturing it. Another technique that is especially useful when starting larger intravenous catheters or doing blind sticks is to initially puncture the overlying skin with an 18- or 20-gauge needle. Stretching the skin to the side of the vessel makes inadvertent puncture of the vein unlikely. The skin should be released after puncture, and then the over-the-needle catheter can be advanced easily through the puncture site and into the vein.

Heel stick

Heel sticks are appropriate for removal of small volumes of blood from newborns and very young infants. The following steps detail this procedure:

1. Warm the heel with a warm towel for several minutes before the procedure.
2. Clean the heel with alcohol and allow it to dry completely.
3. Place the heel in a dependent position.
4. Puncture the heel on the lateral or medial portion with a lancet. Avoid the middle portion of the posterior heel because the calcaneus is too close to the skin at that point and can be inadvertently punctured.
5. Wipe off the first drop of blood with a sterile gauze pad.
6. Squeeze the foot very gently to improve blood flow.
7. Collect subsequent drops in a microtainer with a collection cap or in a capillary tube.
8. Hold pressure to stop bleeding when blood collection is completed.

Blood cultures and large volumes of blood cannot be obtained by this method.

Simple peripheral

1. After restraining the child, place a tourniquet that is tight enough to occlude venous flow but that will not occlude arterial flow. A rubber band may be used as a tourniquet in infants.
2. Find a vein by lightly tapping two fingers over the selected site and wiping with an alcohol pad.
3. Clean and prepare the site.
4. Give local anesthesia when appropriate.
5. If only venipuncture for laboratory analysis is being performed, attach an appropriately sized syringe to a butterfly catheter (23- or 25-gauge).
6. Puncture the skin over the vessel.
7. While aspirating gently on the syringe, advance into the vessel.
8. When blood return occurs, stop advancing the needle and withdraw enough blood to perform necessary laboratory tests.
9. Release the tourniquet before withdrawing the needle.
10. After removing the needle, hold pressure over the site for at least 3 minutes and until bleeding has stopped.

If starting an intravenous catheter, use an over-the-needle catheter. Small catheters (22- or 24-gauge) are used in infants and young children. Larger catheters (16- to 20-gauge) are used in older children and when rapid volume delivery is needed.

1. Stretch the skin over the vessel.
2. Puncture the skin several millimeters distal to the site in which you wish to enter the vessel.
3. Advance slowly at a 15- to 30-degree angle until a blood flash appears. With small catheters, the flash can be subtle and delayed, so the catheter should be advanced slowly.
4. Once a flash has appeared, lower the catheter to a position level with the skin and advance the entire catheter apparatus 1 or 2 mm more, then immobilize the needle with one hand while advancing the catheter over the needle with the other hand.
5. Secure the catheter with tape.
6. If obtaining blood samples, attach a syringe with T-connector to the catheter and gently aspirate the necessary amount of blood.
7. Release the tourniquet.
8. Flush the catheter with saline while being careful not to introduce air into the circulation.
9. Apply antibiotic ointment at the entrance site and place a dressing over the catheter.
10. Secure the extremity to an arm board in the younger or uncooperative child.

Complex peripheral

The blind saphenous approach to venous sampling is a good alternative when other sites cannot be found. The most easily accessed site is located 1 cm anterior and 1 cm superior to the medial malleolus at the ankle.

1. Apply the tourniquet at the proximal calf below the knee and place the leg in a dependent position.
2. Clean and prepare the site. The skin in this area is thick, so it is helpful to puncture the overlying skin with an 18-gauge needle first.
3. Proceed in a fashion similar to that used in other intravenous sites.

The external jugular vein is often overlooked as a site for access.

1. Restrain the child in a mild Trendelenberg position, with the head turned to either side. The external jugular vein will be visible midway between the clavicle and the mandible, lying above the sternocleidomastoid muscle.
2. Clean and prepare the site. The external jugular vein is highly mobile, making cannulation sometimes difficult.
3. Stretch the overlying skin taut and puncture it with an 18-gauge needle.
4. While continuing to stretch the skin, advance the intravenous catheter through the puncture site and into the vein in a fashion similar to that used in other intravenous sites.

Scalp

Scalp vein cannulation is appropriate for young infants without other easily identified sites for peripheral access; however, once the infant becomes mobile with agile hands, scalp cannulas are difficult to maintain. For older infants, alternative sites should be chosen if at all possible. Veins will be located in the temporal, frontal, and posterior auricular regions. When attempting to puncture the temporal vein, remember that the temporal artery is located close to the vein and may be inadvertently punctured. Any blanching during infusion or any suggestion of pulsatile blood flow should prompt removal of the catheter.

1. Place a snug-fitting rubber band around the head as a tourniquet. Removal of the rubber band after the procedure will be facilitated by attaching a small piece of tape around the rubber band before placing it on the infant's scalp. This tape can be grasped to remove the rubber band when the procedure is completed.
2. Appropriately restrain the infant in a slight Trendelenberg position.
3. Shave the site if necessary.
4. Clean and prepare the site.
5. Enter the vessel with a small over-the-needle catheter or a butterfly needle.
6. Secure the intravenous catheter with tape and remove the rubber band.

Interpretation of Results

The normative values for the various laboratory tests are available in all major texts or from the laboratory performing the analysis. Catheter patency can be confirmed by the easy flushing of saline into the catheter without noticeable swelling or blanching in the subcutaneous tissue around the catheter. Smaller catheters may not have free-flowing blood even when they are in proper position. Any difficulty flushing the catheter suggests improper placement.

What the Patient and Family Should Know

Venous sampling is never completely pain free. Children should never be told that a procedure does not hurt when indeed it will. Children should be informed that the procedure will feel like a pinch or a sting. Parents and children should be advised that even in experienced hands venous sampling sometimes requires several attempts before success is achieved. Parents occasionally are concerned about papoosing or restraining their child. These concerns can be addressed by explaining to them that appropriate restraint not only maximizes the chances of successfully completing the procedure but also minimizes the risk of children harming themselves while struggling.

Possible Complications

Discomfort and hematomas at the sites of puncture are the primary complications. Puncture of an underlying artery is possible. Puncture of other underlying structures, such as nerves or tendons, is rare but theoretically possible. Intravenous infusions occasionally infiltrate into surrounding tissues, which can result in deep burns and tissue injury if the fluid or medication is sclerosing or caustic. Intravenous catheters can become infected, resulting in phlebitis or cellulitis. Infants and children can become hypothermic during venous sampling procedures if temperature control is not addressed.

Aftercare Instructions

Pressure should be maintained on the puncture site until all bleeding has stopped. The intravenous site should be checked often for signs of failure, infiltration, or infection. Any excessive pain or swelling of the extremity indicates catheter failure. If concern exists regarding the integrity of the intravenous catheter, it should be removed and replaced at another site.

Modifications for Situations of Limited Resources

Butterfly catheters may be used as intravenous infusion catheters if over-the-needle catheters are not available. These types of catheters must be taped securely in place because they can easily puncture the opposite wall of the vessel and become infiltrated.

PERCUTANEOUS CENTRAL VENOUS CATHETERIZATION

Background and Introduction

There are five methods to access the central vasculature of a pediatric patient: percutaneous central venous catheterization (PCVC), venous cutdown, intraosseous needle insertion, umbilical vessel cannulation, and indwelling ports and catheters. Central venous access provides a path into the venous circulation when it is not feasible through a peripheral approach.

Relevant Anatomy

Femoral vein

The femoral vein is medial and adjacent to the femoral artery (Fig. 2-3). The location is found by palpating for the pulse of the femoral artery and directing the puncture site medial to the pulsation and 1 to 2 cm inferior to the inguinal ligament. If no pulse can be felt, the site can be estimated to fall just medial to the halfway point between the anterior superior iliac spine and pubic tubercle. The benefits of using the femoral vein over another central access site include easily identifiable landmarks, good hemostasis after unsuccessful attempts, and ready access when resuscitation procedures are occurring.

Internal jugular vein

The internal jugular vein lies behind the carotid artery in the upper neck. It courses lateral to the carotid artery in the lower neck. It joins with the subclavian vein immediately behind the medial head of the clavicle (Fig. 2-4). The right side of the neck is preferred because of the presence of the thoracic duct in the left chest. The

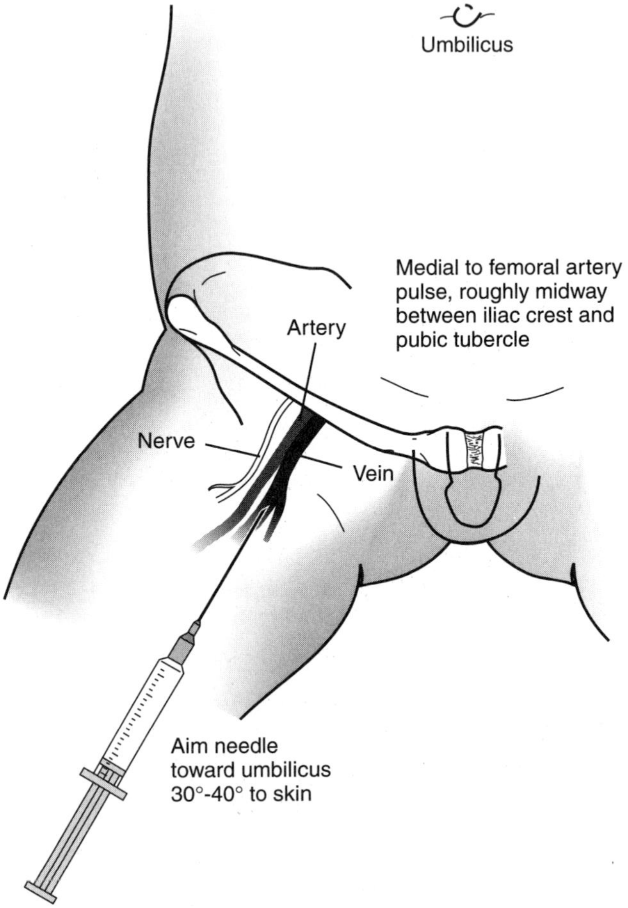

FIG. 2-3. Femoral central catheter placement.

right-side approach has the added advantage of providing a more direct route from the internal jugular vein into the right atrium. The pleural cap is lower on the right side, so there is a smaller possibility of causing a pneumothorax. Venipuncture should be performed in the lower neck where the vein is lateral to the carotid artery.

Subclavian vein

The subclavian vein lies immediately behind the medial portion of the clavicle. Entry is just inferior to the midclavicle where the clavicle bends posteriorly (Fig. 2-5).

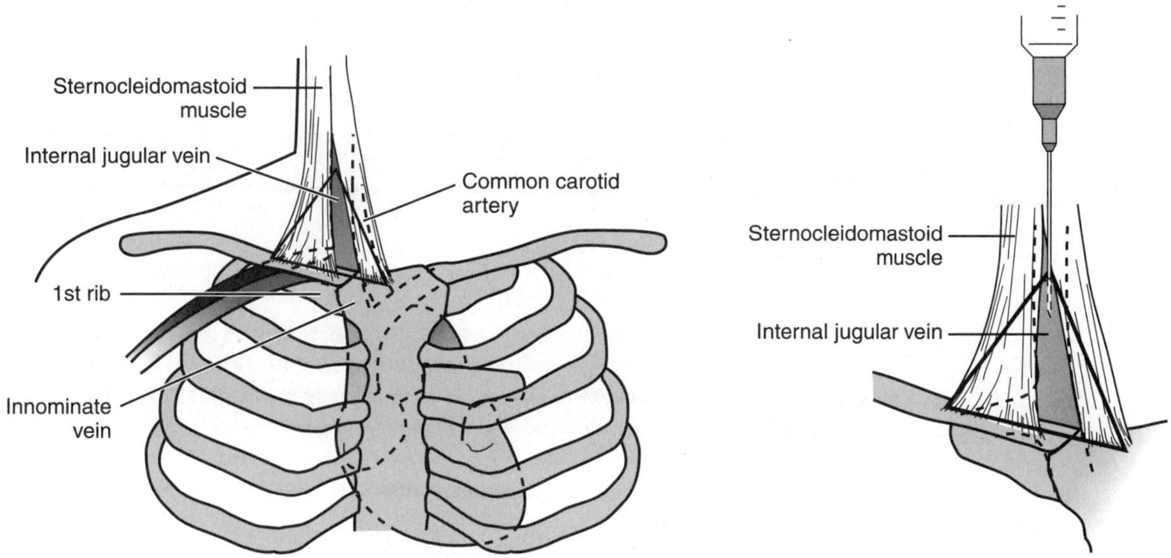

FIG. 2-4. Anatomy of the internal jugular vein.

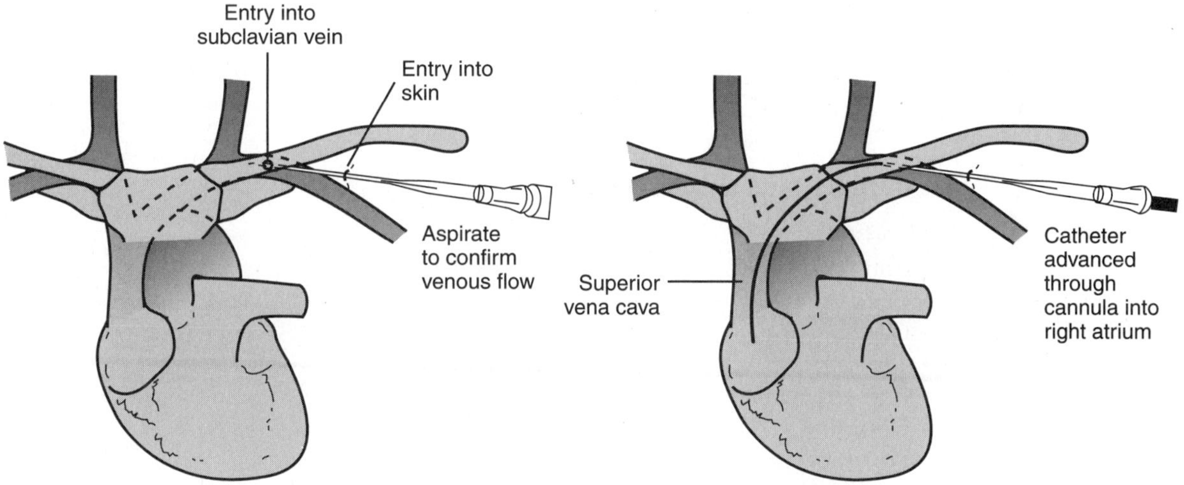

FIG. 2-5. Anatomy of the subclavian vein.

Indications

The primary indication for PCVC is the inability to obtain peripheral vascular access. Certain other clinical situations necessitate central vascular access. The administration of hypertonic fluids, parenteral hyperalimentation, and vasopressors usually requires central access. In an intensive care setting, PCVC is necessary for hemodynamic monitoring purposes.

Contraindications and Reasons for Referral to a Specialist

The only true contraindications to a central venous cannulation depend on the site of placement. A catheter should not be placed distal to or overlying an injured or infected region. A femoral catheterization should not be performed if the patient has any major abdominal or lower extremity injuries. An exception to this contraindication is that a subclavian catheterization may be performed on the side of any chest wall or lung injury if it does not involve the region in which the catheter will be inserted.

A relative contraindication is central line placement in patients with coagulopathies. If PCVC is indicated, any coagulopathy should be corrected with platelet or fresh frozen plasma transfusions as the need indicates before line placement.

Given the risks of central venous cannulation, it should not be performed unless there is a clear indication for its use. If a peripheral intravenous line can function properly to meet the need for vascular access, then central cannulation should not be attempted.

Recommended Nursing Skills and Procedure

The nursing staff caring for a child with a central venous catheter should be well acquainted with the type of catheter and how to maintain it. They should also be familiar with the specific medications being administered through it. If the catheter is for central venous pressure monitoring, the staff needs to be aware of the proper way to calibrate the tracing and how to identify proper waveforms. All central catheters require close monitoring to maintain proper function because they are prone to clotting and infectious complications.

Supplies and Equipment

Need to have

- Antibiotic ointment and dressing material
- Catheter
- Gauze
- Guidewire
- Introducing needle
- Lidocaine (1%)
- Povidone-iodine solution
- Scalpel (No. 11)
- Sterile drapes
- Sterile gloves
- Suture
- Syringe (3-ml with a 25-gauge 1.5-in needle for anesthetizing)
- Syringe (5-ml)

Nice to have

A sedated or cooperative patient makes the procedure easier and safer. At all times, with the possible exception of emergent resuscitation, the person performing the cannulation should do so in as sterile a manner as possible. The operator should be wearing sterile gloves and gown, along with a mask and cap. A variety of catheter sizes and lengths should be available. If time allows, all catheter ports should be flushed before placement. Monitoring equipment should be calibrated and ready to be connected as soon as the line is in place and secured. Depending on the skill of the person placing the central line, an assistant in proper sterile attire should be available to aid in line placement.

Procedure

Several different styles of catheters are available for central venous cannulation. They fall into one of three general types: catheter-over-needle devices, catheter-through-needle devices, and catheters for use with a guidewire.

Over-the-needle catheter

The catheter over the needle is represented by the familiar angiocath or peripheral intravenous devices. These types are rarely used for central venous cannulation because of the limited lengths that are available. The one situation in which they can be used is in emergent femoral vein access. When used, these catheters are placed in a similar fashion to starting peripheral intravenous lines.

Through-the-needle catheter

This method of venous cannulation consists of venipuncture with a needle through which a catheter is passed into the lumen of the vein. The needle is withdrawn over the catheter and is immobilized with a guard device so as not to damage the catheter or injure the patient. These catheters are prone to tearing; therefore they are rarely used. The catheter cannot be withdrawn through the needle without the risk of damage to the catheter and possible creation of catheter emboli. If the catheter does not thread easily through the needle and does not advance into the vein, the needle must be removed before or simultaneously with the catheter. *The catheter must never be withdrawn through the needle.*

Guidewire

This method, which is also known as a *modified Seldinger technique,* is probably the most popular and common method of placing a central venous catheter. Catheters come in a variety of lengths and sizes and with either single or multiple ports. Preassembled kits come prepared with the catheters and all supplies for cannulation and placement.

1. Choose a catheter length to approximate the distance measured over the external body surface from the insertion site to the site where final placement of the catheter tip is desired. Long catheters decrease the flow rate. If medications or fluids need to be infused quickly, a shorter catheter is more appropriate. Catheter diameter depends on patient size and the purpose of catheterization. Generally, for pressure monitoring or resuscitation purposes, infants usually require a 3 or 4 Fr catheter, a young child a 3 to 5 Fr, older children a 5 or 6 Fr, and the vessels of an adolescent can

BOX 2-1 STERILE PREPPING FOR CENTRAL VENOUS CANNULATION

- Position the patient so that the cannulation site is more easily accessible according to the procedure to be performed.
- With a circular sweeping motion, wipe from the center out with povidone-iodine–soaked gauze covering the region over the cannulation site. Repeat the povidone-iodine preparation at least three times. The povidone-iodine must be allowed to dry thoroughly before proceeding with the procedure to provide maximum bactericidal effect.
- Wash hands thoroughly. Dress in cap, mask, sterile gloves, and sterile gown.
- Drape the procedure site with sterile towels or a sterile drape with a precut center, which is provided with most cannulation kits. Provide a wide sterile field when draping to provide adequate room to spread out all needed supplies and to make performing the procedure more comfortable.
- Lay out and check all equipment needed for the procedure. Verify that the proper size needle and catheter are available. Inspect the guidewire. Confirm that there is a scalpel, syringe for aspirating and anesthetizing, dilating catheter, local anesthetic, and suture to secure the line after placement.
- Infiltrate the skin over the vein to be cannulated with a local anesthetic.
- Flush all catheter lumens and ports with the appropriate flush solution.

be cannulated with an adult size 7 or 8 Fr. The number of lumens or ports depend on the number and kinds of medications that will be administered simultaneously.

2. Prepare and drape the field in a sterile manner (Box 2-1).
3. Don sterile gloves, and anesthetize the site with lidocaine where the catheter will be placed.
4. Perform the initial venipuncture using a regular small-bore needle (20- to 23-gauge) attached to a 5- or 10-ml syringe. Make certain the guidewire will pass through the insertion needle.
5. After puncturing the skin, maintain slight negative pressure on the syringe plunger.
6. Slowly insert and then withdraw the needle until free flow of blood is obtained.
7. Stabilize the needle by steadying it with one hand and remove the syringe. Always cover the hub of the needle with a gloved finger when changing syringes or wires to avoid air embolization.
8. After successfully obtaining needle access, introduce the guidewire through the needle into the vein. The preferred end of the guidewire to use is the J-end, which facilitates the passage of the wire through the main venous channel. If the J-end of the guidewire does not pass freely into the vein, the straight end may be tried with caution. When introducing the guidewire either by the J-end or by the straight end, it should pass freely without meeting resistance. *Do not force the passage of the wire.* If resistance is met when passing the guidewire, simultaneously withdraw the wire with the needle. *Never withdraw a guidewire through a needle.* The needle and wire should be removed together to avoid cutting the wire and risking fragment emboli.
9. After the guidewire is threaded into the vein, the needle is withdrawn over the wire while leaving the wire in place. Keep holding a portion of the guidewire

while removing the needle. *The operator must always grasp a portion of the guidewire,* or the entire guidewire can be lost into the circulation. Caution must be taken when a guidewire is advancing toward the heart because dysrhythmias can occur (this is especially a concern for subclavian and internal jugular approaches). If a cardiac arrythmia occurs, immediately pull the guidewire back.

10. Pass a semirigid dilating catheter (also known as an *introducer catheter*) down the guidewire through the skin and into the lumen of the vein. Passage of the dilator through the skin often requires that a small incision be made with a No. 11 scalpel blade at the site where the guidewire enters the skin. The purpose of the dilating catheter is to facilitate passage of the flexible venous catheter through the skin and underlying tissues. Rotating the dilator as it advances through the skin and fascia enables easier entry into the vein than simply pushing it through.
11. Completely remove the dilating catheter over the guidewire while the operator continues to hold the guidewire.
12. Place direct pressure at the insertion site to control bleeding.
13. Thread the venous catheter over the guidewire into the lumen of the vein. Rotating the catheter as you advance it facilitates insertion into the vein and decreases the likelihood of kinking or damaging it. Grasp the guidewire at the skin while threading the catheter. As it passes out through the distal port, grasp the wire at the distal end before releasing it at the skin and completing the insertion of the catheter. *Always have a portion of the guidewire in your grasp while threading the catheter.*
14. After the catheter has been completely inserted, remove the guidewire, check for free-flowing blood return, and confirm that normal saline flushes easily in all ports.
15. Suture the catheter in place and apply a sterile dressing.
16. Obtain a radiograph to confirm placement and to assess for complications in subclavian and internal jugular lines. Central pressure monitoring is best obtained when the catheter tip rests in the inferior or superior vena cava. Avoid having the catheter tip in the atrium of the heart or at the level of the renal arteries. Measuring the pressures via a transducer helps determine if the catheter is properly positioned.

The guidewire technique has certain advantages compared with the previous two methods. The initial venipuncture can be performed with a small-gauge needle. The needle can be as small as will accommodate the smallest guidewire. This technique may minimize the problems of bleeding, hematoma formation, and other complications during venipuncture attempts. Catheter-over-needle and catheter-through-needle devices require large-bore needles to permit cannulation with a catheter of even modest size.

A second advantage of the guidewire technique is the ability to exchange one central venous catheter for another. A guidewire is placed through the distal port of the catheter in the vein. The catheter is removed over the guidewire, leaving it in the vein. A new catheter is threaded over the guidewire into the vein. The guidewire is then removed with the new catheter in position, which is then sutured in place and dressed.

Femoral vein

The femoral vein is the most common site for a central venous catheterization in pediatric patients.

1. Select a side for an insertion site. Perfusion to the distal extremity must be documented before and after the procedure. Avoid sites with overlying infection, surgical scars, or injury. Placing the catheter on the right side usually makes central venous monitoring easier to achieve.
2. Position the leg with the hip slightly flexed, partially abducted, and slightly externally rotated. Placing a towel or folded sheet under the buttocks improves positioning of the pelvis.
3. While palpating the femoral pulse, insert the needle through the skin 2 to 4 cm below the inguinal ligament and 0.5 to 1.5 cm medial to the femoral pulse. Continually palpate the pulse with your free hand during the venipuncture.
4. With the needle at a 30- to 45-degree angle to the skin and aiming toward the umbilicus, advance the needle until blood flow is obtained. If no blood return occurs after advancing the needle, withdraw the needle slowly. Blood return often occurs when the needle is withdrawn.
5. If the artery is inadvertently punctured or the vein is punctured but free flow of blood cannot be achieved, withdraw the needle and apply pressure for a few minutes before attempting venipuncture again. If a hematoma develops, further attempts at central access must be made in another location.

Internal jugular vein

This route is less commonly used for obtaining central vascular access because it is technically more difficult to perform. The limited space and adjacent vital structures give this method a higher chance of causing injury during attempts to cannulate the vein. This site cannot be accessed when other resuscitation procedures are occurring at the patient's head.

1. Position the patient in a 20- to 30-degree Trendelenberg position. Placing a roll under the patient's spine between the scapulae improves positioning.
2. Turn the patient's head to the side 20 to 30 degrees away from the operator.
3. Because of the risk of this procedure, sedate the patient before attempting to place an internal jugular vein catheter. (Although there are three approaches to cannulation of the internal jugular vein, the central approach is the most commonly used and is the only one discussed.)
4. Insert the needle at a 30-degree angle to the skin directed toward the ipsilateral nipple. The entry site is at the apex of the triangle formed when the sternocleidomastoid muscle divides into two portions, one inserting onto the midclavicle and the other onto the sternum. The internal jugular vein is superficial; blood return should be achieved at a depth of 0.5 to 3.0 cm.
5. If no blood return is achieved at a depth of 3 cm, look for blood return while

slowly withdrawing the needle to just below the skin. Attempt the cannulation again while aiming slightly lateral of the ipsilateral nipple.

6. If a hematoma develops, further attempts should be made at alternate sites. Do not use the other internal jugular vein. Bilateral hematomas can cause tracheal compression and asphyxiation.

Subclavian vein

This method is the least common and riskiest for central venous cannulation in pediatric patients because identification of the landmarks is more difficult than in other sites. This approach also has a higher incidence of pneumothorax. Inadvertent subclavian artery puncture, a possible complication, may also cause severe problems because it is a noncompressible vessel.

1. Position the patient in a 20- to 30-degree Trendelenberg position. Placing a roll under the patient's spine between the scapulae improves positioning.
2. Turn the patient's head to the side 20 to 30 degrees away from the operator.
3. Because of the risk of this procedure, sedate the patient before attempting to place a subclavian vein catheter.
4. At the midpoint of the clavicle, roughly the region where it curves, insert the needle 1 to 2 cm lateral to the curvature.
5. Advance the needle until the bone is approached.
6. Walk the needle under the bone and advance it along the back of the medial portion of the clavicle. Aim toward the sternal notch. Keep the needle from pointing toward the spine and inadvertently puncturing the artery.
7. If no blood return is obtained, slowly withdraw the needle until blood return is achieved. Blood return often occurs when the needle is withdrawn.
8. If the artery is inadvertently punctured, or if the vein is punctured but free flow of blood cannot be achieved, withdraw the needle and apply pressure above and below the clavicle for a few minutes before attempting venipuncture again. If a hematoma develops, further attempts at central access must be made at another site.

Interpretation of Results

Proper placement should be confirmed by radiograph after any central line placement attempts in the neck or chest. The ability to obtain free blood return suggests proper placement. Connecting the catheter to a transducer confirms placement by the waveform detected. Any blood sample results are interpreted as needed.

What the Patient and Family Should Know

If performed in a nonemergent situation, the risks and benefits of PCVC should be fully discussed with the family and the patient (if he or she is old enough to understand). Informed consent should be obtained. The indication for central vein cannulation should be described in terms that are easily understood. It should be clear to the family and the patient, as it should be for the person performing the procedure, that the risks are justified by the need for central vein catheterization. If central venous cannulation is performed in an emergency situation, consent need not be obtained.

Possible Complications

Although following proper techniques may decrease the likelihood of complications, it does not exclude them from happening. The rate of complications is proportional to the skill of the operator. Anyone performing central venous cannulation should be aware of the potential complications before proceeding with catheterization. It is also imperative to have knowledge of how a complication occurs and to be prepared with the necessary materials and equipment to handle it.

Complications fall into one of two categories, those that are general for any of the procedures and those specific to a particular method. General complications are typically vascular or infectious. Vascular complications include hemorrhage, local hematoma, vessel injury, inadvertent arterial puncture, and arteriovenous fistula. Infectious complications include local cellulitis, phlebitis, bacteremia, osteomyelitis, septic arthritis, and generalized sepsis. Other general complications involve adjacent nerve injury, dysrhythmias, and catheter malposition. Complications of femoral vein cannulation are intraperitoneal infusion and bleeding, peritonitis, and bladder or bowel perforation. Vascular injuries necessitating amputation have occurred. Inguinal and muscular abscess formation has been reported. Complications from subclavian and internal jugular cannulation are pneumothorax, hemothorax, chylothorax (usually occurs when using the left side), hemomediastinum, hydromediastinum, and tracheal perforation. Central venous pressure monitoring can result in inaccurate measurements, and the catheters themselves may cause dysrhythmias and cardiac or large vascular perforation.

Aftercare Instruction

Central venous catheter care includes maintaining a sterile dressing at the insertion site with regular local wound care. The catheter should be sutured securely in place to decrease the risk of being dislodged. The care for patients with central venous catheters is primarily restricted to a hospital or intensive care setting. All ports should be routinely flushed with saline or a heparinized solution. With the exception of indwelling ports (discussed later), central venous catheters are usually removed before discharge. Applied pressure at the insertion site is necessary when the catheter is removed to prevent hematoma formation and thrombosis of the vessel.

Modification for Situations of Limited Resources

For most situations central venous catheterization is a rather intensive procedure requiring specific materials. The one situation that could be modified when resources are limited is the use of a long peripheral angiocath (catheter-over-needle) device for femoral cannulation. This device can be used for infants and small children without too much difficulty. In larger children and adolescents, the use of a long angiocath becomes technically more challenging.

VENOUS CUTDOWN

Background

Before the development of plastic peripheral vascular catheters and PCVC techniques, intravenous fluids were commonly administered by venous cutdown technique. The procedure involves the placement of a catheter directly into a vein after dissecting through the overlying tissues. This procedure is not commonly used anymore because it takes longer to perform than other vascular access techniques. Even though it is a technically difficult procedure, a cutdown can be life saving in situations when other access is not possible.

Relevant Anatomy

Although several peripheral veins can be utilized for a venous cutdown, the distal saphenous vein is most commonly used and is the only one detailed here. Other potential sites are the proximal saphenous vein in the inguinal area, the basilic vein, and the external jugular vein.

The saphenous vein runs superficially just anterior and superior to the medial malleolus. The saphenous nerve travels adjacent to it. The location of the saphenous vein remains rather constant regardless of age. Because of this consistency in location, the saphenous vein is the easiest vein to access for a cutdown.

Indications

A venous cutdown is indicated when percutaneous peripheral venipuncture is unsuccessful and when other procedures to gain vascular access have been unsuccessful. In the instance of severe hypovolemia, percutaneous access of the venous circulation may be impossible, and a venous cutdown may be beneficial. If the operator is experienced and proficient with cutdowns, the procedure may be used in preference to other central techniques in the critically ill child.

Contraindications

A venous cutdown is contraindicated if a less invasive procedure can be performed to obtain vascular access. Cutdowns should never be performed at sites distal to extremity injuries. Patients with coagulopathies and those with impaired host defenses are considered poor candidates for venous cutdowns.

Reasons for Referral to a Specialist

Many practitioners are not familiar with performing venous cutdowns. Because a cutdown is technically difficult, it should be performed by the most experienced person available. Surgeons, intensivists, and emergency physicians are good sources for consultation.

Supplies and Equipment

Need to have

- Antibiotic ointment and dressing materials
- Curved hemostats (Kelly hemostats) and small mosquito hemostats
- Gauze sponges
- Iris scissors
- Intravenous catheter
- Lidocaine (1%)
- Nylon suture (4-0) on a cutting needle
- Plastic venous dilator or lifter
- Povidone-iodine solution and alcohol prep
- Scalpel (No. 11)
- Silk suture ties (4-0)
- Sterile drapes
- Sterile gloves
- Tourniquet

Nice to have

- Arm board
- IV tubing and fluid ready
- Monitoring equipment calibrated
- Personnel to assist with the procedure
- Sedated patient
- Sterile gown, mask, and cap
- Tape
- Tissue spreaders
- Various size catheters

Procedure

The actual procedure for venous cutdown is similar regardless of the vein. The operator should have a detailed understanding of the local anatomy for the chosen site. This knowledge enables the operator to perform the cutdown rapidly and decreases the risk of possible damage to any surrounding structures.

1. Prepare and drape the site in a sterile fashion (Box 2-1).
2. Infiltrate the incision site with a local anesthetic.
3. Make a superficial transverse incision, crossing the path of the vein.
4. Bluntly dissect parallel to the direction of the vein, isolating 1 to 2 cm of the vessel from the surrounding subcutaneous fat and tissue.

5. Pass the two silk ties beneath the vessel, one distal and one proximal to the free vein segment (Fig. 2-6). The ties help to stabilize the vein segment.
6. Clamp the ends of both ties with a hemostat. Some operators choose to tie off the distal silk suture, but this step is considered optional.
7. Catheterize the vein. There are two methods for cannulating the vein: venipuncture under direct visualization or venotomy. Venipuncture under direct visualization involves placing an over-the-needle catheter into the vein while stabilizing it with a pair of hemostats or by applying traction to the suture ties. An alternative technique is to perform a venipuncture under direct vision with a needle. A guidewire is threaded through this needle into the vein, the needle is removed, and a catheter is passed over the wire into the vein (refer to the guidewire technique in the PCVC section).
8. To perform a venotomy technique, use a No. 11 scalpel blade or a pair of iris scissors to make an incision in the vein (Fig. 2-7). Use extreme care not to tear or transect the vessel.
9. Stabilize the vein with a pair of hemostats passed beneath the vessel or by placing traction on the suture ties.
10. Cannulate the vein using either a catheter or a guidewire technique through the venotomy.
11. Apply traction on the suture ties to help control bleeding.
12. As the catheter is passed through the venotomy, relax traction on the proximal suture to allow the catheter to thread into the vein.
13. Once the catheter has been advanced into the lumen, tie the proximal suture to secure the catheter in the vein. The distal suture can be left untied or tied. Tying the vessel with the distal suture may help control bleeding. Some operators tie the distal suture to the external portion of the catheter to further secure it in place.
14. Close the incision site after placement is confirmed.

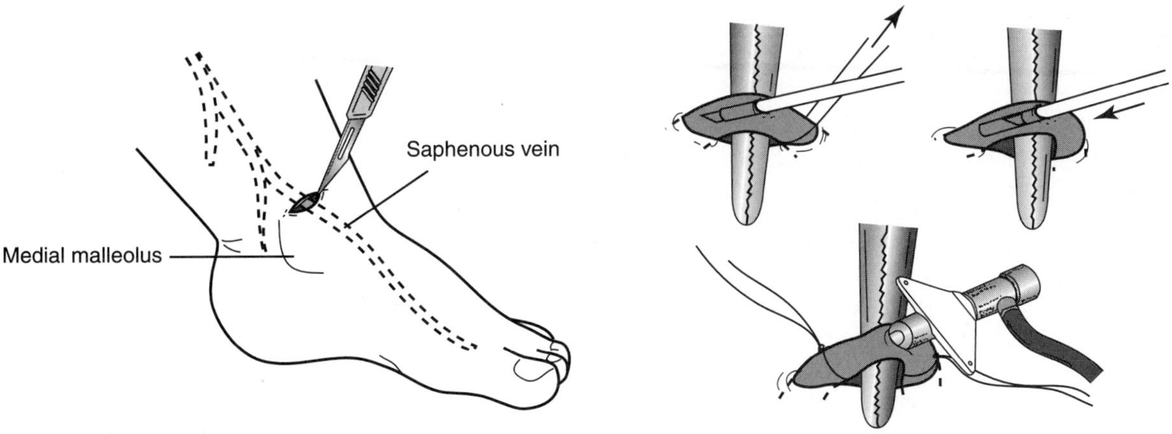

FIG. 2-6. Procedure for venous cutdown.

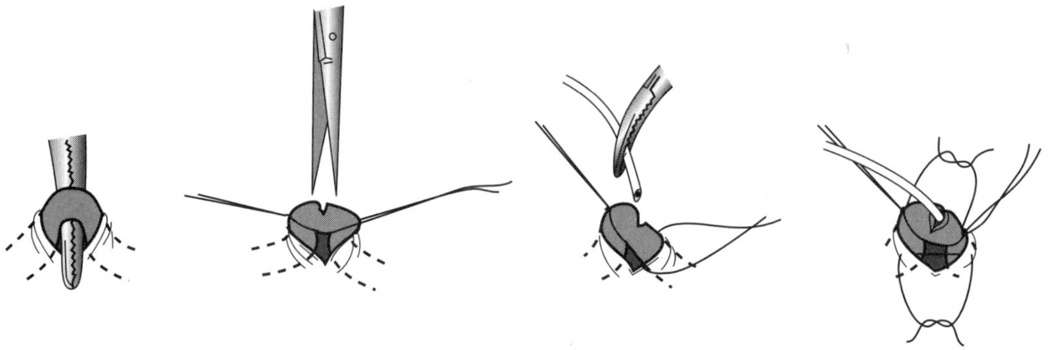

FIG. 2-7. Procedure for venotomy.

With either method, some operators tunnel the catheter beneath the skin 1 to 2 cm distal to the incision site before entering the vein. This variation is believed to reduce the risk of infection and allow for better suture closure of the incision site.

Interpretation of Results

Placement is confirmed by having good blood return and being able to flush with minimum resistance. Any testing on blood samples obtained through a catheter placed by venous cutdown should be done according to routine method.

What the Patient and Family Should Know

The need to perform a venous cutdown almost always arises in emergency situations; therefore informed consent is not usually obtained. Inform families that the catheter will be removed as soon as another vascular access site can be found. The families need to be aware of possible short-term and long-term complications of venous cutdowns and how the patient benefits from short-term use of a cutdown.

Possible Complications

Complications of a venous cutdown include bleeding problems such as local hematoma formation and oozing. Infectious complications range from local wound infection to sepsis. The incision site can develop an abscess and wound dehiscence. Phlebitis of the vessel may occur as a possible result of irritation from the catheter. Similar to any catheterization technique, there is a risk of catheter emboli. If the procedure is not done with extreme care, the vessel can be irreparably damaged. Associated structures at the cutdown site can be injured even when the procedure is performed carefully.

Aftercare Instructions

Aftercare instructions for a venous cutdown are primarily for the care of the insertion site and catheter maintenance care. A cutdown is not a means for attaining permanent vascular access. The venous cutdown catheter should be removed once another means of access has been achieved. Local wound care for the insertion site is needed to decrease the risk of infection. Apply pressure at the insertion site when the catheter is removed to prevent hematoma formation and thrombosis of the vessel.

Modifications for Situations of Limited Resources

In situations when high flow rates of large volumes are needed, intravenous tubing placed directly into the vessel can take the place of the catheter. This procedure is normally reserved for extreme situations such as severely dehydrated patients or acute trauma with excessive poorly controlled bleeding.

INTRAOSSEOUS ACCESS

Background

Intraosseous cannulation has been used for vascular access since the early twentieth century. With the introduction of plastic catheters, intraosseous infusion became obsolete for nonemergent venous access. As standards for pediatric resuscitation matured in the 1980s, intraosseous cannulation was recognized as a method for obtaining quick and successful vascular access in emergency situations. The procedure is relatively easy to learn and perform. When peripheral venous access is not rapidly available in the critically ill child, intraosseous cannulation is the standard procedure for emergency access in both the hospital and prehospital setting.

Relevant Anatomy

The principle of intraosseous infusion is based on the fact that the marrow cavity of long bones acts as a noncollapsing vessel. Blood flows into bones via nutrient arteries, which subsequently divide into arterioles and then into capillaries. These capillaries collectively drain into the medullary sinusoids, which in turn drain through the central venous channels and out into the peripheral venous system through the nutrient and emissary veins (Fig. 2-8). Infusions of fluids of any type into the medullary sinusoids will gain rapid access to the circulatory system. Almost any bone could potentially be used for intraosseous infusion. The sternum was the site initially used by investigators of this method, but it was fraught with complications and is no longer used. The proximal tibia, the distal tibia, and the distal femur, all of which have readily identifiable landmarks, are the preferred locations. These three locations

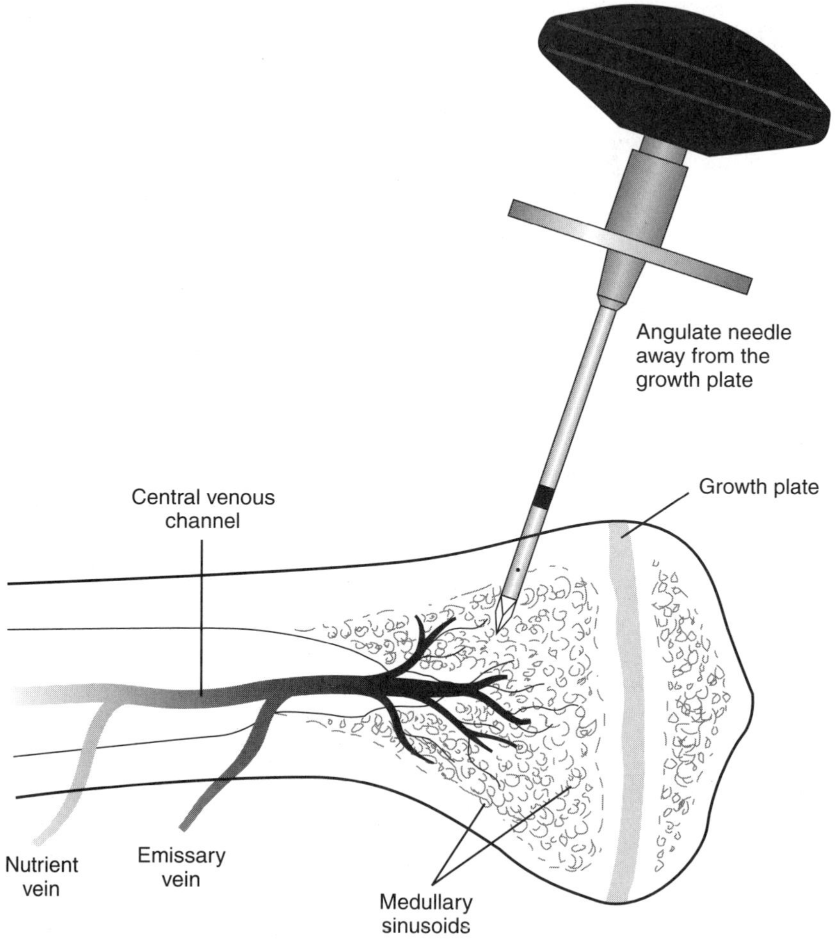

FIG. 2-8. Anatomy of intraosseous infusion.

have the added advantage of being distal to any other resuscitation maneuvers being performed.

Indications

Intraosseous infusion is indicated for situations in which immediate vascular access is required and other means are unsuccessful. Intraosseous cannulation is most easily performed in children under the age of 6 years. This approach has been demonstrated to be quick and reliable. Intraosseous infusion is used for fluid and drug administration in cardiopulmonary resuscitation, fluid resuscitation of shock states, and other emergent conditions that require immediate treatment. Common scenarios for intraosseous infusion are severe dehydration, shock, hypovolemic trauma, status epilepticus, and extensive burns.

Laboratory analysis can be performed on blood obtained from an intraosseous catheter. With the exception of a complete blood count, virtually any test that can be performed on samples obtained through a peripheral venipuncture can be performed on samples taken from an intraosseous site. This includes blood for type and cross-matching, electrolytes, glucose, and chemistry studies. Blood gas samples also give results similar to a central venous sample.

Once vascular access has been obtained through some other method, the intraosseous infusion should be discontinued. When the intraosseous line is removed as soon as possible after placement, the risk of complications such as infection is minimized. The one significant exception to this guideline is when the patient is transported to another facility. In this situation, once intraosseous access has been achieved, the needle should be secured and kept in place as long as the patient is being transported.

Contraindications

Any disruption of the bony cortex in the bone being used leads to the extravasation of infused fluids and medication. Starting an intraosseous line distal to a fracture is contraindicated. Once an attempt at intraosseous placement has been unsuccessful, another site (in another bone) must be chosen because of the risk of extravasation through the previous bony puncture sites. Intraosseous needles should not be placed in children with osteogenesis imperfecta or other fragile bone diseases. Sites with overlying burns, cellulitis, trauma, disruption of the soft tissue, or suspicion of tumor growth should be avoided.

Recommended Reasons for Referral to a Specialist

Referral to a specialist is usually required when complications such as osteomyelitis occur. Any patient requiring an intraosseous infusion should be admitted to a facility capable of delivering a high level of care. The intraosseous line should be secured and remain in place until another access site is attained. If adjacent structures are injured during introduction of the intraosseous needle, appropriate referral should be made for follow-up care.

Supplies and Equipment

Need to have

- Gloves
- Large-gauge needles with a stylette (bone marrow needles are ideal)
- Povidone-iodine solution and alcohol prep
- Syringe

Any large-bore, short, sturdy needle may be used for an intraosseous infusion. The needle sizes usually range from a 20- to 13-gauge. Regular needles and catheters used for blood drawing are not adequate for successful intraosseous placement.

Nice to have

- Board for immobilizing the extremity
- Gauze packing material for securing the needle
- Lidocaine
- Various sizes of needles

Procedure

1. Select a site for needle placement. The most commonly used site is the proximal tibia, 1 to 3 cm (one to two finger widths) below the tibial tuberosity or plateau. This is a good site for placement in children up to the age of 6 years. The distal tibia, the site most commonly used in older children and some adults, is punctured on the medial surface a couple of centimeters proximal to the medial malleolus and posterior to the saphenous vein. An alternative site is the distal femur, 2 to 3 cm proximal to the external femoral condyles in the midline of the bone shaft. Regardless of location, needle insertion is performed the same way.
2. Anesthetize the site with lidocaine if the patient is awake and alert.
3. After the site is prepared in standard fashion, stabilize the extremity using the nondominant hand.
4. Direct the point of the needle in line with the long axis of the bone and angled away from the growth plate.
5. Hold the intraosseous needle with the hub in the palm and the needle with the thumb and index finger 1 to 2 cm from the tip. This positioning decreases the likelihood of the needle being pushed too far into the bone and through the opposite side.
6. Using a rotating, drilling motion, gradually apply a steady, increasing pressure on the needle hub until the bone cortex is penetrated.
7. Use the nondominant hand to stabilize the extremity, but *never* place the hand behind the extremity, where the needle could penetrate if it passes directly through the patient.
8. Avoid rocking the needle from side to side and bending the needle. A sudden loss of resistance will be felt when the marrow is entered. When the needle is in proper position, marrow can often be aspirated, and the needle should be stable enough to stand up on its own without support.
9. Secure the needle so it will not be dislodged accidentally.

More pressure is required to infuse fluids via the intraosseous route than for intravenous infusion. Fluid can be infused manually with a syringe or can be instilled from a pressure bag. To reduce the risk of dislodging the needle, a short extension tubing may be placed between the hub of the needle and the syringe used for infusing the initial fluid.

Interpretation of Results

Fluid flushing easily through the needle into the marrow space indicates proper positioning. There will be a mild degree of resistance. A hand placed on the side of the extremity opposite to the insertion site should feel no swelling when fluid is forcibly injected. If such swelling is felt, the needle should be removed. Frequent subsequent evaluation of the soft tissue surrounding the site where the bone is punctured is essential. Any swelling of the surrounding tissue indicates that the needle has been dislodged. Swelling will also be evident if the bone cortex has any disruptions from fractures or previous intraosseous attempts.

What the Patient and Family Should Know

The need to use intraosseous infusion arises in emergency situations. Informed consent is not needed in these cases. Inform families that the needle will remain in place only until another vascular access method can be obtained. The families need to be aware of possible short-term and long-term complications of intraosseous infusions and how the patient benefits from short-term use of the infusion.

Possible Complications

Complications arise in one of two ways: technical difficulties or latent problems. The most common pitfall is inserting the needle all the way through the bone or not placing it far enough into the cortex to completely penetrate it. Once a bone has been punctured, either through to the backside or if the needle has become dislodged, that bone can no longer be used for intraosseous infusion. A properly placed and secured needle is unlikely to become dislodged and extravasate into the tissue. Intraosseous line placement is more difficult in younger patients with smaller bones. The needle may slip off the bone and enter the soft tissues of the patient or impale the operator.

Latent problems are either infectious or growth related. Infection risk is directly related to the length of time the catheter remains in the bone. Infections of the skin, soft tissue, and bone are possible. Bone growth can be impaired, especially if growth-plate injury occurred during placement.

Aftercare Instructions

Local wound care for the insertion site is essential. Applied pressure at the insertion site is necessary to prevent bleeding when the needle is removed. Close observation of the insertion site is needed to watch for signs of infection or infiltration.

Modifications for Situations of Limited Resources

Intraosseous infusion can be performed with virtually any sturdy large-bore needle. A styleted needle is preferable to prevent it from plugging. If a plug does occlude the needle, a forceful injection of fluid may be needed to clear it. Fluids can be infused by hand with a syringe if a pressure bag is not available.

INDWELLING PORTS AND CATHETERS

Background and Introduction

Children with medical conditions that require prolonged fluid or medication support often have long-term central venous catheters placed. Examples of medical illnesses that might require prolonged central venous access include malignancies that require chemotherapy, short gut syndrome with a need for parenteral nutrition, and osteomyelitis (for intravenous antibiotics). Although these catheters are usually placed as a surgical procedure under general anesthesia, these patients need to have their indwelling line accessed for venous sampling and intravenous therapy. Practitioners in the primary care setting must understand how to properly and safely access these lines.

There are three basic categories of indwelling catheters: the partially implanted external catheter (Broviac, Hickman, Groshong), the fully implanted catheter (Infus-A-Port, Port-A-Cath), and the peripherally inserted central catheter (PICC line). The partially implanted catheter is tunneled under the chest wall and anchored by a Dacron cuff before exiting the skin. Once exiting the skin, the catheter may have up to three ports representing the separate lumens of the catheter. Each port will be covered with a special cap, which is fitted over a Luer-lock adapter. Proximal to the ports are reinforced areas where clamps can be placed when accessing the catheters.

The fully implanted catheter is tunneled into a reservoir that lies beneath the chest wall in the subcutaneous tissue. The reservoir is covered with a self-sealing silicone membrane, which will not be damaged as long as it is punctured with the correct needle. The PICC line is placed in the brachial vein of the arm and threaded into the central circulation. Each kind of line is accessed in a specific fashion. The patency of the indwelling central catheters is maintained by various types of heparin or saline flush regimens. The manufacturer's instructions should be consulted to determine the specific recommendations for flushing and maintaining a specific catheter. Most catheters are flushed regularly with heparin, but some of the newer catheters are flushed with saline only.

Relevant Anatomy

The proximal tip of all of the central catheters should be located at the junction of the superior vena cava and the right atrium. When these lines are placed, they are normally threaded through the subclavian vein, the jugular venous system, or the cephalic vein. When evaluating for proper positioning of the catheter, the position can be confirmed by chest radiography. The reservoir of the internalized catheter is easily palpated immediately under the skin in the anterior chest wall. The tunnel and cuff of the external catheter can be palpated along its course in the chest wall.

Indications

The central venous catheter is accessed whenever blood sampling or intravenous therapy is needed in a patient who has an indwelling catheter. The indwelling catheter is accessed preferentially over peripheral sites to minimize discomfort to the patient with a chronic illness; however, when blood cultures are being obtained, they should be drawn both peripherally and from the indwelling catheter.

Contraindications

Indwelling central lines should not be accessed if catheter migration or breakage is suspected. If, after accessing the line, the catheter does not have both easy return of several milliliters of blood and easy flushing of saline solution, then catheter malfunction should be strongly suspected and catheter use should be discontinued until the problem is clarified and corrected. The patient should be referred to the surgeon who placed and manages the catheter if complications are suspected or if the line is not functioning normally.

Recommended Nursing Skills

The nurses who access indwelling catheters should be thoroughly trained in aseptic technique to minimize the risk of introducing contamination into the central line. Manufacturer's protocols for the specific management of each catheter should be followed.

Supplies and Equipment

Need to have

- Central venous catheter caps
- Hemostat without teeth
- Heparin flushes (100 u/ml)
- Intravenous extension tubing
- Noncoring (Huber) needles (19-, 20-, 22-gauge)
- Normal saline flushes
- Povidone-iodine solution
- Sterile gauze
- Sterile towels
- Syringes (10 ml)
- Tape
- Transparent dressings
- Universal precaution supplies (sterile gloves, drapes, and gown, mask, goggles)

Procedure

Because indwelling catheters communicate directly with the central circulation, sterile technique must always be utilized, and the introduction of air into the circulation should carefully be avoided. The provider's hands must be washed thoroughly, and sterile gloves, gown, and mask must be worn. Sterile towels are placed under the catheters when performing the procedure. All necessary supplies should be arranged on sterile towels before the procedure is begun.

For external catheters, blood samples may be drawn from the cap that fits over the terminal end of the largest lumen of the catheter. Blood cultures should not be drawn through the cap. To draw blood, the following procedures should be used:

1. Clean the cap with povidone-iodine and wait for it to dry.
2. Attach a 22-gauge needle to a 10-ml syringe and insert the needle through the cap.
3. Gently aspirate 5 ml of blood and discard the syringe.
4. Enter the cap with a new 10-ml syringe and needle and aspirate the needed amount of blood.
5. Flush the catheter with 5 ml of saline followed by the recommended flush of heparin solution.

When blood cultures are being drawn or when intravenous access is desired, the following procedures are used:

1. To avoid the risk of introducing air into the circulation, clamp the catheter any time the connection at the port is being changed.
2. After preparing all equipment, including carefully flushing the intravenous tubing, clean the cap with povidone-iodine and allow it to dry.
3. Clamp the catheter several inches proximal to the port in the reinforced portion with a toothless hemostat.
4. Remove the cap and attach a 10-ml Luer-lock syringe to the port.
5. Release the clamp and withdraw 5 ml of blood, reclamp the catheter, and discard the syringe.
6. Attach a new 10-ml syringe and aspirate the needed amount of blood and then reclamp the catheter.
7. Attach a syringe with saline solution, unclamp the catheter, and gently flush 5 ml of saline.
8. Clamp the catheter again, disconnect the syringe, and place a new LAP on the port.
9. Unclamp the catheter.

If intravenous fluids are being started, the following procedures are used:

1. Clamp the catheter, attach the prepared intravenous tubing, unclamp the catheter, and begin the infusion.
2. When the infusion is complete, clean the attachment at the port with povidone-iodine.
3. Clamp the catheter, remove the tubing, and attach a 10-ml flush syringe.
4. After unclamping the catheter, flush according to the recommended guidelines.
5. Clamp the catheter again, disconnect the syringe, and place a new cap on the port.
6. Unclamp the catheter and place a dressing over the site.

To access an internal port, a special noncoring (Huber) needle must be used to avoid damaging the membrane of the reservoir. These needles normally have a 90-degree bend to assist in stabilizing them when they are in place. The following procedures should be used:

1. When time allows, place EMLA over the reservoir site because the puncture through the skin overlying the reservoir is painful.

2. Using sterile technique, attach extension tubing to the noncoring needle and flush both with saline.
3. Prepare the skin over the reservoir with povidone-iodine and allow it to dry.
4. After localizing and stabilizing the reservoir with the thumb and first two fingers, puncture through the skin and the membrane of the reservoir until the resistance of the bottom of the reservoir is felt.
5. Similar to external catheters, clamp the tubing any time the connection is changed to avoid entraining air.
6. Aspirate 5 ml of blood to confirm patency.
7. If drawing blood, clamp the extension tubing and attach a new syringe.
8. Withdraw the necessary amount of blood after unclamping the tubing.
9. Clamp the tubing, attach a saline flush, unclamp the tubing, and flush with 5 ml of saline.
10. Observe for infiltration in the subcutaneous tissue when flushing. The intravenous tubing can be attached, and the infusion can begin.
11. When the infusion is complete, flush the port according to the manufacturer's instructions. The site of puncture does not need a special dressing unless bleeding is noted.

Interpretation of Results

Assuming that the first 5 ml of blood was discarded, the laboratory results are valid for most tests drawn through a central catheter. Coagulation studies are the exception to this rule. The heparin that is used to maintain catheter patency often causes erroneous coagulation profiles, even when large amounts of blood are discarded initially.

The practitioner must confirm that the catheter is patent and is performing normally. Blood should be easily aspirated, and the catheter should flush readily. Some catheters can function positionally. When blood is not easily aspirated or if the catheter is not flushing smoothly, move the child and his or her arms into different positions. If positional changes do not affect the function, then the catheter must be assumed to be nonfunctioning. Never forcefully inject or aspirate the catheter. Several protocols exist for reestablishing catheter patency; however, discussion of these protocols is beyond the scope of this chapter. The surgeon who placed the catheter should be consulted if suspicion of catheter failure exists.

What the Patient and Family Should Know

The family should know that any time the catheter is accessed, damage or infection can occur; however, this is unlikely when the catheter is accessed carefully with sterile technique. When catheter infections are being evaluated, families need careful explanation of the need for obtaining both peripheral and central cultures. Many families become very skilled in managing their child's catheters and can provide invaluable assistance to the staff, especially with managing temperamental lines.

Possible Complications

Infectious complications, such as infected catheters, cellulitis along the catheter tunnel, and bacteremia, are common of indwelling lines. Utilizing strict sterile technique when accessing central lines reduces the rate of this complication but does not eliminate it. Air embolism can occur if air is allowed to enter the catheter when syringes or tubing are connected and disconnected. Careful attention to clamping the line minimizes this risk. Catheter thrombi can be dislodged, especially if forceful injection or aspiration is used in a poorly functioning line.

Aftercare Instructions

Patients will have strict flushing and dressing regimens, which are determined by the specialist who placed the catheter. Families should continue this regimen and be instructed to follow up promptly for any sign of infection or catheter failure.

Modifications for Situations of Limited Resources

Indwelling central lines must always be accessed with strict sterile technique and attention to detail. If all of the appropriate equipment is not available, the central line should not be accessed given the risk of contamination and catheter failure.

SUGGESTED READINGS

Aoki BY, McCloskey K: *Evaluation, stabilization, and transport of the critically ill child,* St Louis, 1992, Mosby.

Bhende MS: Venipuncture and peripheral venous access. In Henretig FM, King C, editors: *Textbook of pediatric emergency procedures,* Baltimore, 1997, Williams and Wilkins.

Chameides L, Hazinski MF, editors: *Textbook of pediatric advanced life support,* Dallas, American Heart Association, 1997.

Cunningham FJ, Spivey WH: Intraosseous infusion. In Roberts JR, Hedges JR, editors: *Clinical procedures in emergency medicine,* Philadelphia, 1998, WB Saunders.

Dyer BJ, Weiman MG, Ludwig S: Central venous catheters in the emergency department: access, utilization, and problem solving, *Ped Emerg Care* 11:112, 1995.

Fuchs SM: Accessing indwelling central lines. In Henretig FM, King C, editors: *Textbook of pediatric emergency procedures,* Baltimore, 1997, Williams and Wilkins.

Strauss RH: Pediatric vascular access. In Fuhrman BP, Zimmerman JJ, editors: *Pediatric critical care,* St Louis, 1992, Mosby.

Webster PA, Salassi-Scotter MR: Peripheral vascular access. In Dieckmann RA, Fiser DH, Selbst SM, editors: *Pediatric emergency and critical care procedures,* St Louis, 1997, Mosby.

CHAPTER 3

Urine Sampling and Access

C. Jean Ogborn

BACKGROUND AND INTRODUCTION

The pediatric practitioner has many reasons to collect and analyze urine samples from patients. The reason dictates the method. For instance, urine obtained in nearly any fashion is adequate to sample for specific gravity, glucose, ketones, protein, or blood; however, urine must be obtained in specific and sterile ways to assess for nitrites and leukocytes or to sample for bacteriological culture. This chapter discusses the reasoning and procedures for obtaining urine by random voided specimen, clean-catch midstream sample, urethral catheterization, and suprapubic aspiration.

RANDOM VOIDED AND BAGGED SPECIMEN COLLECTION

Relevant Anatomy

Anatomical considerations are trivial in all patients except those with unusual anatomy as a result of either congenital defects or surgical intervention. In the case of bagged specimens, the bag must be placed so that urine enters it directly from the urethra and does not spill out into the diaper or onto the bed.

Indications

A *random voided specimen* is urine obtained without any special technique or preparation of the patient. This can be urine pressed from a diaper, caught in a container at home, caught in a nonsterile container in the office, or obtained from a urine bag placed on an infant's perineum. Urine obtained in these fashions is never suitable for culture or nitrite and leukocyte esterase testing because it is subject to contamination from many sources. Random and bagged urine specimens are perfectly adequate for testing for specific gravity, glucose, protein, ketones, bilirubin, pH, blood, some drugs or toxins, and human chorionic gonadotropin.

Contraindications

There are no absolute contraindications to this procedure. The risk of contamination by nonsterile surfaces must always be borne in mind.

Required/Recommended Nursing Skills

No special nursing skills are required beyond the recognition that these specimens are inadequate for culture.

Supplies and Equipment

- Labels
- Sterile or clean specimen container
- Urine collection bag

Procedure

The only techniques involved for the practitioner regarding urine collection are as follows:

1. Ensure that the infant's perineum is clean and dry.
2. Firmly press the adhesive rim of the urine bag against the skin around the perineum (anterior to the rectum) to make a good seal and to prevent leakage of the sample around the edges of the bag.
3. As soon as possible after the child has voided, carefully remove the bag, with attention to avoiding spillage.
4. Remove urine from the bag by inserting a small-gauge needle on a syringe into the blue port at the bottom of the bag or by pulling open the flap on the port and pouring the urine into a container.
5. Clearly indicate the specimen as a "bag" or random sample on the laboratory requisition to avoid misinterpretation of results. Bagged and random voided specimens must never be sent for culture.

Interpretation of Results

As previously discussed, these specimens are appropriate only for very specific tests, and these tests should be interpreted in light of institutional standards. Information that appears on certain standard tests (such as urine dipsticks) and that pertains to infection or inflammation (such as leukocyte esterase, nitrites, or the presence of red or white blood cells) should be ignored.

What the Patient and Family Should Know

Although sterility is not an issue for these specimens, an uncontaminated container should be used, and the specimen should be delivered to the office or laboratory as rapidly as possible. Families should also clearly understand the rationale for obtaining the urine by a nonsterile method.

Possible Complications

There are no direct complications. Inappropriate use of a random or bagged urine specimen for culture can result in false-positive or otherwise misleading information.

Aftercare Instructions

No specific aftercare instructions are needed after obtaining a bagged specimen. Skin reddening may occur as a reaction to the adhesive on the urine bag, but this condition should subside within minutes to a few hours. Swelling, blistering, or persistent redness of the site may indicate an allergic reaction and may necessitate discussion with the physician and avoidance of the use of such bags or adhesives in the future.

CLEAN-CATCH MIDSTREAM SPECIMEN COLLECTION

Relevant Anatomy

Again, anatomical considerations are trivial. The main objective is to transfer urine from the urethra to the sterile specimen container with minimum risk of contamination en route. Age and gender of the patient determine if this is a realistic possibility. If not, an alternative, more invasive means must be chosen when a sterile specimen is necessary.

Indications

Specimens obtained by clean-catch midstream collection are adequate for any of the purposes listed previously and for microscopic examination, cell count, and culture.

Contraindications

There are no absolute contraindications. Children who are not toilet trained are obviously inappropriate candidates for specimen collection in this fashion.

Required/Recommended Nursing Skills and Procedures

None are necessary.

Supplies and Equipment

- Labels
- Soap towelettes
- Sterile urine cups (preferably wide mouthed and with detachable handles)
- Toilet

Procedure

The only significant difficulty arises in ensuring that the patient (and parent, in the case of young children) understands how to correctly prepare for and perform this maneuver because, if done incorrectly, the specimen is no more useful than a randomly voided specimen. The technique varies for males and females.

For a male, the patient (or assistant) should follow these procedures:

1. Cleanse the periurethral area. This involves gently retracting the foreskin (if present, and if possible) and cleansing the glans penis and coronal sulcus with a soap towelette.
2. Initiate voiding and waste the first few milliliters of urine into the toilet.
3. Place a sterile container into the urine stream to catch a portion of the urine.
4. Remove the sterile container and finish the void into the toilet or urinal (thus the term "midstream").

For a female, the process is similar but potentially more cumbersome. The patient (or assistant) should follow these procedures:

1. Cleanse the periurethral area by spreading the labia minora apart, using a separate soap towelette to wipe front to back on each side of the urethra and front to back centrally.
2. Continuously retract the labia after cleansing while the patient initiates voiding into the toilet (wasting the first few milliliters of urine) and while the patient (or assistant) places the sterile container under the urine stream to catch a portion of the urine.
3. Remove the container, release the labia, and complete voiding into the toilet. This sequence can be difficult for a very young child to accomplish, and some practitioners find it easier to have the female straddle the toilet seat facing backward so that a larger portion of the seat opening is accessible to enable the assistant to maneuver the cup under the urine stream.

In each case, the patient and assistant should be cautioned against touching the inside of the container, and the lid should be applied tightly from the outside only. For results interpretation, please see the common section at the end of this chapter.

What the Patient and Family Should Know

Careful attentiveness to sterile technique and the avoidance of contamination are critical for this procedure.

Possible Complications

There are no complications to this procedure. Again, contamination of the specimen may lead to false-positive culture results.

Aftercare Instructions

Occasionally, patients may experience discomfort from the soap used to cleanse the periurethral area, but this irritation should generally respond to rinsing the offending agent off the mucosal tissue. Swelling, persistent irritation, or burning may indicate a more serious allergy and may require attention by the physician.

URETHRAL CATHETERIZATION

Relevant Anatomy

No attempts should ever be made to catheterize the urethra without direct visualization of the external urethral meatus. In circumcised males this procedure is relatively straightforward. In uncircumcised males and in females the urethra can be surprisingly difficult to see. In uncircumcised males the foreskin is gently retracted, revealing the meatus at the tip of the glans. Care must be taken not to pass the catheter into the space between the foreskin and the glans, which at best results in contamination and at worst can produce a "false track."

In females the urethra is located just inferior to the clitoris and generally cannot be seen without retraction of the labia minora. Two pits just lateral to the urethra help identify it, but these glandular orifices must not be mistaken for the urethra itself.

Indications

Urethral catheterization is considered the gold standard method for obtaining urine for culture and rigorous analysis. This technique is indicated if a clean-catch specimen is not obtainable (e.g., menstruating female, infant or child unable to perform this technique), if a previous clean-catch urine specimen has yielded equivocal results, or if urine must be obtained emergently or from an unconscious or uncooperative patient. For a neonate or very young infant, suprapubic aspiration of the bladder may be the preferred technique in these circumstances (see next section).

Contraindications and Reasons for Referral to a Specialist

Absolute contraindications to urethral catheterization include known or suspected urethral disruptions (usually traumatic), absolute neutropenia, and profound thrombocytopenia or other hypocoagulable states. Relative contraindications exist when the urethra is difficult to see directly or when repeated attempts at catheterization have failed.

Required/Recommended Nursing Skills and Procedures

In many settings, nurses perform catheterizations of the urethra, in which case they must be conversant with all of the skills outlined in this section. When functioning in a supportive role, nurses should understand the relevant anatomy and the fundamentals of sterile technique. Finally, an understanding of how to restrain a child for the procedure is critical.

TABLE 3-1
Appropriate catheter sizes by age

Age	Catheter size
0-3 months	5 Fr
4-12 months	5-8 Fr
1-4 years	8 Fr
5-8 years	10 Fr
9-12 years	12 Fr
>12 years	14 Fr

Supplies and Equipment

- Appropriate-sized catheter
- Lubricating jelly (water-soluble)
- Povidone-iodine solution
- Soap towelettes
- Sterile specimen container and label
- Sterile gloves
- Sterile swabs

Size 5 Fr feeding tubes are appropriate for newborn infants; size 8 Fr catheters are appropriate for ages 1 to 4 years; and size 10 to 14 Fr catheters are appropriate for the older child and adolescent (Table 3-1). Latex-free materials are preferable for urethral catheterization to reduce the risk of sensitization or allergic reaction.

Procedure

Preparation for catheterization includes selection of the appropriate catheter, correct positioning and restraint of the patient, and adequate cleansing of the periurethral area.

1. Choose a catheter that approximates the size of the urethral lumen for best results. A catheter that is too small can fail to withdraw urine or can allow leakage around the tubing, and a catheter that is too large can cause pain and possible urethral damage.
2. Position the patient in a supine position, with knees and hips slightly flexed for the male, and legs in frog-leg position for the female. For the cooperative patient, no restraint is required, but many patients need assistance remaining still once the catheter approaches the urethra. One to four assistants may be necessary.
3. For the male, extend the penis gently but firmly in the practitioner's gloved, nondominant hand, with the shaft pointing downward at approximately a 45-degree angle from the plane of the abdomen (Fig. 3-1).
4. For the female, retract the labia majora and minora laterally away from the urethra using the practitioner's nondominant hand (Fig. 3-2).
5. Cleanse the periurethral area, including removing any visible material (e.g., mucous, secretions, discharge) with soap towelettes, followed by sterilizing with povidone-iodine solution.

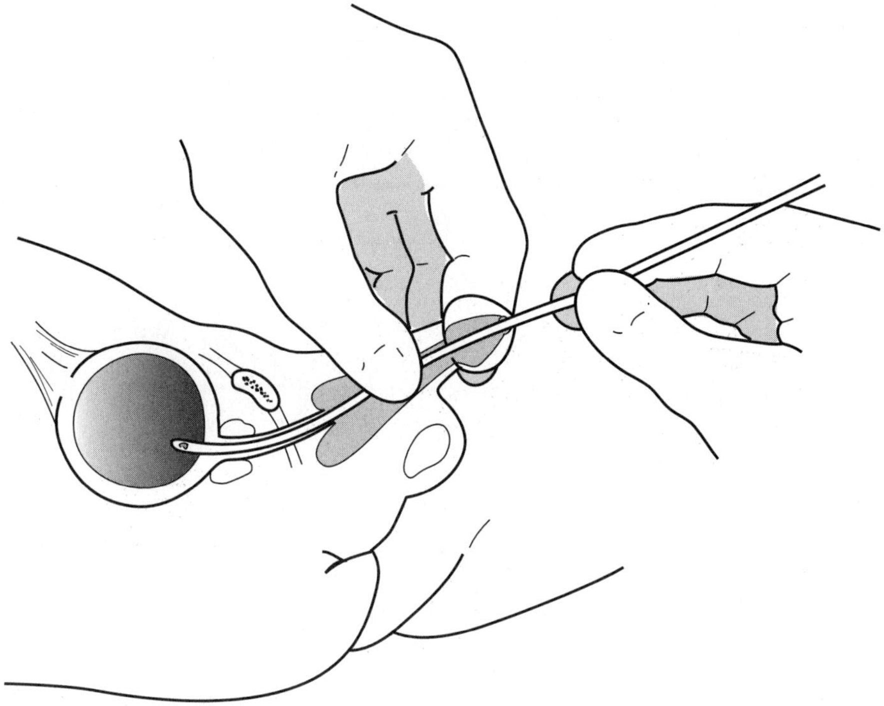

FIG. 3-1. Urethral catheterization of the male.

6. For the circumcised male and the male with a retractable foreskin, swab the entire glans penis down to the coronal sulcus. For the uncircumcised male with a tight foreskin, do not attempt to forcibly retract it, but align the urethral meatus with the foreskin meatus, if possible, and swab the entire area with povidone-iodine solution.
7. For the female, retract the labia majora and minora and swab from anterior to posterior on each side of the urethra, and then centrally, using a fresh povidone-iodine swab each time.
8. Using sterile technique, pass the catheter (lubricated with water-soluble sterile jelly) into the urethra until the balloon enters the bladder and free flow of urine is obtained.
9. If no urine appears immediately, pass the catheter a little farther, aiming toward the spine, and aspirate with a sterile syringe attached to the end of the catheter or feeding tube.
10. Once urine has been obtained and collected into the sterile container, gently withdraw the catheter and discard the urine remaining in the catheter.
11. If the catheter is to be left in place, inflate the balloon with saline or water and pull back gently to snug the balloon up next to the bladder neck to prevent leakage.

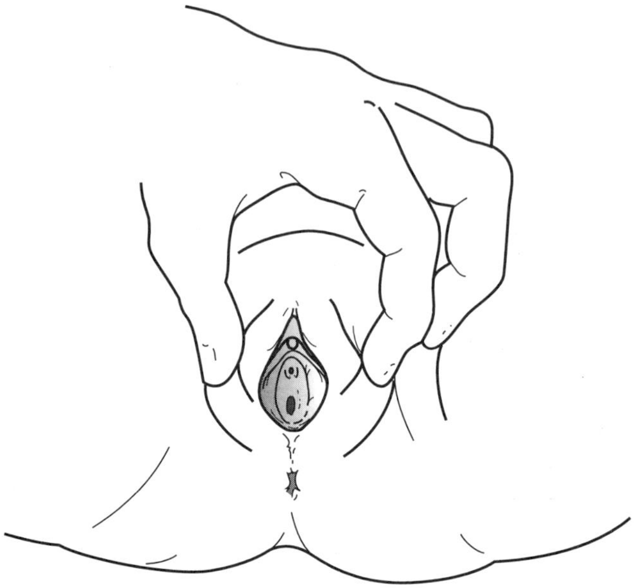

FIG. 3-2. Female perineal anatomy with retraction of labia.

12. Secure the tubing with tape and connect it to a sterile urinary collection system. Only urine obtained from the initial catheterization should be sent for culture and microscopic analysis; colonization of the catheter and bladder occurs within hours of catheter placement. For interpretation of results, please see the common section near the end of this chapter.

What the Patient and Family Should Know

Urethral catheterization is uncomfortable and threatening, especially for the young child. When caring for a verbal child, the procedure should be explained in simple terms. If the intent is to leave an indwelling catheter in place, this should be made explicit to both the child and family members. Care should be taken not to pull or dislodge an indwelling catheter. Occasionally, a small amount of bleeding may accompany passage of the catheter; explanation of this reaction before the procedure can allay many concerns.

Possible Complications

Significant complications of urethral catheterization include urethral tears and contusions. Extremely careless technique can introduce pathogens into the bladder, although this complication is rare. Also on rare occasions, a catheter can form a true knot in the bladder, which can be avoided by inserting the catheter only just far enough to obtain urine. Should significant resistance be met while withdrawing the catheter, a knot should be suspected and confirmed radiologically. If a knot is confirmed, prompt consultation with a urologist is indicated.

False tracking of the catheter can produce local mucosal tears of little significance. Contamination of the catheter tip with fecal, vaginal, or skin flora can produce false-positive cultures. Vaginal catheterization is common, especially in small children, and is generally apparent when the tip of the catheter is observed returning toward the operator, or when resistance is met before urine is obtained.

Aftercare Instructions

Parents should be instructed that children may experience some urgency or dysuria after bladder catheterization. If this condition persists beyond the first void after catheterization, the parents should notify the practitioner and ask for advice. Frank hematuria is always a reason to consult a physician.

SUPRAPUBIC BLADDER ASPIRATION

Relevant Anatomy

This technique is usually reserved for children under 2 years of age because the bladder in these young infants rises above the symphysis pubis and is an abdominal organ, whereas it is contained within the pelvis in older children and adults and is thus not readily accessible.

Indications

In neonates or some infants, it may be difficult or impossible to perform catheterization of the urethra because of the extremely small size of the infant, congenital abnormalities of the genitourinary tract, or other technical considerations. In these cases, and in some instances of practitioner preference or institutional tradition, it is possible to obtain urine for culture by suprapubic bladder aspiration, or "bladder tap." Advantages of this technique include minimal risk of specimen contamination, allowing for confidence in culture results. Obtaining an informed consent from the parents is advisable.

Contraindications

Coagulopathies and leukopenia represent relative contraindications to direct bladder aspiration.

Required/Recommended Nursing Skills

Familiarity with the technique to be performed and with general sterile procedures are required nursing skills, along with the ability to adequately position and restrain the child.

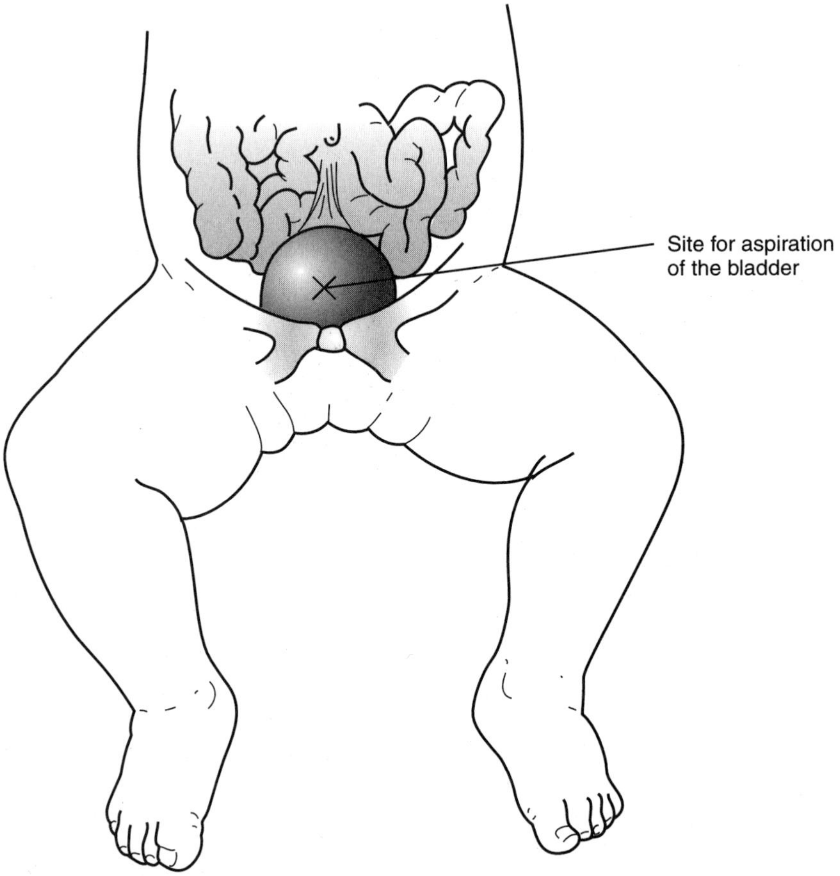

FIG. 3-3. Anterior view showing intraabdominal location of the bladder in an infant.

Supplies and Equipment

- Adhesive bandages
- Needles (22- or 25-gauge, 1.5-in length)
- Povidone-iodine solution
- Sterile alcohol swabs (optional)
- Sterile gloves
- Sterile specimen containers
- Sterile swabs
- Sterile syringes (3 or 5 ml)

Procedure

1. Restrain the infant in the supine position, with hips in the frog-leg position. The landmarks are the midabdominal line, 1 to 2 cm above the symphysis pubis (Fig. 3-3).

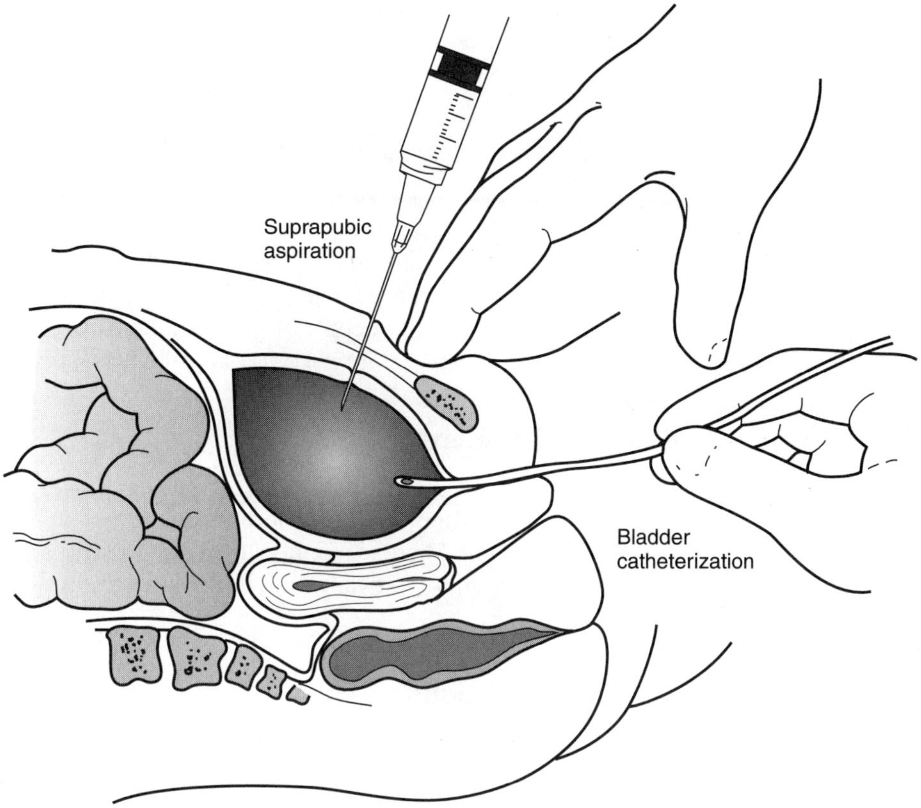

FIG. 3-4. Lateral view showing urethral catheterization of female and suprapubic bladder aspiration.

2. Swab the skin of the abdominal wall with povidone-iodine solution and allow it to air dry, after which the solution may be wiped off with a sterile alcohol pad, if desired.
3. Using sterile technique, hold the syringe like a pencil and firmly insert a 22- or 25-gauge needle attached to a 3- to 5-ml syringe through the skin and into the bladder one half to 1 inch at an angle of 15 to 20 degrees from true vertical (Fig. 3-4).
4. After insertion, pull back on the plunger to aspirate urine.
5. If no urine is forthcoming, withdraw the needle slightly while steadily pulling back on the plunger.
6. If urine still does not appear in the syringe, change the angle of the needle in the bladder by 10 to 20 degrees caudad and aspirate again.
7. If no urine is aspirated, change the angle one more time to a more cephalad position and aspirate a third time.
8. If these attempts are unsuccessful, withdraw the needle and consider waiting 1 hour or so until the bladder has accumulated more urine.

9. After urine is successfully aspirated, cleanse the skin with water to remove the iodine and place a bandage over the needle puncture site. Please see the common section for interpretation of results.

What the Patient and Family Should Know

Suprapubic bladder aspiration is a remarkably simple and rapid procedure. It is only performed in infants, and the procedure should be explained to the family before performing it, with documentation of informed consent advisable or even required at some institutions. The procedure is obviously painful but appears to be no more so than a venipuncture or intravenous catheter placement. A small spot of blood at the puncture site is common; otherwise, few sequellae occur.

Possible Complications

Possible complications of this technique include bowel perforation, bladder wall or abdominal wall hemorrhage, and introduction of infection into the bladder or the abdominal wall. Microscopic hematuria is not rare. If bladder catheterization is performed subsequent to a failed attempt at aspiration, some hematuria should be anticipated.

Aftercare Instructions

Infants may have microscopic hematuria after suprapubic bladder aspiration, but any visible blood in the urine should be brought to the attention of the physician immediately. The bandage can be removed after several hours.

INTERPRETATION OF RESULTS: URINE SPECIMENS

Local laboratory standards for interpretation of the results of dipstick urinalysis, microscopic urinalysis, Gram stain, cell count, and culture results should be consulted. As a general rule, colony counts of more than 10^5 colony-forming units (cfu)/ml are considered positive for urine obtained by the clean-catch midstream technique, although some authorities consider colony counts of more than 50,000 cfu/ml positive. Colony counts of more than 10,000 cfu/ml are considered positive for urine obtained by sterile catheterization. For a suprapubic aspirate specimen, most authorities consider any bacterial growth to be significant. Equivocal results may require obtaining additional urine (perhaps using a more rigorous technique) and clinical correlation with the patient's condition.

MODIFICATIONS FOR SITUATIONS OF LIMITED RESOURCES

Because of the intrinsic simplicity of these procedures, few modifications can be made to further simplify them. Suprapubic aspiration may be substituted for bladder catheterization in infants if small catheters are unavailable.

SUGGESTED READINGS

Broselow Pediatric Emergency Tape, 1991, Broselow Medical Technologies.

Burns M, Burns J, Krieger J: Pediatric urinary tract infection: diagnosis, classification, and significance, *Ped Clin North Am* 24:1111, 1987.

Hellerstein S: Urinary tract infections: old and new concepts, *Ped Clin North Am* 42:1433, 1985.

Hoberman A: Infection of the urinary tract. In Burg FD, Crellis SS, Kagan BM, editors: *Gellis and Kagan's current pediatric therapy,* ed 16, Philadelphia, 1999, WB Saunders.

The Johns Hopkins Children's Center Kids Kard, 1997, The Johns Hopkins University.

Morrell RE, Duritz G, Oltorf C: Suprapubic aspiration associated with hematuria, *Pediatrics* 69:455, 1982.

Polnay L, Fraser AM, Lewis JM: Complications of suprapubic bladder aspiration, *Arch Dis Child* 50:80, 1975.

Rushton HG: Genitourinary infections: non-specific infections. In Kelalis PP, King LR, and Belman AB, editors: *Clinical pediatric urology,* ed 3, Philadelphia, 1992, WB Saunders.

Shaw K, Gorelick MH: Urinary tract infection in the pediatric patient, *Ped Clin North Am* 46:1111, 1999.

CHAPTER 4

Lumbar Puncture

Joseph J. Zorc

BACKGROUND AND INTRODUCTION

Lumbar puncture (LP) is a common procedure used to (1) obtain cerebrospinal fluid (CSF) for investigation of suspected central nervous system (CNS) infection, inflammation, hemorrhage, or malignancy; (2) measure and treat elevated CSF pressure in cases of suspected benign intracranial hypertension (*pseudotumor cerebri*); or (3) administer intrathecal dye or medications for diagnosis or treatment of CNS disorders.

RELEVANT ANATOMY

Lumbar puncture is usually performed at or below the interspace between the third and fourth lumbar (L3-L4) vertebrae. This location prevents injury to the spinal cord, which ends at the L3 level in infants and higher in older children and adolescents. A needle passing through the midline at this location will intersect the following, in order: skin, subcutaneous fat, supraspinal and interspinal ligaments, ligamentum flavum, dura mater, and arachnoid mater (Fig. 4-1).

INDICATIONS

Lumbar puncture is indicated as a diagnostic evaluation for the following suspected disorders:

- Meningitis or encephalitis based on signs and symptoms, including:
  - — Fever: LP has been recommended as part of the routine workup for fever without source in infants less than 3 months old. In older children, a more selective approach is appropriate, based on the presence or absence of other signs and symptoms.
  - — Meningismus (may be absent in infants and toddlers with meningitis)
    - Brudzinski's sign: pain with neck flexion
    - Kernig's sign: pain with knee extension with the hip flexed at 90 degrees
  - — Altered mental status, irritability
  - — Bulging fontanel

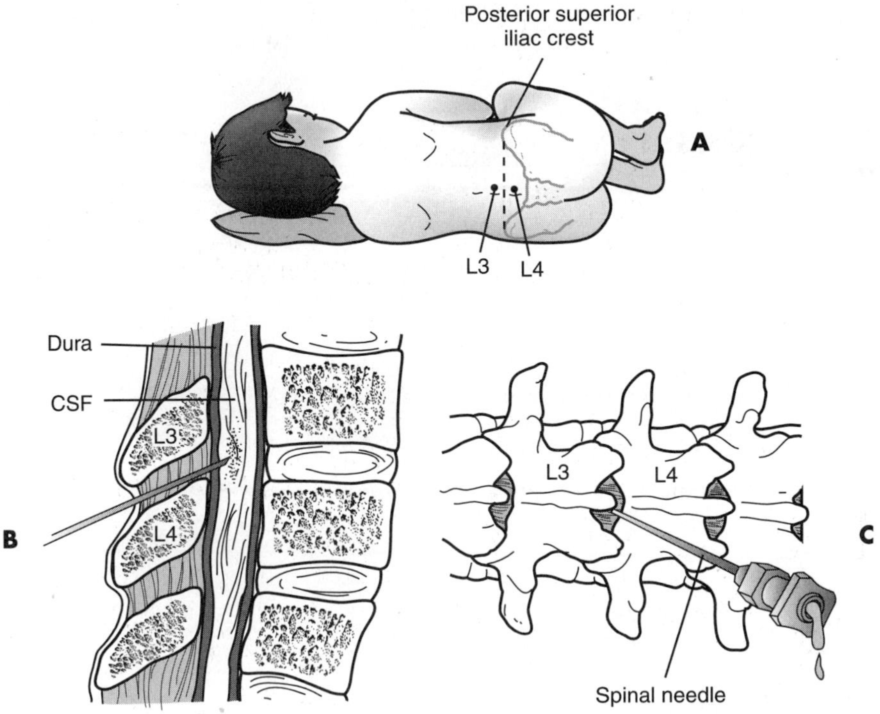

FIG. 4-1. Performing a Lumbar Puncture. The patient is positioned in the lateral decubitus or seated position. The L2-3 or 3-4 interspace is chosen, and the patient's legs and hips are flexed to maximally open the interspaces. **A,** It is not necessary to flex the neck with good hip flexion. Using strict aseptic technique, prepare and drape the back. Infiltrate the skin, subcutaneous tissue, and superficial ligaments with local anesthetic. Insert the spinal needle into the prepared space. **B,** The approach should be in the midline and perpendicular to the patient's spinal axis. **C,** Deviations from the perpendicular plane result in needle tip placement lateral to the midline, not into the subarachnoid space. Needle lengths range from 1.5 in for neonates to 3.5 in for adults; a 22-gauge needle is a good size for both collection of cerebrospinal fluid and measurements of opening pressure.

— Complex febrile seizure
— Systemic infection with potential CNS involvement (e.g., bacteremia, syphilis)

- Subarachnoid hemorrhage: Evidenced by sudden, severe headache with or without meningismus. Imaging is usually performed first to detect a large hemorrhage, but LP may detect small amounts of blood not seen on radiographic studies.
- *Pseudotumor cerebri:* Evidenced by chronic headaches with papilledema on physical examination. Benign intracranial hypertension is a primary condition, and a focal mass lesion should first be ruled out by careful neurologic examination and CNS imaging.
- Inflammatory diseases of the CNS, including Guillain-Barré syndrome, multiple sclerosis, and collagen vascular diseases (e.g., systemic lupus erythematosus)

Lumbar puncture is also used as a means for administration of intrathecal medications (e.g., chemotherapy, antibiotics, spinal anesthesia) or dye for imaging procedures (e.g., myelography or cystography).

CONTRAINDICATIONS

- Elevated intracranial pressure: If focal neurologic findings or papilledema are present, a space-occupying intracranial lesion should be ruled out by radiographic imaging before performing LP. If signs of impending cerebral herniation (e.g., pupillary changes, decerebrate posturing, coma) or Cushing's Triad (i.e., hypertension, bradycardia, bradypnea) are present, LP should be deferred and appropriate therapy initiated.
- Uncorrected coagulopathy or thrombocytopenia (platelet count less than $50{,}000/mm^3$)
- Local skin infection in the lumbar area
- Respiratory or cardiovascular instability that may worsen with positioning in flexion

SUPPLIES AND EQUIPMENT

- Sterile gloves
- Povidone-iodine solution
- Items usually included in commercial lumbar puncture tray:
  - Sterile drapes
  - Sterile sponges or gauze
  - Lidocaine (1%) without epinephrine
  - Sterile 3-ml syringe and 25- to 30-gauge needle for lidocaine infiltration
  - Sterile collecting tubes
  - Sterile spinal needle, 22-gauge, 1.5-in length for infant or toddler, 2.5-in length for older child, 3.5-in length for adolescent or adult
- Additional items for pressure measurement
  - Manometer and stopcock

PROCEDURE

Good positioning is the key to successful lumbar puncture in pediatric patients. Infants and toddlers require positioning by an experienced and knowledgable assistant. For older children and adolescents, local anesthesia and reassurance usually provide adequate conditions for the procedure. A topical anesthetic such as the eutectic mixture of local anesthetics (EMLA) can be applied in advance if a delay is acceptable before the procedure. For anxious children who are not able to cooperate, sedation should be considered (see Chapter 8), avoiding agents such as ketamine, which may increase intracranial pressure.

Monitoring of cardiorespiratory status and oximetry is important in sedated patients or those (such as young infants) for whom positioning in flexion may potentially impair respiration. For uncooperative or sedated children, the patient is usually placed in the lateral decubitus position with neck flexed and knees drawn upward. The assistant can place one arm behind the neck and another behind the knees and lock both hands to stabilize this position. Cooperative patients can sit on the side of the bed and voluntarily bend forward to flex the spine and open the lumbar interspaces. The following steps detail this procedure:

1. Before prepping the back, examine the area and identify the site for the procedure; this will usually be the L3-L4 or L4-L5 interspace.
2. Draw an imaginary line between the posterior superior iliac crests intersecting the spine just above the L4 level (Fig. 4-1, *A*).
3. Press firmly with a thumbnail at the anticipated puncture site, leaving a mark for several minutes to help ensure proper location after skin preparation and draping.
4. Prepare the lumbar area at least three times with povidone-iodine solution from top to bottom; allow the area to dry and cover it with sterile drapes.
5. Again locate the interspace to inject lidocaine locally, first raising a skin wheal and then infiltrating superficially to the level of the spinal ligaments, taking care not to inject into the spinal canal. Local anesthetic should be used in all age groups; in newborns, it has been shown to decrease pain response without reducing the success of the procedure.
6. After ensuring that the patient is well-positioned, again recheck landmarks and identify the appropriate site. It may be helpful to place the tip of the nondominant thumb on the spinous process above the interspace as a landmark during the procedure.
7. Insert the spinal needle in the midline with the bevel parallel to the long axis of the spine; the needle should point slightly cephalad, aiming at the umbilicus (Fig. 4-1, *B* and *C*).
8. Support the needle at the level of the skin with one hand to prevent movement during the procedure.
9. Advance the needle slowly with the stylet in place; resistance may be felt as the needle passes through the ligamentum flavum and again as it passes through the dura. Gentle pressure will overcome this resistance, resulting in a "pop" as the needle passes into the next space.
10. Remove the stylet to check for fluid return. Rotating the hub 90 degrees may improve fluid flow if the bevel is partially obstructed.
11. If no CSF returns, reinsert the stylet and advance the needle another few millimeters. The depth of the spinal canal is quite superficial in young infants (1 to 2 cm) but can be more than 5 cm in adolescents, requiring the use of a 3.5-in needle. If the needle passes through the spinal space into the epidural venous plexus or laterally into a radicular vessel, blood may return. The blood may clear with CSF flow; if this does not happen, remove the needle and reattempt the procedure at another interspace.
12. Once CSF begins to flow, attach the manometer to the spinal needle and measure the column of fluid to obtain an opening pressure. Accurate measurement of opening pressure requires the patient to be lying on his or her side with legs extended. Interposition of a short (3-in) extension tubing

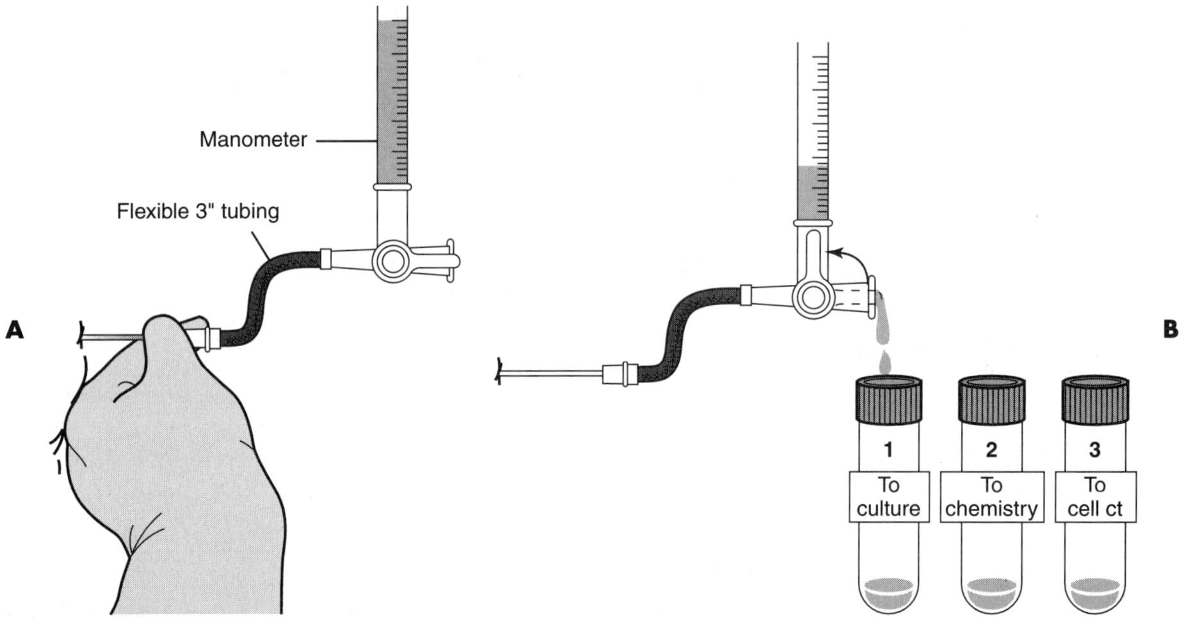

FIG. 4-2. Measurement of Opening Pressure. **A,** The opening pressure is measured immediatedly after obtaining cerebrospinal fluid (CSF) flow. This is most easily done by connecting the manometer and stopcock to a short, flexible piece of tubing. This tubing is connected directly to the spinal needle. (All pieces of the system must be sterile.) The stopcock is turned so that CSF travels up the manometer. Allow the flow to continue until it stops and the level varies with respirations. This is then the patient's opening pressure, measured in mm or cm H_2O. (The conversion of cm H_2O to mmHg is 10 cm H_2O to 7.5 mmHg.) **B,** After obtaining the opening pressure, turn the stopcock so that CSF from the manometer flows into collection tubes. Turn the stopcock again so that CSF drips from the patient into the collection tubes. Note: An accurate opening pressure can be obtained only in a quiet, noncrying child.

between the hub of the needle and the stopcock reduces the chances of dislodging the needle during manipulation of the stopcock (Fig. 4-2).

13. Turn the stopcock away from the needle initially to divert flow upward into the column (Fig. 4-2, *A*).
14. Drain fluid off for laboratory studies (Fig. 4-2, *B*). Usually, the first tube is sent for Gram stain and culture; intermediate tubes are sent for glucose and protein and any additional studies such as bacterial antigen tests (not cost effective unless partially treated meningitis is suspected) or polymerase chain reaction for suspected viral infections; and the last tube is sent for cell count and differential. If bleeding has occurred, there may be value in sending the first and last tubes for cell count to document a declining red blood cell count suggestive of a traumatic tap.
15. At the completion of the procedure, remove the needle with the stylet in place, apply pressure, and clean the area and cover it with a sterile dressing.

TABLE 4-1
Evaluation of cerebrospinal fluid

	Preterm infant	Term infant	Child
Cell count, WBC/mm^3			
mean	9.0	8.2	
range	0-25.4	0-22.4	0-7
Differential, %PMNs	57%	61%	0%
Glucose, mg/dl			
mean	50	52	
range	24-63	34-119	40-80
CSF/blood ratio	55-105%	44-128%	50%
Protein, mg/dl			
mean	115	90	
range	65-150	20-170	5-40
Opening pressure, mm H_2O	Newborn: 80-110	Infant/child: < 200	

INTERPRETATION OF RESULTS

Normal values for standard CSF parameters by age are listed in Table 4-1. For a traumatic tap, the interpretation of cell counts using ratio of white blood cells to red blood cells is unreliable.

INSTRUCTIONS FOR THE FAMILY

Before the procedure, family members should be informed of indications and potential complications of lumbar puncture, including infection, bleeding, and pain (during the procedure as well as postprocedure headache). Parents should be reassured that with local anesthesia and standard precautions the procedure is generally well-tolerated and safe.

POSSIBLE COMPLICATIONS

- Local pain and paresthesia: Superficial discomfort can be reduced with adequate local anesthesia. The LP needle may touch spinal nerves, causing transient neurologic symptoms, although permanent sequellae are not expected if the procedure is done below the level of the cauda equina.
- Post-LP headache and backache: This complication is thought to be caused by ongoing leakage through a dural hole, resulting in reduced CSF volume and epidural fluid collection. Using a small-gauge needle and removing as little CSF as possible can reduce the likelihood of headache. Patients are often instructed to lie prone for several hours after the procedure to reduce CSF hydrostatic pressure, although the efficacy of this advice is unproven. Blood patching using

5 to 15 ml of fresh blood injected into the epidural space can be attempted if CSF continues to leak.

- Infection: Iatrogenic meningitis can occur as a result of poor sterile technique or local cellulitis at the area of the procedure. If the patient is bacteremic at the time of LP, subsequent seeding of the meninges may occur, but the LP procedure does not appear to increase the likelihood of this occurrence.
- Bleeding: Subdural or epidural spinal hematoma presents with pain and neurologic symptoms hours to days after the procedure. These complications are usually associated with thrombocytopenia or coagulopathy and can be avoided by replacing clotting factors and platelets before the procedure.
- Cerebral herniation: This life-threatening complication has been reported after LP in the presence of elevated intracranial pressure both with and without an intracranial mass lesion. The causal relationship between LP and herniation is debated, but if focal neurologic findings or papilledema are present, the procedure should be deferred until a mass lesion has been excluded by imaging. In patients with clinical findings of early herniation (i.e., pupillary abnormalities, posturing, or coma), the risks of the procedure may outweigh its benefits. In a patient with clinical signs of meningitis, a delay for imaging or other reasons should not postpone treatment with antibiotics; other tests (e.g., CSF pleiocytosis, antigen tests, blood culture) can be used to make the diagnosis after empiric treatment.
- Epidermoid spinal cord tumor: Implantation of epidermis into the spinal canal can be avoided by using a spinal needle with a stylet.

AFTERCARE INSTRUCTIONS

After the procedure, patients should rest in bed for several hours, if possible. The LP site should be kept covered and clean; local pressure should be applied if bleeding or leakage of fluid occurs.

SUGGESTED READINGS

Atabaki S, Ochsenschlager D, Vezina G: Post-lumbar puncture headache and backache in pediatrics: a case series and demonstration of magnetic resonance imaging findings, *Arch Pediatr Adolesc Med* 153:770, 1999.

Baraff LJ et al: Practice guideline for the management of infants and children 0 to 36 months of age with fever without source, *Pediatrics* 92:1, 1993.

Cronan, KM, Wiley JF: Lumbar puncture. In Henretig FM, King C, editors: Textbook of pediatric emergency procedures, Baltimore, 1997, Williams and Wilkins.

Maxson S, Lewno MJ, Schutze GE: Clinical usefulness of cerebrospinal fluid bacterial antigen studies, *J Pediatr* 125:235, 1994.

Pinheiro JMB, Furdon S, Ochoa LF: Role of local anesthesia during lumbar puncture in neonates, *Pediatrics* 91:379, 1993.

Shapiro ED et al: Risk factors for development of bacterial meningitis among children with occult bacteremia, *J Pediatr* 109:15, 1986.

Shetty AK et al: Fatal cerebral herniation after lumbar puncture in a patient with a normal computed tomography scan, *Pediatrics* 103:1284, 1999.

Siberry GK, Iannone R: The Harriet Lane Handbook, ed 15, St Louis, 2000, Mosby.

Ward E, Gushurst CA: Uses and technique of pediatric lumbar puncture, *Am J Dis Child* 146:1160, 1992.

CHAPTER 5

Cerebrospinal Fluid Shunt Evaluation

Joseph J. Zorc
Ann-Christine Duhaime

BACKGROUND AND INTRODUCTION

Cerebrospinal fluid (CSF) shunts are used to treat hydrocephalus and related conditions by draining fluid from the central nervous system (CNS) to locations elsewhere in the body. CSF shunt placement has become the most common neurosurgical procedure, with pediatric diseases (including congenital conditions such as meningomyelocele and acquired conditions such as intraventricular hemorrhage related to prematurity) among the most common indications. Although shunting has dramatically improved mortality for these diagnoses, longitudinal studies of patients with CSF shunts have documented a high rate of shunt malfunctions, with approximately 80% of patients requiring revision by 12 years after placement.

Shunt obstruction, the most common complication, results in elevation of intracranial pressure (ICP) that may progress to cerebral herniation and death. Although potentially life-threatening, shunt obstruction may present initially with nonspecific symptoms such as vomiting and headache. Shunt infection, usually occurring after an operation on the shunt, may present with fever with or without symptoms of shunt obstruction. Therefore practitioners caring for children with CSF shunts should be familiar with indications and procedures for shunt evaluation.

RELEVANT ANATOMY

CSF shunts are hollow tubes that carry fluid from areas of impaired absorption within the CNS (e.g., ventricles, cysts, subdural collections, lumbar space) to areas that can absorb CSF in other parts of the body (e.g., peritoneum, pleura, right atrium). Made out of flexible plastic, the type of shunt is anatomically identified by its proximal and distal end, such as ventriculoperitoneal (VP), ventriculoatrial (VA, also called ventriculojugular, VJ), or lumboperitoneal (LP). Assessment of potential

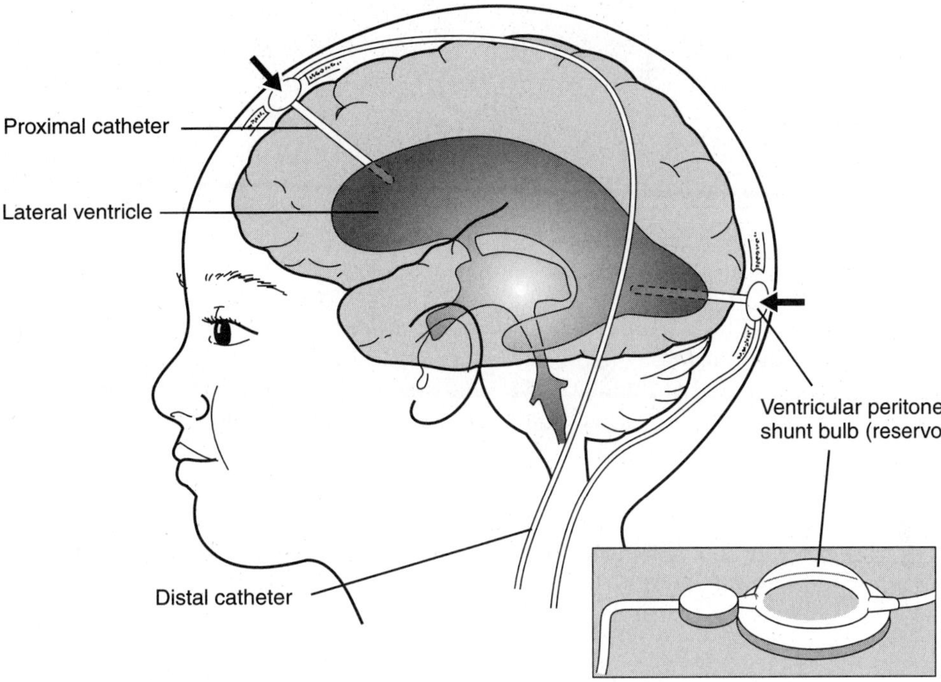

FIG. 5-1. Aspiration of an obstructed ventricular shunt anatomy.

shunt problems requires a basic understanding of their function, which can be divided into four main components (Fig. 5-1):

1. *Proximal catheter:* Drains fluid from the proximal CNS site. For hydrocephalus this is most commonly the lateral ventricle; other sites may include cysts or other fluid-filled spaces. The catheter then passes through brain tissue, through a burr hole in the skull, and out to the subcutaneous space.
2. *Reservoir:* Usually a single or double bulb, button, or cylinder that contains CSF for assessment of flow and makes it accessible for sampling. The reservoir is often located near the burr hole on the side of the head. Many, but not all, reservoirs are compressible and can be assessed manually (see following section, Pumping a Shunt).
3. *Valve:* Controls the rate of CSF flow to prevent overshunting. This may be located within or adjacent to the reservoir or may be a slit valve at the end of the distal catheter.
4. *Distal catheter:* Carries fluid from the reservoir through a subcutaneous tunnel to the distal site.

Other specialized shunt components may also be present, including devices to modify flow (such as antisiphon devices) or to measure or change pressure using special equipment. The physical examination of a patient with suspected shunt malfunction should include inspection and palpation of the reservoir, most often located in the parietal area, and the distal catheter, assessing for disconnections, fluid extravasation, or overlying erythema.

INDICATIONS

Shunt Obstruction

Shunt obstruction or malfunction can present with various signs and symptoms and requires a high level of clinical suspicion. Similar to all chronic pediatric conditions, family members can provide a valuable resource for diagnosis because they may be familiar with the specific symptoms that have heralded shunt malfunction for this child in the past. The signs and symptoms of shunt malfunction include the following:

- Headache
- Vomiting
- Lethargy, irritability, or more subtle changes in behavior or personality
- Bulging anterior fontanel or increasing head circumference in infants
- Persistent or enlarging fluid extravasation around the burr hole reservoir or tubing
- Apnea
- Seizure: usually not alone but in association with other signs and symptoms
- Papilledema: may be absent in obstructed patients
- New cranial nerve or other neurologic findings: for example, upward gaze palsy (sunsetting, usually seen in infants), inability to look laterally (sixth nerve palsy), gait disturbance, or blurry vision
- Signs of impending cerebral herniation: Cushing's triad (i.e., bradycardia, hypertension, bradypnea) or another vital sign instability, posturing

Infection

For shunts that are not located in the bloodstream, the most common source of infection is contamination at the time of surgery. Therefore greater than 90% of infections present within 6 months of shunt placement or revision. For shunts that terminate in the bloodstream (VA shunts), infections can occur at any time from hematogenous seeding. VP shunts can be infected as a result of intraabdominal processes such as ruptured appendicitis or significant bladder infections. Signs or symptoms of shunt infection include the following:

- Fever without other source
- Meningeal signs
- Peritonitis or abdominal tenderness (VP shunts)
- Pseudocyst: a walled-off CSF collection around the peritoneal catheter best seen on ultrasound examination of the abdomen
- Protrusion of shunt tubing through the skin or erythema overlying the shunt
- Nephritis: a rare complication of intravascular shunts

CONTRAINDICATIONS AND REFERRAL TO A SPECIALIST

Because of the complex nature of CSF shunts and the risks of misdiagnosis, a neurosurgeon should be consulted early in the evaluation of suspected malfunction or infection. The course of action may vary depending on the level of concern and available resources. If the patient is stable, further procedures may be deferred while the patient is transported to a tertiary care center. Radiographic studies such as computed tomography (CT) and plain films of the shunt (shunt series) may be used to make the diagnosis noninvasively, avoiding the risk of infection associated with shunt puncture. Radiographic studies should be interpreted carefully by practitioners experienced with shunt assessment because high rates of misdiagnosis have been reported. Comparison of CT scans to baseline studies is often necessary for correct interpretation.

If the diagnosis remains unclear or if the patient's condition is deteriorating, the shunt may need to be tapped to measure ICP, assess flow, obtain fluid for Gram stain and culture, and relieve elevated pressure by withdrawing fluid in the case of a distal obstruction. This procedure is usually performed by a neurosurgeon but in some instances may need to be carried out by other medical personnel. On rare occasions, a child with a proximal shunt obstruction presents with symptoms of life-threatening ICP elevation (e.g., unresponsiveness, bradycardia, extensor posturing) that cannot be relieved with a shunt tap. In these cases, a burr hole puncture may be attempted after initial stabilizing procedures have been completed (i.e., airway stabilization, hyperventilation, initiation of medical management for elevated ICP). Shunt tap or burr hole puncture should not be attempted when a local skin infection overlies the area.

SUPPLIES AND EQUIPMENT

Procedures for suspected shunt malfunction should be performed with monitoring and resuscitation equipment on hand because ICP shifts caused by removal of fluid may be associated with cardiorespiratory instability. Necessary supplies include the following:

For shunt bulb compression: none

For shunt puncture:

- Butterfly needle (23-gauge) and syringe
- Povidone-iodine solution and isopropyl alcohol
- Razor (if hair is dense)
- Sterile collection tubes
- Sterile gloves

For burr hole puncture:

- Povidone-iodine solution and isopropyl alcohol
- Razor
- Spinal needle (21-gauge, 3.5-in)
- Sterile collection tubes
- Sterile gloves and drapes

PROCEDURE

Pumping a Shunt

Many shunt reservoirs are designed to be compressed manually to help assess shunt function. This procedure varies depending on the location and type of reservoir.

For reservoirs with a single chamber or bulb:

1. Compress the bulb followed by observation of refill to provide some information about the presence of an obstruction.
2. Compress and release the shunt bulb gently to minimize suction in the proximal catheter, which may pull choroid tissue into the catheter, potentially causing an obstruction. Resistance to bulb compression suggests an obstruction in the distal catheter. Slow or absent bulb refill suggests a proximal obstruction or, alternatively, the absence of fluid in the ventricles because of small ventricles.

For double reservoir systems:

1. Compress the proximal bulb closest to the burr hole.
2. Keeping the proximal bulb compressed, compress the distal reservoir, with resistance suggesting a distal obstruction.
3. Release the proximal bulb, with slow refill suggesting a proximal obstruction or small ventricles.

Although shunt bulb compression is routinely used to assess shunt bulb function, a study of 200 consecutive shunt patients reported a sensitivity of less than 40% and a negative predictive value of 65% to 90% for this test. Therefore interpretation of shunt pump may require other studies (such as a CT scan to assess ventricular size), and a normal shunt compression test should not preclude further evaluation if the clinical scenario suggests shunt obstruction.

Ventricular Shunt Puncture

A shunt puncture requires particularly careful antiseptic technique because it accesses an indwelling foreign body. Local anesthetic is not generally used because the discomfort created by the procedure is minimal.

1. Place the child in the lateral position for a posterior shunt and supine for a frontal shunt.
2. Cleanse the hair and scalp surrounding the shunt with alcohol. If the hair is dense, shave or clip it to expose the reservoir.
3. Prepare the skin thoroughly with povidone-iodine solution in an outward spiraling fashion.
4. Identify the reservoir bulb and insert the butterfly needle into the reservoir bulb to a depth of a few millimeters (Fig. 5-2). Button-type reservoirs that are situated in the burr hole are accessed straight down, perpendicular to the scalp. Cylindrical valves (Holter-type) should not be punctured except under emergency situations because puncture may damage the valve. A "pop" should be felt as the needle punctures the reservoir dome; if the needle is inserted too far, it may hit the back wall of the reservoir and impair CSF flow.
5. Once flow begins, hold up the tubing vertically and obtain an opening pressure

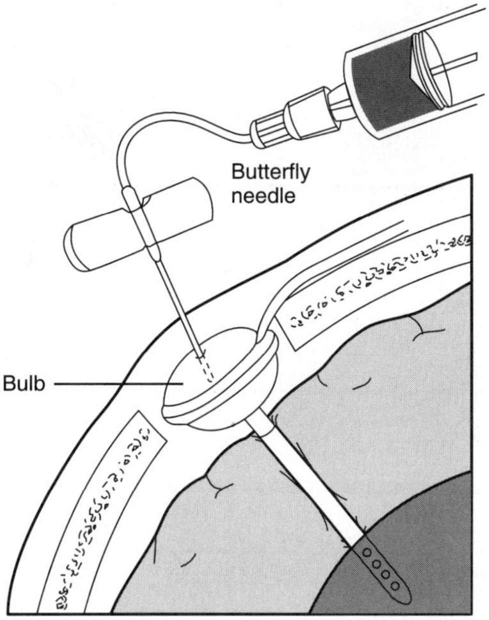

FIG. 5-2. Aspiration of an obstructed ventricular shunt through the proximal shunt chamber.

by measuring the height of the column above the ear when the child is calm. Normal shunt puncture is usually demonstrated by slow flow with variation of the height of the column with respiration. Rapid flow under high pressure (more than 20 cm of water) suggests a distal catheter obstruction.

6. If flow is sluggish or absent, apply gentle suction with a syringe and adjust the position of the needle slightly. An inability to obtain flow or collapsing of the bubble with suction suggests a proximal obstruction or small ventricles.
7. If the shunt is obstructed and fluid can be removed, withdraw at least 10 ml of fluid over a few minutes to acutely decrease the ICP.
8. After completing the procedure, apply gentle pressure with sterile gauze until bleeding ceases.
9. If fluid cannot be withdrawn because of complete proximal obstruction and the patient shows evidence of herniation despite medical management (hyperventilation and mannitol), perform a burr hole puncture.

Burr Hole Puncture

1. After preparing and shaving the scalp as described previously, identify the burr hole and insert a 21-gauge, 3.5-in needle perpendicular to the skull along the path of the proximal catheter (Fig. 5-3). If a reservoir occupies the burr hole, the needle punctures through the bulb on its path.
2. Advance the needle in 0.5-cm increments and remove the stylet at each depth to check for CSF flow. Usually the ventricle is reached by a depth of 5 cm.

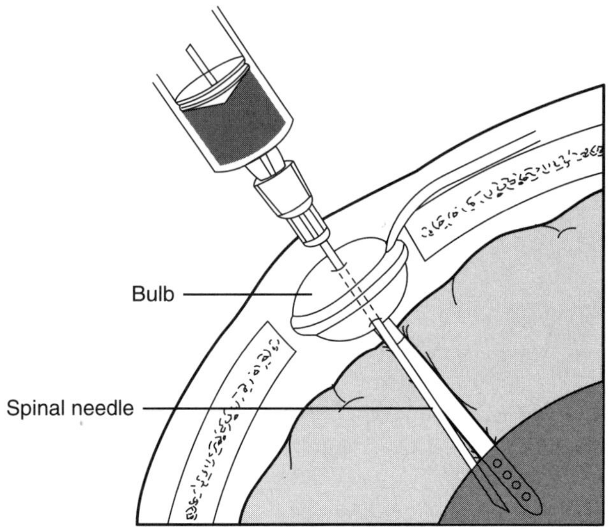

FIG. 5-3. Aspiration of an obstructed ventricular shunt directly into the lateral ventricle.

3. After CSF drainage slows, replace the stylet and slowly withdraw the needle. Because a burr hole puncture will likely injure the shunt and may cause intraparenchymal damage, close monitoring and emergent neurosurgical evaluation is required after this procedure.

INTERPRETATION OF RESULTS

Gram stain and cell culture can be interpreted in the same fashion as lumbar puncture (see Chapter 4). Postoperatively after shunt placement a CSF pleiocytosis may be seen without infection.

INSTRUCTIONS FOR THE FAMILY

The family should be informed of the risks of shunt puncture, including infection and local bleeding. Parents and children should be reassured that pain caused by the procedure is minimal.

POSSIBLE COMPLICATIONS

Complications of shunt pumping are minimal. If the ventricles are collapsed, overzealous compression of the shunt bulb can create suction and potentially trap choroid tissue in the proximal catheter, resulting in obstruction.

Shunt tap is an invasive procedure with potential complications, including the following:

- Infection: reported in 0.5% to 1% of shunt punctures, usually from skin organisms
- Mechanical damage to the shunt or obstruction with choroid or other cellular material
- Rapid pressure shifts as a result of relief of high ICP can cause brain injury and bleeding
- Local bleeding at the puncture site

Burr hole puncture has a much higher likelihood of similar complications and should be viewed as a procedure of last resort to treat herniation as a result of proximal obstruction.

AFTERCARE INSTRUCTIONS

If shunt obstruction or infection is diagnosed, definitive care should be provided by a neurosurgeon in a hospital environment that affords appropriate monitoring and access to resuscitation equipment. If shunt function and CSF studies are normal, further evaluation to determine the cause of presenting symptoms should be performed. Because shunt malfunction can be intermittent, "ruling out" this possibility with a single evaluation is difficult. If the diagnosis remains unclear, the patient should be watched closely for progression of symptoms; hospitalization may be warranted in these cases.

MODIFICATIONS FOR SITUATIONS OF LIMITED RESOURCES

Because of the moderate complexity and urgency of these procedures, shunt punctures of any kind should not be attempted in settings in which adequate and appropriate equipment is not available. Rather, patients who may require these procedures should be expeditiously transferred to an appropriate environment after consultation with the receiving physician, whenever possible.

SUGGESTED READINGS

Bondurant CP, Jimenez DF: Epidemiology of cerebrospinal fluid shunting, *Pediatr Neurosurg* 23:254, 1995.

Guertin SR: Cerebrospinal fluid shunts: evaluation, complications, and crisis management, *Pediatr Clin North Am* 34:203, 1987.

Hack Ch et al: Seizures in relation to shunt dysfunction in children with meningomyelocele, *J Pediatr* 116:57, 1990.

Iskandar BJ et al: Pitfalls in the diagnosis of ventricular shunt dysfunction: radiology reports and ventricular size, *Pediatr* 101:1031, 1998.

Kanev PM, Parks TS: The treatment of hydrocephalus, *Neurosurg Clin North Am* 4:611, 1993.

Piatt JH: Physical examination of patients with cerebrospinal fluid shunts: is there useful information in pumping the shunt? *Pediatrics* 89:470, 1992.

Renier D et al: Factors causing acute shunt infection. Computer analysis of 1171 operations, *J Neurosurg* 61:1022, 1984.

Saint-Rose C et al: Mechanical complications in shunts, *Pediatr Neurosurg* 17:2, 1991.

Sekhar LN, Moossy J, Guthkelch N: Malfunctioning ventriculoperitoneal shunts: clinical and pathological features, *J Neurosurg* 56:411, 1982.

CHAPTER 6

Arterial Sampling and Access

Anne F. Brayer

BACKGROUND AND INTRODUCTION

Arterial sampling is often indicated in seriously ill or injured children. It is often performed to obtain vital information about the status of the child's oxygenation, ventilation, perfusion, and acid-base status. It is a procedure of moderate complexity, but in execution it differs little from the procedure in adult patients.

Arterial access (i.e., cannulation) is less commonly necessary in emergency management but may be useful for children who require repeated blood gas sampling or for blood pressure monitoring.

RELEVANT ANATOMY

Similar to adults, arterial blood is most often obtained from the radial artery in children. Arterial blood supply to the hand and digits comes from the superficial and deep palmar arches (Fig. 6-1). In most individuals, the arches are supplied by collateral flow from the ulnar and radial arteries. Because this flow may not be adequate in up to 12% of adults, the presence of collateral flow should be established using the Allen test or Doppler flow test before accessing the radial artery (see following section).

The radial artery is accessed at its most superficial point in the wrist, where its pulse can usually be felt on the volar surface, medial to the styloid process of the radius and just proximal to the transverse skin crease (see Fig. 6-1). Although the pulse may be felt more distal to this crease in young infants, the artery courses deeper here under the flexor tendons on its way to the anatomical snuffbox region.

Other sites appropriate for arterial blood sampling include the dorsalis pedis artery and the posterior tibial artery in the lower extremity. The dorsalis pedis artery courses superficially along the dorsum of the foot as a continuation of the tibial artery (Fig. 6-2). Its strongest pulse is usually felt on the dorsum of the midfoot, just lateral to the extensor hallucis tendon. The posterior tibial artery courses in the posterior ankle. It is accessed at the point of maximal pulsation, between the medial malleolus and the Achilles tendon (Fig. 6-3).

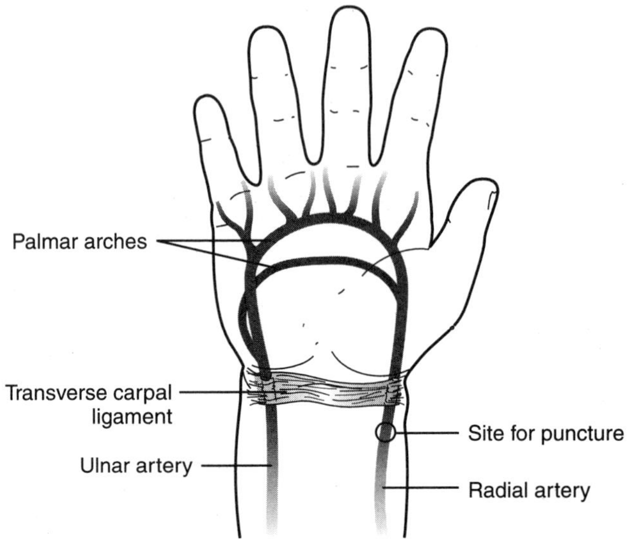

FIG. 6-1. Anatomy of the radial artery.

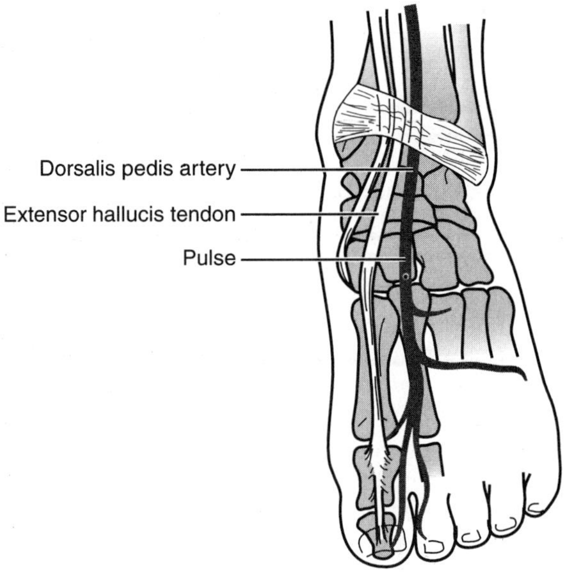

FIG. 6-2. Anatomy of the dorsalis pedis artery.

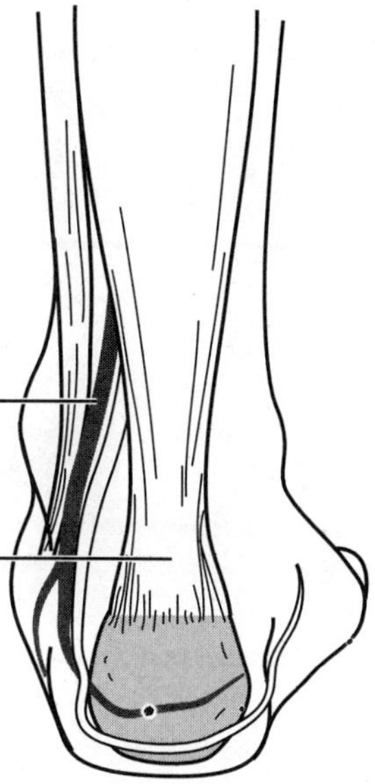

FIG. 6-3. Anatomy of the posterior tibial artery.

The femoral artery may also be used for arterial line placement but is less commonly used for routine sampling. The most common access point of the femoral artery is in the proximal anterior thigh in the femoral triangle (Fig. 6-4). This triangle is bordered superiorly by the inguinal ligament, laterally by the sartorius muscle, and medially by the adductor longus muscle. It is generally located at the midpoint between the anterior superior iliac spine and the pubic symphysis. The femoral vein is located just medial to the artery, and the femoral nerve is positioned just lateral to the artery. The femoral head is deep to the femoral triangle, so care must be taken to avoid bone penetration during arterial access.

INDICATIONS

Arterial blood sampling is indicated to ascertain oxygenation and ventilation (carbon dioxide levels) in children with severe respiratory disease, such as asthma, aspiration, near drowning, bronchiolitis, or pneumonia.

Arterial blood sampling is also often helpful in determining the acid-base status in patients with severe dehydration, diabetic ketoacidosis, toxic ingestions (e.g., aspirin, tricyclic antidepressants), or another metabolic derangement. Arterial blood sampling may be indicated in cases in which venous blood cannot be obtained or is inadequate in volume.

Arterial cannulation and line placement is indicated when frequent repeat blood gases are necessary or when continuous blood pressure monitoring is desired.

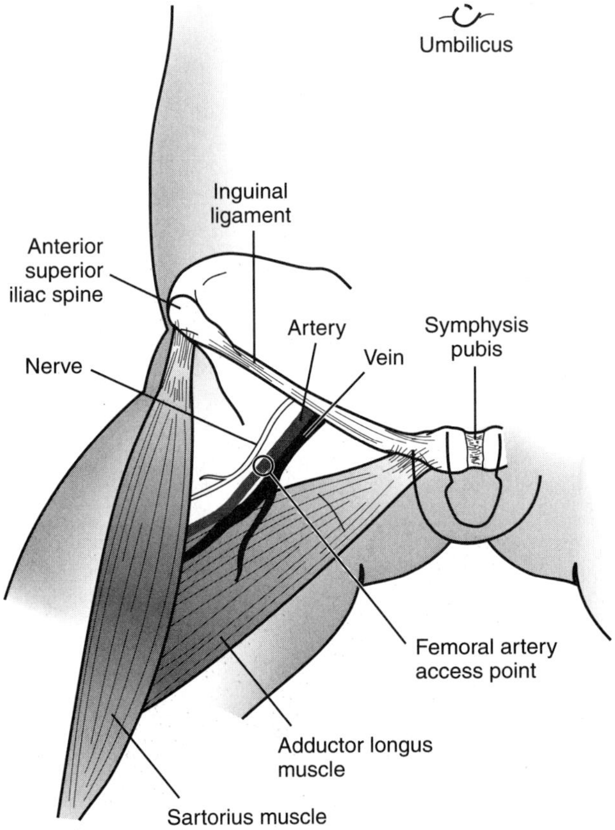

FIG. 6-4. Anatomy of the femoral artery.

CONTRAINDICATIONS

Arterial puncture is relatively contraindicated in patients with a known coagulation disorder or ongoing anticoagulant therapy. Cannulation of the radial artery is contraindicated if the presence of sufficient collateral flow to the hand cannot be established (see following discussion).

REQUIRED/RECOMMENDED NURSING SKILLS AND PROCEDURES

Arterial sampling can be performed by a single practitioner in an older cooperative child or if adequate immobilization of the limb can be obtained. It is helpful to have a second person position the child and maintain pressure on the puncture site after the procedure while the practitioner prepares the sample for the laboratory.

When arterial cannulation is being obtained for continuous blood pressure monitoring, nursing or technical support staff are required to set up the pressure transducer.

SUPPLIES AND EQUIPMENT

Arterial Blood Sampling

Need to have

- Antiseptic solution
- Bandage
- Cap for syringe or stopper for end of needle
- Crushed ice solution
- Gauze pads (2 × 2 in)
- Heparin solution (1000 u/ml)
- Latex gloves (nonsterile)
- Needle or butterfly needle (23- to 25-gauge)
- Sterile syringe (1- or 3-ml)

Nice to have

- Arm board and tape to immobilize wrist for radial puncture
- Prepared blood gas kit, with heparinized syringe
- Transillumination light source for small infants

Arterial Line Placement

Need to have

- Antibiotic ointment
- Antiseptic solution
- Catheter-over-needle device (22- to 24-gauge Intracath) for peripheral line placement
- Catheter-over-wire device (Seldinger technique) for central (femoral) line placement
- Infusion pump with tubing
- Saline solution with 2 u/ml heparin
- Sterile gloves and drapes
- Suture material (nylon or silk 4-0 or 5-0)
- Transducer for continuous blood pressure monitoring

Nice to have

- Prepackaged central line kit for femoral line placement
- Saline-filled stopcock to allow repeated sampling without disconnecting line
- Saline-filled T-piece connector

PROCEDURE

Arterial Puncture and Sampling

In preparation for the procedure, the necessary equipment listed previously should be obtained and packaging should be opened. If necessary, the syringe should be heparinized by drawing heparin into the barrel of the syringe and fully ejecting it because excess heparin in the sample leads to inaccurate results.

1. Before puncturing the radial artery, establish collateral circulation to the hand through the ulnar artery, most commonly with the Allen test. To accomplish this, compress the radial and ulnar arteries with digital pressure for 1 minute.
2. Hold the patient's hand closed in a fist to facilitate blood drainage from the hand.
3. Open the patient's hand with care not to hyperextend the digits or wrist.
4. Assess perfusion of the hand by releasing pressure over the ulnar artery while retaining compression of the radial and watching for color return to the hand. With adequate collateral circulation, color should return within 6 seconds.
5. Alternatively, use a Doppler probe to assess flow through the palmar arch from the ulnar artery by compressing the radial artery and listening with the Doppler device in the space between the third and fourth metacarpal heads on the palm of the hand.
6. To access the radial artery, palpate the pulse just proximal to the transverse wrist crease. Alternatively, when pulses are weak or with a very small infant, the "rule of twos" may be used:
   a. Draw an imaginary line dividing the long axis of the wrist in two equal parts. A second longitudinal imaginary line divides the radial half of the wrist. Where this second line intersects with the second (proximal) palmar crease, enter the skin for the arterial puncture (Fig. 6-5). A mark can be made with a fingernail over the designated access site.
   b. In neonates, a transilluminator placed under the wrist may help in identifying the radial artery.
7. With the wrist fully supinated and extended about 30 degrees, immobilize the forearm either by using an assistant or by taping to an arm board (Fig. 6-6).
8. Prepare the area with sterile betadine solution.
9. Raise a skin wheal over the designated puncture site with 1% lidocaine solution (without epinephrine) using a 25- or 27-gauge needle, if desired.
10. Using the butterfly needle attached to a heparinized syringe, enter the skin over the artery at a 30- to 45-degree angle to the flexor surface of the wrist. Advance the needle until a flash of blood is seen in the tubing. If the needle is in the artery, blood in the catheter should be pulsatile. In larger children, the blood may fill the syringe without withdrawing the plunger, but in infants, it is often necessary to apply gentle back pressure to the plunger to fill the syringe (0.3 to 1 ml is usually necessary for arterial blood gases).
11. If no blood is obtained on the first attempt, slowly withdraw the needle (which may have gone through the artery), with gentle suction on the plunger until blood flows into the syringe.

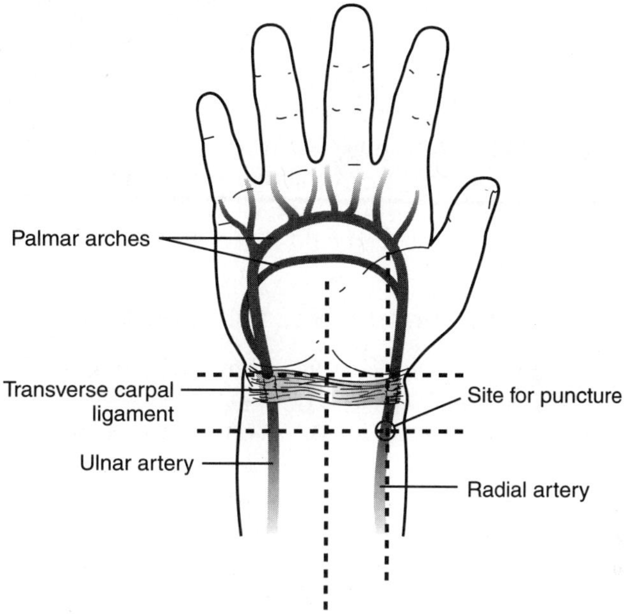

FIG. 6-5. The "rule of twos." Puncture the skin at the intersection of the second palmar crease and the imaginary line halfway between the middle of the wrist and the radial margin.

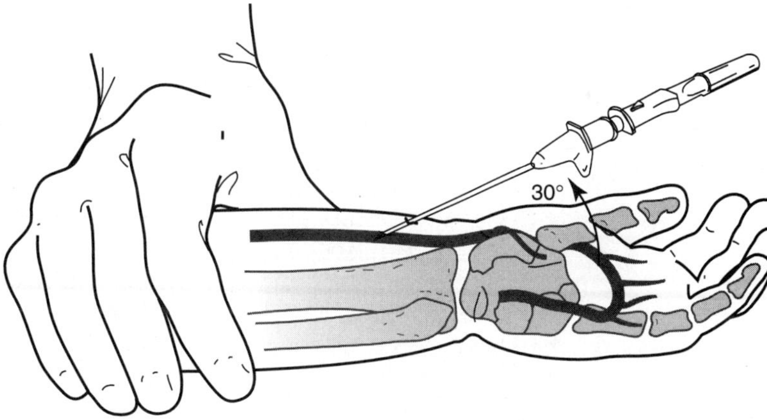

FIG. 6-6. Radial artery puncture.

12. If no blood is obtained on withdrawal, withdraw the needle until it is just under the skin surface, redirect it slightly, and make a second attempt. Care should be taken not to hyperextend the wrist, which may impede free blood flow through the artery.

The dorsalis pedis and posterior tibial arteries can be accessed in a similar fashion. For the dorsalis pedis, hold the foot with the ankle comfortably plantar-flexed. To access the posterior tibial artery, hold the ankle in dorsiflexion. Insert the needle at the point of maximal pulsation, at a 30-degree angle to the skin, aiming proximally along the course of the artery.

13. After the needle is withdrawn, apply firm pressure over the puncture site with gauze for several minutes to minimize hematoma formation.
14. Eject any air in the sample syringe; cap the syringe and place it in crushed ice before sending it for analysis.

Peripheral Arterial Catheter Placement

Arterial catheter placement can be achieved in the radial artery using similar technique.

1. Advance a 22- or 24-gauge catheter-over-needle device until pulsatile blood is seen in the hub of the catheter.
2. Lower the angle of the needle to about 10 degrees, and advance the needle slightly (1 mm) to ensure that the catheter end has also entered the artery (Fig. 6-7, *A*).
3. Advance the catheter while stabilizing the needle.
4. If no blood flow is achieved in the catheter, withdraw it slightly until flow is achieved, in case it has penetrated the posterior wall of the artery (Fig. 6-7, *B*).
5. Remove the needle once the catheter is fully advanced.
6. Hold pressure over the artery to prevent flow from the catheter until it is attached to the prepared setup.
7. Assess distal arterial flow after line placement by checking for cyanosis or pallor of the fingers or hand.
8. Secure the catheter with suture material though the skin, tie the suture, and then wrap the suture around the catheter or through the fenestrations on the wings of the catheter (Fig. 6-7, *C*).
9. Apply antibiotic ointment at the insertion site, and place a transparent dressing over the catheter hub. The line is further secured using tape and an arm board.
10. Attach a saline-filled T-piece connector tubing and stopcock to the catheter and then to transducer tubing to allow repeated blood sampling.
11. Attach the line to a pump, and run heparinized saline continuously through the line at 1 to 2 ml/hour. The line should not be used for administration of maintenance fluids, blood products, dextrose, or medications.

Central Arterial Access

Central arterial access is most commonly obtained in the femoral artery. Technique for line placement is similar to central venous access in the femoral vein.

1. Position the patient with the hip comfortably flexed and the leg externally rotated. The artery lies lateral to the vein in the femoral triangle.
2. Obtain access using a catheter-over-wire technique as described in detail in the venous access chapter.

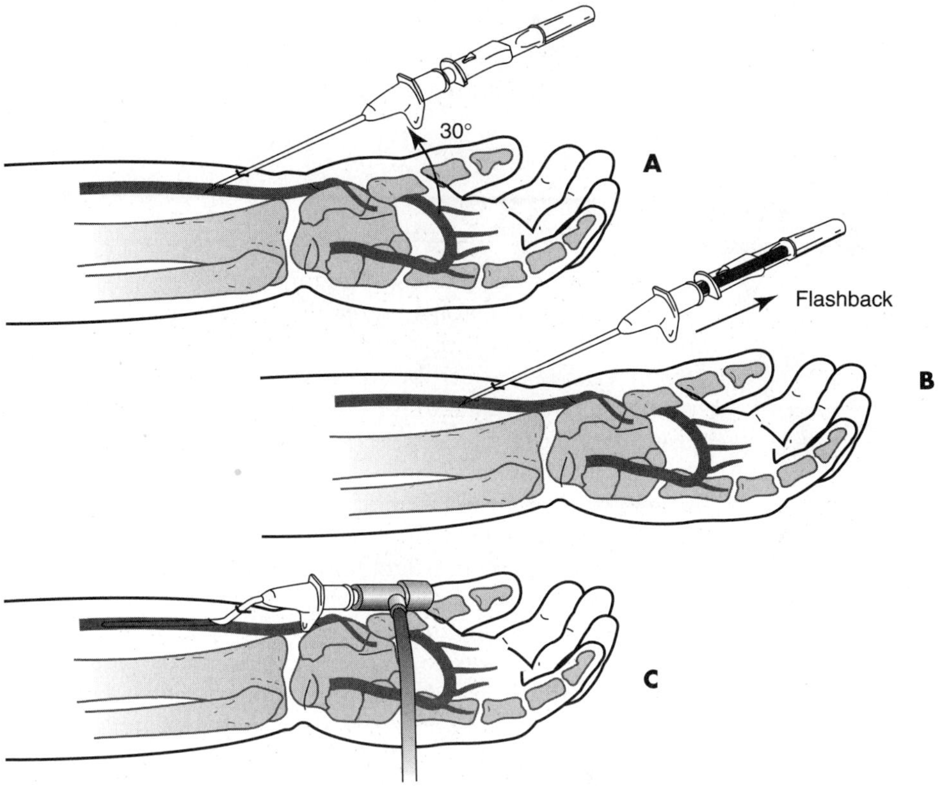

FIG. 6-7. Peripheral arterial line placement. **A,** Advancing catheter-over-needle device 1 mm into arterial lumen. **B,** Pull back slightly and advance catheter into lumen, while stabilizing needle. **C,** Catheter secured in artery.

INTERPRETATION OF RESULTS

Arterial blood gases are obtained to assess oxygenation (PaO_2), ventilation ($PaCO_2$), and acid-base status (arterial pH). It is important to keep in mind the patient's status when the sample was obtained. For example, if the patient was receiving supplemental oxygen at the time of the procedure, the PaO_2 value obtained will reflect this. In some patients, breath holding at the time of the procedure causes an elevated $PaCO_2$ and a depressed PaO_2. If blood is mistakenly obtained from a vein rather than from an artery, or if the sample is mixed arterial and venous, the measured PO_2 will be significantly lowered, and to a lesser extent, the PCO_2 may be raised. Noting the saturation by pulse oximetry at the time of arterial sampling may help differentiate between true hypoxia and venous sampling. Heparin has a very low pH, so presence of excess heparin may significantly lower the measured pH. Air in the syringe may lead to a falsely high PaO_2 and low $PaCO_2$ reading because the sample equilibrates with the air. A delay in sample processing or failure to cool the blood adequately may lead to spurious results because ongoing cellular metabolism leads to lowering of the PaO_2 and pH.

POSSIBLE COMPLICATIONS

Complications of arterial puncture are generally few but include infection, hemorrhage, hematoma, arterial thrombosis, arterial spasm, and damage to underlying structures. Hematoma and hemorrhage are the most common complications and can be minimized by prolonged application of pressure after needle withdrawal. Skin infection is uncommon when proper sterile technique is used. Localized infections can be treated with warm compresses or soaks and appropriate antibiotic therapy. Nerve damage can result from the needle itself or from pressure from a hematoma. Femoral head osteomyelitis and avascular necrosis have been reported as a complication of femoral artery puncture. Arterial spasm is generally transient and requires no specific treatment. Thrombosis can occur with arterial puncture but is more common with arterial line placement. Thrombosis that results in ischemia of the distal extremity may require surgical evaluation and treatment. Loss of digits and extremities has been reported. With indwelling lines, vasculitis, catheter tip infections, and systemic infections are also possible and may require parenteral antibiotic treatment after line removal.

AFTERCARE INSTRUCTIONS

Securing and labeling an arterial line before transferring the patient to another health care facility is essential. The line should be labeled to prevent misuse, such as administration of fluids or medications. The line must also be protected from dislodgment by securing the extremity to a board with tape and covering the catheter with gauze bandaging or a modified plastic cup.

MODIFICATIONS FOR SITUATIONS OF LIMITED RESOURCES

When arterial blood cannot be obtained, or in cases when information on $PaCO_2$ or pH is most essential, venous or capillary blood may be sampled. Studies comparing simultaneous venous, capillary, and arterial gases generally show a reasonable correlation between pH and, to a lesser extent, PCO_2 values. Several studies have shown a correlation between venous pH and PCO_2 and simultaneous arterial measurements. Venous blood may be drawn via venipuncture with a heparinized syringe and sent for analysis on ice, similar to arterial sampling.

To obtain capillary blood for analysis, blood may be obtained from the medial or lateral side of the distal fingerpad or heel, using a lancet. Warming the body part before lancet puncture improves capillary blood flow and increases the correlation with arterial measurements. The initial drop of blood should be wiped away before specimen collection. The blood should be collected in heparinized capillary tubes, which should be held as close as possible to the puncture site to minimize equilibration with air. To get accurate results, the blood must be free flowing without squeezing the body part. Approximately 0.2 ml of blood in a single capillary tube should be adequate for blood gas analysis.

SUGGESTED READINGS

Allen EV: Thromboangiitis obliterans: methods of diagnosis of chronic occlusive arterial lesions distal to the wrist with illustrative cases, *Am J Med Sci* 178:237, 1929.

Brandenburg MA, Dire DJ: Comparison of arterial and venous blood gas values in the initial emergency department evaluation of patients with diabetic ketoacidosis, *Ann Emerg Med* 31:459, 1998.

Chameides L, Hazinski MF, editors: *Pediatric advanced life support,* Dallas, 1997, American Heart Association.

Courtney SE et al: Capillary blood gases in the neonate: a reassessment and review of the literature, *Am J Dis Child* 144:168, 1990.

Cunningham FJ et al: Pediatric vascular access and blood sampling techniques. In Roberts JR, Hedges JR, editors: *Clinical procedures in emergency medicine,* Philadelphia, 1998, WB Saunders.

Harrison AM et al: Comparison of simultaneously obtained arterial and capillary blood gases in pediatric intensive care unit patients, *Crit Care Med* 25:1904, 1997.

McGillivray D et al: Clinical decision making based on venous versus capillary blood gas values in the well-perfused child, *Ann Emerg Med* 34:58, 1999.

Saladino R, Bachman D, Fleisher G: Arterial access in the pediatric emergency department, *Ann Emerg Med* 19:382, 1990.

Torrey SB, Saladino R: Arterial puncture and catheterization. In Henretig FM, editor: *Textbook of pediatric emergency procedures,* Baltimore, 1997, Williams and Wilkins.

CHAPTER 7

Microbiology Procedures for the Office Setting

James A. Wilde
John T. Benjamin
John C.H. Steele, Jr.

BACKGROUND AND INTRODUCTION

Most primary care pediatricians who practice in an office setting do not perform a wide variety of microbiologic tests in their office laboratories. Routine blood, cerebrospinal fluid, or wound cultures for bacteria or other microorganisms are usually completed in a highly specialized laboratory setting by people who have extensive training in performing and interpreting the tests. In addition, susceptibility testing is also well beyond the scope of most small outpatient laboratories.

A few microbiology procedures can be readily performed in an office setting, particularly those that focus on simple "positive" or "negative" results. Among these tests are cultures for group A streptococcus and screening urine cultures. In addition, several rapid antigen detection systems have been developed for use in office laboratories; of particular utility are those designed to detect the presence of group A streptococcus and Epstein-Barr virus, the primary cause of infectious mononucleosis. Finally, light microscopy with or without Gram stains is readily performed in an office setting and can provide valuable information to the practitioner to help guide therapeutic decisions. This chapter presents these microbiologic techniques and how they can be incorporated into the primary care office setting.

The Office Laboratory and CLIA '88 Legislation

The Clinical Laboratory Improvement Amendments of 1988 (CLIA, 1988) established three levels of complexity for office-based tests: (1) waived tests, (2) moderately complex tests, and (3) highly complex tests. In 1993, the provider-performed microscopy (PPM) category was added as a subgroup within the moderately complex category. All office laboratories and laboratories not associated with a hospital that perform tests in any of these four categories must have proper certification in order to operate. Although all office laboratories are subject to inspection, those facilities performing only waived tests and/or PPM are usually not routinely inspected. Waived tests are defined as simple tests with negligible risk to the patient from an erroneous result. Originally limited to 8 tests, additions since 1988 have brought the current total of waived tests to 26.

No personnel requirements are mandated for a laboratory that is certified to perform waived tests. PPM procedures must be performed personally by a physician, dentist, or midlevel practitioner under the supervision of a physician. Laboratories performing moderately complex or highly complex tests must meet specific personnel requirements for positions from laboratory director to testing personnel. These laboratories also must submit to unannounced inspections conducted on at least a biennial basis, use test systems approved by the Food and Drug Administration (FDA), maintain procedure manuals, and keep records of all quality control activities. As of 1999, 72% of all office laboratories were classified as either waived or PPM.

SPECIFIC MICROBIOLOGIC TESTS

Box 7-1 is a complete list of microbiologic tests that fall within the waived, moderately complex, or PPM categories. Box 7-2 lists some selected moderately complex microbiologic tests. A few examples of waived and moderately complex tests are discussed in the following sections.

Group A Strep Rapid Tests

Many rapid tests are now available for detecting group A streptococcus antigens from throat swabs. Nine of these tests are in the waived category, including ICON Fx, Biostar Acceava, Abbott Signify Strep A test, Surestep Strep A Test from Applied Biotech, Meridian Diagnostics ImmunoCard STAT Strep A, Jant Pharmacal

BOX 7-1 MICROBIOLOGY TESTS: WAIVED AND PROVIDER-PERFORMED MICROSCOPY

Waived

Some *Helicobacter Pylori* tests
Some rapid group A streptococcus tests
Infectious mononucleosis tests

Provider-Performed Microscopy

Wet mounts
All KOH preparations
Pinworm examinations
Urinalysis, microscopic examination
Fecal leukocyte examination
Nasal smear for eosinophils and granulocytes

BOX 7-2 MICROBIOLOGY TESTS: SELECTED MODERATELY COMPLEX TESTS

Throat culture
Urine culture: Identification of positive or negative only
Limited Gram stain
Some rapid streptococcal antigen tests
Some rapid infectious mononucleosis tests
Rapid *Helicobacter Pylori* antibody tests
Influenza A and B tests
DNA probe tests for Gardnerella, Candida, Trichomonas

AccuStrip Strep A, Mainline Technology Strep A Dots Test, Link 2 Strep A Rapid test, and the Quidel One-Step. Other tests in the moderately complex category include ICON from Smith-Kline, Biostar OIA Max, Abbott Strep Plus, and the BD Directogen. Most rapid streptococcal antigen tests can be performed in 5 minutes, are inexpensive to run, and have reported sensitivities in the 90% to 95% range, although sensitivities tend to be lower in routine use. All of the available tests are less sensitive with low bacterial colony counts. The American Academy of Pediatrics recommends that if the rapid test is negative in a child with suspected group A strep pharyngitis, a culture should also be performed.

Several different methodologies exist for performing rapid tests, but all involve detection of antigen-antibody complexes formed by group A streptococcus antigens in the throat swab and the corresponding antibodies supplied in the test kit. A positive result is indicated by a color change or by a symbol such as a "plus" sign in the test window. Instructions for performing the tests vary by manufacturer and should be carefully followed to ensure optimal results. The ImmunoCard STAT Strep A (Fig. 7-1) is an example of a streptococcal antigen test from the waived category. The appearance of two horizontal lines in the test window indicates the presence of group A streptococcus; a single line appears at the completion of the incubation period if no group A streptococcus is present.

Infectious Mononucleosis Tests

Tests for infectious mononucleosis are similar to tests for group A streptococcus. Nine waived rapid tests are currently available, including the Genzyme Contrast Mono, Color Q, Biostar Acceava Mono Test, LifeSign UniStep Mono, Princeton BioMeditech BioSign Mono WB, Quidel CARDS O.S. Mono, Seradyn Color Q Mono, and Wampole Mono-Plus WB. Several moderately complex tests include the Wampole Mono-Plus Serum Test, Seradyn Color Slide Mono II test, and Card QS Mono/Quidel test. The waived tests use whole blood, whereas the moderately complex tests use serum. These tests can be completed in approximately 5 minutes and are all comparable in their performance characteristics. Instructions for completing the tests vary by manufacturer and should be followed closely to ensure optimal results.

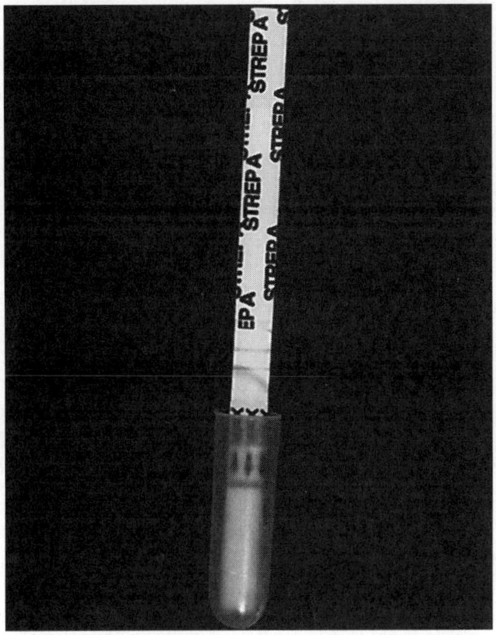

FIG. 7-1. Positive group A strep rapid test, using ImmunoCard STAT Strep A from Meridian Diagnostics. Two horizontal (red) lines indicate the presence of group A strep; a single line indicates a negative test.

Throat Culture for Group A Streptococcus

Because of the excellent specificity of the rapid tests for group A streptococcus, many office laboratories do not rely on throat cultures to make the diagnosis of strep throat; however, the sensitivities of the rapid strep tests are somewhat lower, and false-negative results may occur. The current strategy employed by many office laboratories, and recommended by the American Academy of Pediatrics, is to use the throat culture as a backup test in the event of a negative result from a rapid test. Throat cultures are easily performed in an office setting using blood agar plates and bacitracin disks. The technique is quite simple, as follows:

1. Rub the tonsils and posterior pharynx with a cotton-tipped swab.
2. Streak a blood agar plate with the sample, being careful to sample the tip as well as the side of the swab.
3. "Stab" the agar so that some of the sample is within the agar layer itself.
4. Place a bacitracin disk within the streaked area on the plate.
5. Incubate overnight at 35° to 37° C in air.

More than 90% of Gram-positive cocci that are in chains, that produce beta-hemolysis on blood agar, and that are inhibited by bacitracin are streptococcus pyogenes (group A streptococcus). Fig. 7-2 shows a typical culture plate with group A strep. Note the clear appearance of the agar around the isolates indicating beta-hemolysis and the lack of beta-hemolysis adjacent to the bacitracin disc because of inhibition of bacterial growth. This finding is enough information to make a presumptive diagnosis of group A strep; no microscopy is required to confirm the presence of Gram-positive cocci in chains.

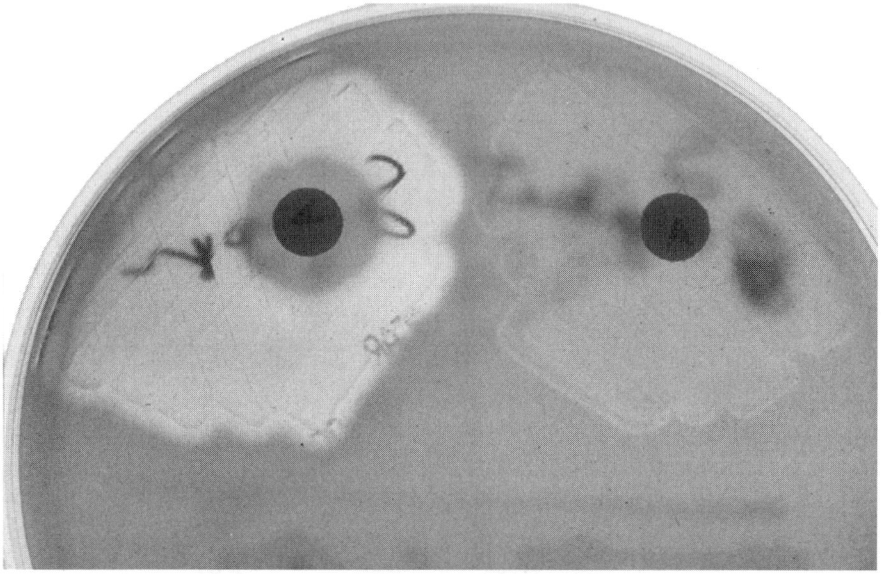

FIG. 7-2. Positive culture for group A strep (upper left of photo). Note the clear appearance of the agar, indicating beta hemolysis, and the lack of beta hemolysis immediately adjacent to the bacitracin disk. The culture on the right side of the plate shows no beta hemolysis, indicating a negative result for group A strep.

Urine Culture

Many office laboratories perform quantitative urine cultures to diagnosis a urinary tract infection. The advantage to the practitioner is that the sample can be incubated immediately after it is obtained, the test can be performed without the need for a fully equipped microbiology laboratory, and the result can be easily interpreted within 24 hours. Some tests provide only confirmation or rejection of the diagnosis of urinary tract infection, but relatively simple products are available that also provide information about the identification of the organism and even sensitivity to various antimicrobials. The sensitivity and specificity of these tests, which are classified as moderately complex, have been reported to be excellent.

One example of a kit for office-based urine cultures is the Uri-three, from Culture Kits, Inc. This kit utilizes a single petri dish divided into three sections, with various agars that allow for accurate estimation of colony counts and identification of the organisms. Samples are streaked onto the surface of the agars, and the plate is incubated at 35° C for 18 to 24 hours. A color chart is used as a standard to estimate the colony count and to presumptively identify the organism. A variety of paddle systems that contain different agars on either side of the paddle are also available. A particularly popular paddle system is the Uricult from Medical Technology Corporation. The paddle is dipped into the urine sample, incubated overnight, and read in a manner similar to the Uri-three with the use of color charts.

To avoid erroneous results, the manufacturer's instructions must be followed carefully. For example, a delay in inoculating the culture system may result in falsely elevated colony counts, and excessively prolonged incubation times may allow reactions to occur that lead to misinterpreted test results.

Gram Stain

The Gram stain is another moderately complex test that can be essential in establishing a diagnosis. For example, the differentiation of a bacterial paronychia from herpetic whitlow can be difficult based on physical examination alone. In this situation, use of the Gram stain on the material obtained from the infected site provides valuable added information. This test is easily performed and interpreted and requires only a few reagents and a light microscope.

The technique for the Gram stain is quite simple but requires proper preparation of the sample on the slide. The sample should be smeared in a thin film on the glass slide using a Dacron-tipped swab; cotton-tipped swabs should be avoided. The sample is air-dried, then heat-fixed. If heat fixation is not completed, the sample may be washed off the slide during the staining process. Heat fixation is performed by applying a flame from a match or Bunsen burner to the bottom of the slide on which the sample has been applied. Care must be taken not to overheat the slide, which could cause destruction of cells or bacteria. One method to avoid overheating is to apply the flame to the slide for several seconds, then place the slide on the back of your hand. If the slide is too hot for your hand, it is too hot for the material on the slide. Repeat this sequence two to three times for proper fixation.

Methanol fixation is an alternate method that can be used in place of heat fixation. The sample slide is air-dried, immersed in 100% methanol for 30 seconds, and allowed to fully air-dry once again. This method is superior to heat fixation for viewing cells and equivalent for viewing bacteria. Another advantage is that if the immersion step is done for a full 5 minutes, all viruses in the sample are inactivated, with the exception of Jakob-Creutzfeld virus. The primary disadvantage is potential contamination of the methanol, but this can be avoided by changing the solution after 20 to 50 slides have been processed.

The materials necessary for a Gram stain include crystal violet, Gram's iodine, acetone-ethanol, safranin counterstain, and slowly running water. The details of the process are as follows:

1. Place the slide on a flat surface, preferably on a wire rack over a sink.
2. Apply the crystal violet stain to the top of the slide and allow it to stay in a puddle for 30 to 60 seconds (Fig. 7-3, *A*).
3. Pour the crystal violet off the slide, and apply the Gram's iodine in a puddle for 30 to 60 seconds (Fig. 7-3, *B*).
4. Pour off the iodine, and with the slide tipped at a 45-degree angle, drip the acetone-ethanol decolorizer over the stained sample for several seconds. Caution should be used to prevent overdecolorization, which can wash the crystal violet out of the Gram-positive bacteria and result in misinterpretation of the test (Fig. 7-3, *C*).

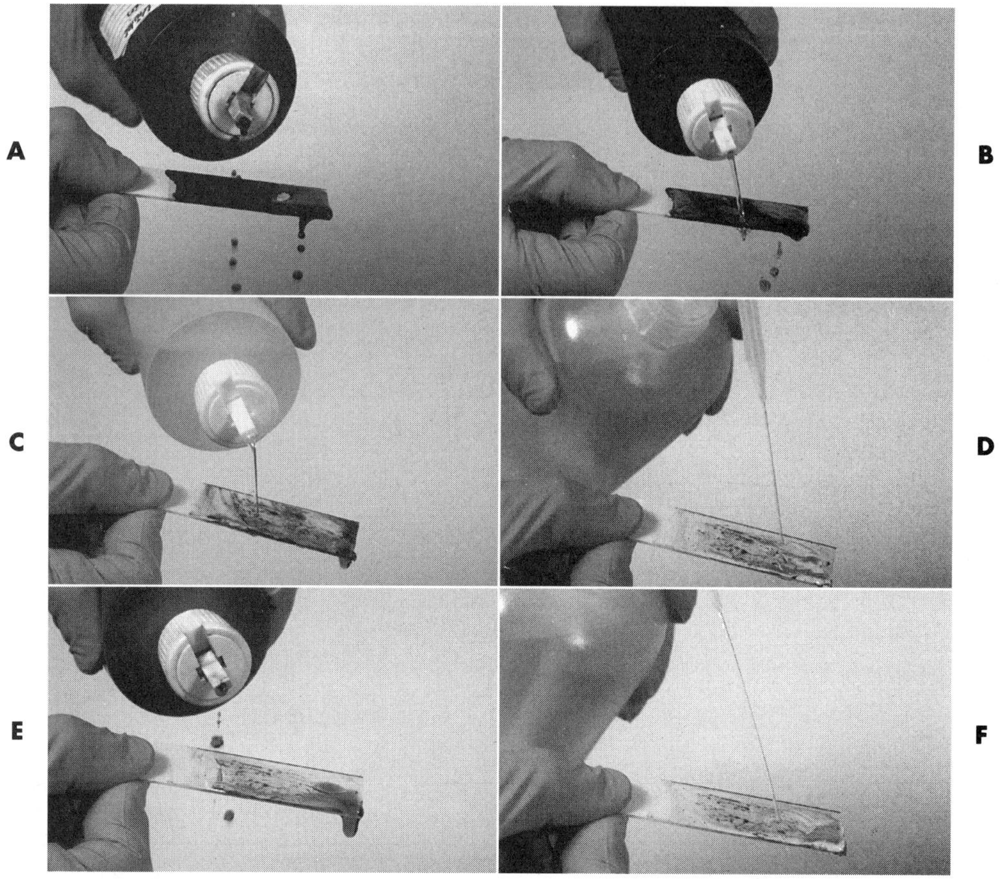

FIG. 7-3. Steps involved in Gram stain.

5. Rinse the slide briefly in a stream of water to remove any remaining acetone-ethanol (Fig. 7-3, *D*).
6. Apply the safranin counterstain in a puddle and allow it to stand for 30 to 60 seconds (Fig. 7-3, *E*).
7. Rinse the safranin off the slide with a gentle stream of water. The slide can be air-dried or blotted dry with a paper towel (Fig. 7-3, *F*).
8. Examine the sample using the microscope. Bacteria can be seen under the high-power objective ("high dry" lens) but are much better seen with an oil immersion technique. Gram-positive organisms are blue, and Gram-negative organisms are red.

SPECIMEN HANDLING

Many physicians collect specimens for blood and urine cultures in their offices but do not actually perform the tests in the office laboratory. These samples are usually sent to a central, better-equipped laboratory for further testing. If this option is chosen, it is essential that the samples be collected and stored properly.

To avoid contamination of blood cultures by skin flora, the skin should be cleansed with an antibacterial solution such as povidone-iodine before venipuncture. This solution kills as it dries, so the skin should not be punctured with the needle until after the povidone-iodine has completely dried. Ideally, blood should be inoculated into an aerobic blood culture vial, then kept in a 37° C incubator until transferred. Anaerobic vials can be reserved for clinical situations in which anaerobes are suspected. The optimal blood volume to be inoculated is at least 1 to 2 ml. Growth of some fastidious organisms such as Haemophilus influenzae type B may be inhibited if the blood sample is kept at room temperature for prolonged periods.

Urine samples should be obtained by the "clean-catch" method or by bladder catheterization; specimens obtained by placing a plastic bag over the perineum are likely to be contaminated and should not be used for culture. Because the actual number of organisms present in the culture is critical for interpreting a urine culture, growth in the urine sample must be inhibited before inoculation into the growth media or an artificially high colony count will result. This step is accomplished by storing the sample for up to 12 hours in a refrigerator set at 4° C until it is ready for further manipulation. Alternatively, the urine sample may be added to a commercially available borate solution that acts as a preservative.

CONCLUSION

Primary care pediatricians can perform several microbiological tests in their office laboratories. Performing these tests in the office laboratory benefits both the physician and the patient in a variety of ways. By getting a rapid result in their own laboratories, physicians can make quicker definitive diagnoses, start appropriate therapy earlier, and improve "customer satisfaction." Depending on the volume of tests done, physicians may even reap economic benefits because reimbursement for these tests is provided by most payors.

SUGGESTED READINGS

Bisno AL: Streptococcus pyogenes. In Mandel, Bennet, Dolin, editors: *Principles and practice of infectious diseases,* ed 4, Philadelphia, 1995, Churchill Livingstone.

Federal Register, Public Law 100-578, October 31, 1988, Clinical Laboratory Improvement Amendments of 1988.

Isaacman DJ et al: Effect of number of blood cultures and volume of blood on detection of bacteremia in children, *J Pediatr* 128:190, 1996.

McAllister TA et al: *Nephrology* 11:111, 1973.

Schelonka RL et al: Volume of blood required to detect common neonatal pathogens, *J Pediatr* 129:275, 1996.

Schwartz B et al: Pharyngitis—Principles of judicious use of antimicrobial agents, *Pediatrics* 101(Suppl):171, 1998.

CHAPTER 8

Analgesia and Sedation

Mark A. Hostetler

BACKGROUND AND INTRODUCTION

Health care workers must remain sensitive to the pain and anxiety experienced by children in the course of undergoing medical procedures. Although adults are generally capable of verbalizing and coping with their pain and anxieties, children often cannot. When performing medical procedures, practitioners must always assume that children will have pain and anxiety. Because they act as children's advocates, practitioners should ensure that children have adequate analgesia and sedation in order to cope with pain. This chapter provides an overall approach to analgesia and sedation that is both safe and effective.

INDICATIONS

- Sedative and analgesic agents minimize the pain and anxiety suffered by children during painful procedures and often provide amnesia of the painful event.
- Parents and families benefit by knowing that although a procedure may be painful, their children are being made as comfortable as possible.
- Procedures are technically much easier to perform when patients are sedated and not moving.
- Sedation decreases the length of time necessary to perform a procedure and reduces the potential risk of injury to patients or health care workers as a result of uncontrolled movements.
- Patients, families, and health care providers all benefit from providing adequate analgesia and sedation.

KEY CONCEPTS

- When performing a procedure, practitioners must distinguish between the relative needs for pain control (analgesia) and those for behavioral control (sedation).

- In general, the need for pain control varies by procedure, and the need for behavioral control varies by the patient (age, developmental stage).
- Physicians should consider and address separately the individual needs of analgesia and sedation when planning a procedure.

DEFINITIONS

- *Pain* is a complex subjective experience defined as any unpleasant sensory or emotional experience that results from actual or potential injury.
- *Analgesia* refers to the lessening of pain.
- *Anesthesia* refers to the absence of sensation.
- *Sedation* refers to a reduced level of awareness. For our purposes, it generally refers to a reduced level of anxiety (anxiolysis) or a state of behavioral control that facilitates performing a procedure.

LEVELS OF SEDATION

- Sedation occurs along a continuum from lighter to deeper.
- The three stages of sedation are sedation, deep sedation, and general anesthesia (Table 8-1).
- Physicians must remain vigilant because patients may inadvertently progress to a deeper level of sedation, and increasing depth is associated with increasing risk of complications.

RELEVANT ANATOMY AND PHYSIOLOGY

Anatomy

- *Nociceptors* are specialized pain receptors composed of both type A and C nerve fibers.

TABLE 8-1
Levels of sedation

Sedation	Deep sedation	General anesthesia
Controlled lessening of a patient's awareness of the environment and/or pain perception while maintaining stable vital signs, an independent airway, and adequate spontaneous respirations.	Profound depression of awareness to any stimuli. This state is frequently accompanied by a loss of protective reflexes and requires active attention to appropriate airway and ventilatory management and blood pressure control.	Complete loss of awareness of the environment accompanied by loss of protective reflexes.

- *A fibers* are myelinated and conduct impulses rapidly. They are most prevalent in the skin and mucous membranes and transmit sharp, localized pain.
- *C fibers* are unmyelinated and conduct impulses more slowly. They tend to be most prevalent in deep tissues and skin and transmit dull, poorly localized pain.
- *Mechanoreceptors* and *thermoreceptors* are composed of A fibers located in the skin and carry the sensations responsible for light touch and pressure.
- Afferent impulses enter the spinal cord via the *dorsal root ganglia,* synapse with the ascending neurons in the *dorsal spinal horn,* and ascend as the *ventrolateral funiculus* or *spinothalamic tract.*

Physiology of the Perception and Modulation of Pain

- *Origin:* Impulse transmission may be blocked at the site of origination by local anesthetics.
- *Spinal cord:* Intense stimulation of A fibers by electrical stimulation, vibration, or pressure may raise the threshold of C fiber firing and decrease the amount of pain perceived.
- *Midbrain:* Endogenous and exogenous opioids cause presynaptic inhibition.
- *Cerebral cortex:* Pain can be modulated by a wide variety of developmental and psychological factors: cognitive ability, previous experience, fear, rationalization, and biofeedback mechanisms.

Developmental Changes Associated with Pain and Anxiety Perception

- Developmental changes affect children's ability to understand and cope with the pain and anxiety associated with medical procedures (Table 8-2).
- Preverbal children have visible physiological responses such as crying and increased heart and respiratory rate but are unable to verbalize their fear.
- As children grow older, they can speak and are better able to describe their fears. They remain, however, incapable of logical thought.

TABLE 8-2
Developmental changes associated with pain perception

Age	Developmental stage
< 6 mo.	Physiologic response (unknown memory/psychological response)
6-18 mo.	Stranger anxiety (early localization and language development for pain)
18 mo. to 6 yrs.	Prelogical, egocentric (magical thinking, distortion of reality)
6-10 yrs.	Concrete operational (behavioral coping mechanisms)
> 10 yrs.	Formal logical (cognitive coping strategies)

- Older children gain the cognitive ability to understand cause and effect and eventually are able to accept not only the rationale for procedures but also the consequences of their behavior.

IMPORTANT CONSIDERATIONS

Safety

Safety must always retain utmost priority when planning or assisting in providing analgesia and sedation. Although the goals are to reduce pain and suffering in pediatric patients and to control behavior to better facilitate performing a procedure, these goals should never be pursued at the risk of additional injury. Knowledge has increased greatly in recent years as technology, training, and pharmacology have progressed. Although this increased knowledge has resulted in reducing many of the inherent risks, risks remain nonetheless. A team approach that utilizes careful attention to detail in preparation, patient selection, pharmacology, and monitoring further decreases these risks.

Preparation

Preparation is the single most important step in providing safe analgesia and sedation. Thorough preparation helps ensure that patient selection is appropriate, that agents are appropriate, and that nursing staff members are comfortable and capable of assisting in the sedation. Preparation occurs long before the sedation begins and provides for the worst possible outcome. If the worst happens, mechanisms need to have been in place well before the procedure begins.

- *Physician* preparation includes thorough training with the agents that are intended for use.
- *Nursing* preparation includes thorough training of what can reasonably be expected of the agents being used, as well as a working knowledge of appropriate monitoring and resuscitation equipment and advanced life support.
- *Patient* preparation varies according to the developmental stage of the children.
- *Family* preparation includes education on what to realistically expect during and after the procedure. It allows for discussion of their expectations and potential fears associated with the procedure. It also includes addressing the risks and benefits of sedation and obtaining informed consent.

Team Approach

A team approach is mandatory to the success of the sedation and the procedure. Roles and responsibilities for all participants, including the sedating physician, nurse, procedural physician, and ancillary personnel, should be well established. Success of the sedation does not depend on the drug given or the expertise of the

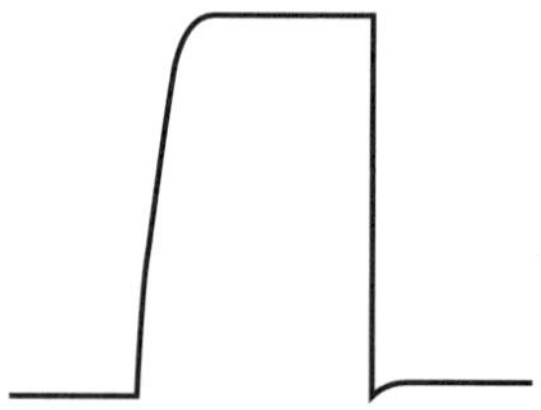

FIG. 8-1. Typical representation of the pain induced by a procedure such as fracture reduction. This type of pain can be most closely matched with intravenous titration of agents.

sedating physician, but rather it depends on the team of health care workers providing care, their ability to work toward a common goal in a safe and efficient manner, and their appropriate preparation for all possible outcomes.

CONSIDERATIONS FOR DECIDING WHICH AGENT TO USE

- The ideal agent has potent analgesic and sedative properties that are rapid, titratable, and reversible, with minimal side effects.
- No single agent, or combination of agents, can be recommended for all children or every procedure.
- All agents have varying degrees of advantages and disadvantages, side effects, and contraindications.
- Potential risks and benefits need to be weighed when deciding which set of medications to use, and vary depending on the combination of drugs used.
- Choice of agents varies depending on procedure, patient, and physician familiarity and training.

Procedure Characteristics

- Different procedures vary in the type and amount of pain produced.
- Reduction of a fracture, for example, generally causes an intense, although relatively brief, salvo of pain.
- Suturing a complex laceration causes very little pain (if appropriately anesthetized with local anesthetics), yet the procedure may last for a considerable amount of time and require significant sedation in order for patients to cooperate with and facilitate the procedure.
- It is useful to think of the pain and anxiety induced by a procedure in terms of a curve and then try to imagine the analgesia and sedation as a complementary curve that approximates the pain as closely as possible.
- Intense, short procedures are best suited to ultra-short-acting powerful analgesics (Fig. 8-1), whereas long, less painful procedures are perhaps better suited to smooth, longer-lasting sedative agents with amnestic properties (Fig. 8-2).

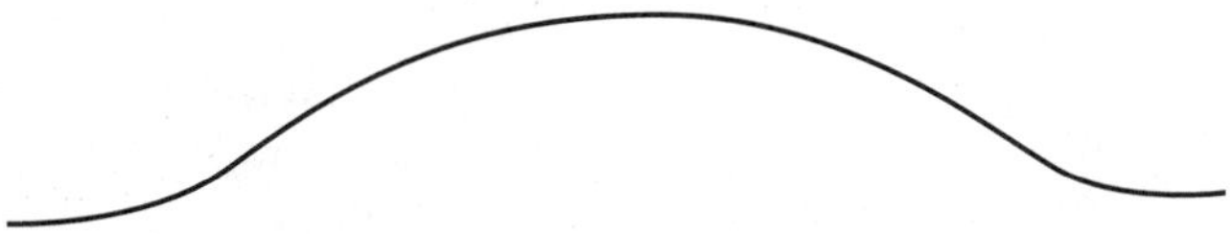

FIG. 8-2. Typical representation of effects provided by intramuscular or oral dosing with gradual onset and resolution.

Patient Characteristics

- *Age:* Children of different ages have varying abilities to understand and cooperate with procedures. Younger children generally tend to require more sedation than do older children.
- *Co-morbid conditions:* Children with cardiac disease or craniofacial malformations are particularly at risk and should usually be referred to a pediatric anesthesiologist.
- *Past history:* Children may have had similar procedures done in the past. Taking a detailed history from the parents and thoroughly reviewing the medical record may provide important insight into which modalities have either worked particularly well or have been associated with untoward reactions.

Physician Familiarity and Training

- There are numerous medications and modalities available to physicians with innumerable possible combinations.
- Physicians should use only those agents that they have been trained to use and are comfortable working with.
- It is generally more advisable to become extremely familiar with a few agents rather than attempting to master many.

NONPHARMACOLOGIC METHODS

- *Education:* For older children with the cognitive capacity to understand, thorough explanation of the procedure may aid greatly in decreasing anxiety. Child life workers are particularly skillful at developmentally appropriate age-based explanations of procedures.
- *Distraction:* Purposely distracting patients may decrease anxiety by focusing their attention on other things. Child life workers are particularly skillful at distraction techniques.
- *Hypnosis and guided imagery:* Hypnosis and guided imagery runs the spectrum from general relaxation via comforting speech and conversation to formal training on induction into altered states of consciousness. Guided imagery may be particularly helpful in patients undergoing ketamine sedation as they are extremely receptive to suggestion.

- *Physical restraint:* Physical restraint may occasionally be necessary in order to provide safety for the patient and to facilitate the procedure. Physical restraint is not a substitute for analgesia, however, and should always be instituted in as humane a manner as possible.

PHARMACOLOGIC METHODS

Topical/Local Agents

The following methods are less invasive modes of providing analgesia/anesthesia.

- *Eutectic mixture of local anesthetics (EMLA):* Applied topically under an occlusive dressing, best results occur after a minimum of 30 minutes and last approximately 2 hours. EMLA may be safely applied to both intact and nonintact skin. EMLA contains prilocaine and has been associated with methemoglobinemia in neonates. EMLA does cause some degree of vasoconstriction. When used for venipuncture, some physicians advocate combining three-quarters EMLA with one-quarter Nitropaste to provide vasodilation and counteract the vasoconstriction.
- *Lidocaine, epinephrine, tetracaine (LET)* and *Tetracaine, adrenalin, cocaine (TAC)*: LET and TAC are the two most common topical anesthetics used today. Both can be made using a gel or combined with cellulose to make the consistency more viscous and adherent to the wound. LET is favored by many physicians because of its lack of side effects. TAC is used less often because of case reports describing cocaine toxicity. TAC is usually made by individual institutions and, therefore, comes in a variety of concentrations. The toxic dose of cocaine is considered to be 3 mg/kg. TAC should not be applied to mucous membranes as absorption and the potential for toxicity increase.
- *Lidocaine/Bupivacaine infiltration:* Anesthetics such as lidocaine and bupivacaine may be infiltrated to provide local or regional anesthesia. Care should be taken with dosing because toxicity may occur (Table 8-3). Local and regional blocks are discussed in detail in a separate chapter.

Routes of Administration

- Nonparenteral routes (i.e., oral, nasal, rectal) are less invasive; however, absorption can be somewhat erratic, and this method does not allow for the ability to titrate agents.

TABLE 8-3
Local anesthetics and maximum recommended dosages

Anesthetic	Max dose	Onset	Duration
Bupivacaine	2 mg/kg	5-10 min.	4-8 hrs.
Lidocaine plain	5 mg/kg	2-5 min.	1-2 hrs.
Lidocaine w/epinephrine	7 mg/kg	2-5 min.	1-3 hrs.

- Intramuscular (IM) injections allow for more precise absorption than do mucous membranes; however, they do not allow for titration. IM dosing may be particularly useful in cases lasting longer periods in which analgesia is not as great a concern, such as complex laceration repair. IM dosing is not recommended in cases of shock or potential shock (e.g., severe trauma or burns).
- Intravenous (IV) dosing of medications allows for precise titration of effects and ensures that venous access is available in the event that an untoward reaction occurs.

Dosing Considerations

- Appropriate dosing requires balancing the relative needs of analgesia and sedation with the specific patient and procedure.
- When using IM dosing, shorter or less painful procedures may often be accomplished with doses on the lower end of the dosing range; however, remember that titration is not possible and, if necessary, would require additional injections.
- When using IV dosing, start low and titrate to effect. Also, be certain to *flush* the medication entirely through the tubing and allow the medication enough time to take effect *before* redosing.
- Younger children have higher volumes of distribution, higher rates of metabolism, and may require somewhat higher doses. Attention to the maximum recommended dose is required because older children may receive too much medication if the full mg/kg dose is given.

Specific Agents (see Appendices 8-1 and 8-2)

- *Chloral hydrate* is a sedative/hypnotic agent used commonly for painless procedures. Chloral hydrate is available in an oral solution as well as in rectal suppositories. It has no analgesic properties. Care should be taken when combining it with other agents. Chloral hydrate requires the same monitoring as other sedative agents.
- *Codeine* may be given orally in an elixir with Tylenol 1 hour before a procedure. It provides useful analgesia for regularly scheduled procedures, such as burn dressing changes, that are only mildly to moderately painful.
- *Ketamine* (*Ketalar*) is a dissociative anesthetic with potent sedative, analgesic, amnestic, and anesthetic properties. Ketamine acts by causing a dissociation between the limbic and cortical areas of the brain and has an excellent safety record. Ketamine acts as a bronchodilator, does not cause respiratory depression, and has a minimal effect on protective airway reflexes. The only exception is that when given rapidly in an IV push, ketamine may cause apnea. Ketamine causes the release of endogenous catecholamines and is therefore not associated with hypotension. Ketamine may be given by the rectal, IM, or IV routes and has gained increasing popularity for painful procedures in the pediatric emergency department. Given rectally or intramuscularly, ketamine provides excellent analgesia and sedation for procedures of moderate duration, such as laceration

repair. Given intravenously, ketamine provides excellent sedation and analgesia for intensely painful, short procedures, such as fracture reduction. Ketamine is a secretory agent associated with sialorrhea and bronchorrhea. Therefore most physicians recommend using it in conjunction with either atropine or glycopyrrolate. Ketamine is chemically related to phencyclidine and has historically been associated with unpleasant hallucinations or behavioral reactions (so-called emergence reactions). Many physicians advocate using low-dose (0.035 to 0.05 mg/kg) midazolam in hopes of blunting this response. Some evidence suggests that the occurrence of unpleasant behavioral reactions (emergence reactions) are most closely associated with the patient's presedation level of anxiety. Those children with the least amount of anxiety going into the sedation are at the least risk for having an unpleasant reaction. For this reason, I recommend prehypnotic suggestion in combination with low-dose midazolam 5 to 10 minutes before administering the ketamine. For the prehypnotic suggestion, I determine children's favorite places, foods, and activities. I then tell children that they are going to go to sleep and dream about being at their favorite place, and that when they wake up we will be finished, they won't remember anything, and it won't hurt. Contrary to popular belief, ketamine is safe in older children and not associated with unusually higher rates of emergence reactions. Ketamine is contraindicated in patients with increased intraocular or intracranial pressure. No reversal agent is available.

- *Meperidine* (*Demerol*), *promethazine* (*Phenergan*), and *chlorpromazine* (*Thorazine*) in combination was historically used almost exclusively for pediatric sedation. This combination has been almost completely abandoned because of unusually high rates of complications and the availability of newer and better agents.
- *Methohexital* (*Brevital*) is an ultra-short-acting barbiturate used for sedation that does not have any analgesic properties. Methohexital is most commonly given by either the rectal or IV routes but may be given by the IM route as well. Respiratory depression may occur with any route of administration but is most commonly associated with IV bolus administration. Apnea may occur and is most commonly caused by head positioning causing airway obstruction. Seizures have been reported; however, they are usually in patients with known seizure disorders. Methohexital is becoming increasingly popular for sedation involving painless procedures, such as imaging in the radiology suite. No reversal agents are available.
- *Midazolam* (*Versed*) is widely used for its sedative and amnestic properties, but it does not provide any analgesia. Midazolam may be given orally, nasally, or rectally; is relatively short acting; and is reversible with *flumazenil* (*Romazicon*). Significant respiratory depression can occur, particularly when midazolam is combined with an opioid. This agent should be used only with continuous pulse oximetry in place. When using an opioid and a benzodiazepine, the initial dose of each agent should be reduced by 25%.
- *Morphine* and *fentanyl* (*Sublimaze*) are two opioids with reasonably good safety records that are commonly used for analgesia. Respiratory depression can occur, particularly when combined with benzodiazepines (midazolam). When using an opioid and a benzodiazepine, the initial dose of each should

be reduced by 25%. Sedation may also become more pronounced when the painful procedure is completed and children are no longer being stimulated. Opioids are reversible with naloxone (Narcan) or nalmefene (Revex). Chest wall rigidity may occasionally occur following opioid administration. This reaction results in the mass contraction of the thoracic musculature, making ventilation nearly impossible, but may be remedied either by directly reversing the opioid with naloxone (Narcan) or by using pharmacologic muscle relaxation (succinylcholine).

- *Nitrous oxide* may be effective for those children able to participate with mask inhalation. A dual-tank system that guarantees a 50:50 mixture with oxygen is recommended. A scavenger collection system is also recommended to prevent leakage into the ambient air and intoxication of health care workers. A demand-valve system is commonly used, wherein the patient holds the face mask and inhales deeply when feeling pain to trigger the release of nitrous oxide gas. Care should be taken when combining nitrous oxide with other agents.
- *Propofol (Diprivan)* is a potent IV anesthetic with extremely rapid titrating characteristics. Patients may be bolused with 1 mg/kg and/or have a continuous IV infusion at 50 to 200 μg/kg per minute. Lower doses provide excellent sedation with rapid recovery; however, when given alone, they may not provide complete analgesia. Local anesthesia should be used if possible. Higher doses may be associated with hypotension and produce a complete loss of protective airway reflexes. The induction dose for intubation and general anesthesia is 2 to 4 mg/kg. This agent is particularly useful for hemodynamically stable patients requiring painless imaging procedures. Propofol burns as it is infused. The pain is easily ameliorated, however, by either using a larger vein such as the antecubital or with a small dose of IV lidocaine before infusion. Propofol is contraindicated in persons with egg or soy allergy. No reversal agents are available.

POSSIBLE COMPLICATIONS

Side effects are associated with any of these medications. Some risks such as nausea or somnolence are relatively minor, whereas others such as respiratory depression or hypotension may be life-threatening. Potential risks and benefits need to be weighed when deciding which set of medications to use and vary depending on the combination of drugs used.

- *Allergic hypersensitivity reactions* may occur and range from brief urticarial reactions to true anaphylaxis.
- *Airway:*
  - — *Loss of protective airway reflexes* may result from oversedation with opioids, benzodiazepines, or propofol. Reversal agents are available for opioids and benzodiazepines, but not for propofol.
  - — *Upper airway obstruction* may result from oversedation and relaxation of the upper airway musculature; it can usually be remedied by repositioning.
  - — *Respiratory depression* may result from oversedation and may require a reversal agent.

— *Laryngospasm* is one of the most feared complications. It occurs when the vocal cords go into spasm and results in the inability to ventilate. It is often self-limited and resolves on its own. If persistent, the physician can attempt to manually ventilate past the obstruction; however, this increases the risk of overdistention of the stomach and aspiration. If still unable to ventilate, pharmacologic muscle relaxation with succinylcholine may be necessary to block the spasm.

— *Chest wall rigidity* may occasionally occur following opioid administration. It results in the mass contraction of the thoracic musculature, making ventilation nearly impossible. It may be remedied either by directly reversing the opioid with naloxone (Narcan) or by using pharmacologic muscle relaxation (succinylcholine).

- *Cardiovascular:*
  — *Hypotension* may result following the administration of many of the sedative or analgesic agents and can usually be remedied by administration of an IV fluid bolus.
- *Behavioral:*
  — *Double vision* may occur for various reasons. It is always self-limited and may occur in conjunction with nausea. Patients may gain some relief by keeping their eyes closed until it resolves.
  — *Dysphoric reactions* may occur while patients emerge from sedation. Reactions include mild moaning, crying or calling out, or may occasionally be severe with feelings of terror or hallucinations. The more severe reactions are sometimes referred to as *emergence reactions;* however, this is a poorly defined term. The only remedy for these reactions is time. Some physicians advocate additional benzodiazepines such as midazolam to blunt this response.
- *Gastrointestinal:*
  — *Nausea and vomiting* are perhaps the most common complications of analgesia and sedation. Results can be disastrous if vomiting occurs early in the sedation when airway reflexes are not intact. Fortunately, however, vomiting usually occurs later during recovery. Standard antiemetics may be beneficial; however, remember that most antiemetics also have additional sedative effects.

CONTRAINDICATIONS AND REASONS FOR REFERRAL TO A SPECIALIST

History

- Patients should be referred to a pediatric anesthesiologist if they have a known history of allergy, hypersensitivity, or a serious problem associated with either analgesia or sedation.
- Children with congenital heart disease and craniofacial abnormalities are at particularly high risk and should also be referred.

TABLE 8-4
ASA physical status classification

Class	Physical status
Class I	A normally healthy patient
Class II	A patient with mild systemic disease
Class III	A patient with severe systemic disease
Class IV	A patient with severe systemic disease that is a constant threat to life
Class V	A moribund patient who is not expected to survive without the operation

Physical Status

- The American Society of Anesthesiology uses a classification system that aids in distinguishing and standardizing the way in which we define the overall physical well-being of patients (Table 8-4).
- In general, patients of Class III or above should be referred to a pediatric anesthesiologist.

Airway Assessment

- Patients should undergo an airway assessment to determine if the potential for a difficult airway exists.
- Components of airway assessment:
  - — Ability to open/close mouth
  - — Tongue size
  - — Neck size and range of motion
  - — Dentition (loose or chipped teeth, dentures)
  - — Morphological features (atypical features consistent with a congenital craniofacial abnormality)
  - — History of snoring, tonsillar hypertrophy, or sleep apnea
- Patients with a potentially difficult airway should be referred to a pediatric anesthesiologist.

Dietary Precautions

- Sedations always carry the risk of vomiting and aspiration.
- Depending on age, the American Academy of Pediatrics recommends between 4 to 8 hours of fasting before sedation. For children younger than 36 months, no milk or solids is recommended for 4 to 6 hours, and for those older than 36 months, no milk or solids is allowed for 8 hours before the procedure.
- The American College of Emergency Physicians' official policy on procedural sedation states that recent food intake is not a contraindication for administering analgesia and sedation but should be considered when choosing the depth and target level of sedation.
- Although it is more desirable to perform sedations only on patients who have

completely empty stomachs, many variables are associated with determining the rate of gastric emptying, and little data are available to support any of the previously recommended time limits.

SUPPLIES, EQUIPMENT, AND MONITORING

Essential Equipment

Minimum supplies that should be readily available *at the bedside* include:

- *Continuous noninvasive pulse oximetry,* which allows for the early detection of hypoxemia before catastrophic events such as cardiac arrest occur. Pulse oximetry is the single most important technological advancement responsible for improving outcomes in sedation and analgesia.
- *Oxygen* and *suction* (connected and in working order *before* sedation begins)
- *Advanced airway equipment* (resuscitation bag and mask)
- *Reversal agents* (naloxone, flumazenil)
- *Blood pressure monitoring* equipment

An appropriately stocked *crash cart* should be *readily available* in all areas in which sedations occur and should include the following equipment:

- Advanced airway equipment: airways, resuscitation bag and mask, laryngoscope, endotracheal tubes (age and size appropriate for pediatric patients)
- Standard resuscitation medications
- Dosing tables for use during resuscitations (age- and weight-based)
- Supplies and equipment for venous access
- Cardiopulmonary monitor with defibrillator

Optional Equipment

End-tidal CO_2 monitors are optional and vary depending on the level of sedation used, institution, and availability of supplies.

PATIENT MONITORING

Sedation

- All patients undergoing sedation should remain on continuous pulse oximetry to provide continuous monitoring of heart rate and oxygen saturations.
- The physician monitoring the sedation may assist in interruptible tasks.
- Vital signs should be taken and recorded a minimum of every 15 minutes.

Deep Sedation

- In addition to pulse oximetry, all patients undergoing deep sedation should have an IV in place and be connected to a cardiopulmonary monitor.

- The physician monitoring the sedation should maintain the sole function of monitoring the sedation. No other tasks should be performed.

REQUIRED NURSING SKILLS

Nursing personnel should be familiar with the following:

- Fundamental principles of sedation
- Monitoring equipment
- Advanced life support protocols (ACLS, PALS, APLS)
- Institutional protocols and forms
- Documentation: Most institutions have standardized nursing forms for sedations, including the following:
  - Presedation Checklist (medications, allergies, past medical history, NPO status)
  - Procedural Flow Sheet (vital signs, level of responsiveness, nursing notes)
  - Recovery Flow Sheet (vital signs, level of responsiveness, nursing notes)
  - Discharge Checklist (discharge criteria, vital signs, instructions, medications, follow-up)

DOCUMENTATION

Before

- History
- Physical examination
- Indications
- Absence of contraindications
- Informed consent

During

- Medication dosages and times given
- Response to medications/modalities
- Response to procedure
- Physiologic monitoring, vital signs, level of sedation

After

- Recovery: Criteria for determining ability to safely discharge patient (Box 8-1)
- Complications
- Instructions and education: Reasonable things to expect
- Detailed follow-up instructions:
  - What to do, what not to do, specific medication instructions
  - When and where to follow up
  - Things to watch out and return for

BOX 8-1 RECOMMENDED DISCHARGE CRITERIA

1. Airway is patent and protective airway reflexes are intact.
2. Cardiovascular status and vital signs are stable.
3. The patient is easily arousable and/or has returned to presedation level of responsiveness.
4. The patient can sit up unaided (if age-appropriate).
5. The child is adequately hydrated.

MODIFICATIONS FOR SITUATIONS OF LIMITED RESOURCES

In situations of limited resources, such as those found in underdeveloped countries, ketamine is the drug of choice. Ketamine has minimal respiratory and cardiovascular effects, has maintained a long track record of safety in underdeveloped countries, and allows for safely providing general anesthesia with a modicum of equipment and personnel.

SUGGESTED READINGS

Algren JT, Algren CL: Sedation and analgesia for minor pediatric procedures, *Pediatr Emerg Care* 12:435, 1996.

American Academy of Pediatrics Committee on Drugs: Guidelines for the elective use of conscious sedation, deep sedation, and general anesthesia in pediatric patients, *Pediatrics* 89:1110, 1992.

American College of Emergency Physicians: Clinical policy for procedural sedation and analgesia in the emergency department, *Ann Emerg Med* 31:663, 1998.

American Society of Anesthesiologists: Practice guidelines for sedation and analgesia by non-anesthesiologists, *Anesthesiology* 84:459, 1996.

Andrews JS: Conscious sedation in the pediatric emergency department, *Curr Opin Pediatr* 7:309, 1995.

Bauman LA et al: Pediatric sedation with analgesia, *Am J Emerg Med* 17:1, 1999.

Broennle AM, Cohen DE: Pediatric anesthesia and sedation, *Curr Opin Pediatr* 5:310, 1993.

Conners GP, Sacks WK, Leahey NF: Variations in sedating uncooperative, stable children for post-traumatic head CT, *Pediatr Emerg Care* 15:241, 1999.

Cote CJ: Sedation for the pediatric patient, *Pediatr Clin North Am* 41:31, 1994.

D'Agostino J, Terndrup TE: Comparative review of the adverse effects of sedatives used in children undergoing outpatient procedures, *Drug Safety* 14:146, 1996.

Hawk W et al: Conscious sedation of the pediatric patient for suturing: a survey, *Pediatr Emerg Care* 6:84, 1990.

Holzman RS et al: Guidelines for sedation by nonanesthesiologists during diagnostic and therapeutic procedures, The Risk Management Committee of the Department of Anaesthesia of Harvard Medical School, *J Clin Anesth* 4:265, 1994.

Ilkhanipour K, Juels CR, Langdorf MI: Pediatric pain control and conscious sedation: a survey of emergency medicine residencies, *Acad Emerg Med* 14:368, 1994.

Innes G et al: Procedural sedation and analgesia in the emergency department, Canadian Consensus Guidelines, *J Emerg Med* 17:145, 1999.

Krauss B, Zurakowski D: Sedation patterns in pediatric and general community hospital emergency departments, *Pediatr Emerg Care* 14:99, 1998.

Litman RS: Sedation and anesthesia outside the operating room: answers to common questions, *Semin Pediatr Surg* 8:34, 1999.

Litman RS: Recent trends in the management of acute pain in children, *J Am Osteopath Assoc* 96:290, 1996.

Lowrie L, Weiss AH, Lacombe C: The pediatric sedation unit: a mechanism for pediatric sedation, *Pediatrics* 102:E30, 1998.

Malviya S, Voepel-Lewis T, Tait AR: Adverse events and risk factors associated with the sedation of children by nonanesthesiologist, *Anesth Analg* 85:1207, 1997.

Petrack EM, Christopher NC, Kriwinsky J: Pain management in the emergency department: patterns of analgesic utilization, *Pediatrics* 99:711, 1997.

Sacchetti A et al: Community hospital management of pediatric emergencies: implications for pediatric emergency medical services, *Am J Emerg Med* 4:10, 1986.

Sacchetti A et al: Pediatric analgesia and sedation, *Ann Emerg Med* 23:237, 1994.

Schweich PJ et al: Pediatric emergency medicine practice patterns: a comparison of pediatric and general emergency physicians, *Pediatr Emerg Care* 14:89, 1998.

U.S. Department of Health and Human Services, Public Health Service, Agency for Health Care Policy and Research, Acute Pain Management Guideline Panel: *Clinical practice guideline—Acute pain management: operative or medical procedures and trauma,* Washington, DC, February 1992, U.S. Government Printing Office.

Weisman SJ, Bernstein B, Schechter NL: Consequences of inadequate analgesia during painful procedures in children, *Arch Pediatr Adolesc Med* 152:147, 1998.

Woolard DJ, Terndrup TE: Sedative-analgesic agent administration in children: analysis of use and complications in the emergency department, *J Emerg Med* 12:453, 1994.

APPENDIX 8-1
Commonly used agents for analgesia and sedation in pediatric emergency medicine

Agent	Route	Dose	Duration	Comments	Reversal agent
Chloral hydrate	PO, PR	50-100 mg/kg (2 g max)	3-5 hr	Sedative agent without analgesic properties. Requires same monitoring as other sedative agents.	None available
Fentanyl (Sublimaze)	PO (Oralet) IV	10-15 μg/kg (400 μg max) 1-2 μg/kg titrated	30-60 min 15-30 min	Child self-medicates by sucking on Oralet until sedated. May be associated with vomiting. May cause respiratory depression, particularly if combined with a benzodiazepine. Sedation may become more pronounced when the painful procedure has been completed and the child is no longer being stimulated.	Naloxone (Narcan), Nalmefene (Revex)
Ketamine (Ketalar)	PR IM IV	4-6 mg/kg 2-4 mg/kg 1-2 mg/kg titrated	30-60 min 30-60 min 15-30 min	Consider antisecretory agent (atropine, glycopyrrolate). Consider benzodiazepine (midazolam). IV ketamine given too rapidly may cause apnea. Bronchodilator without respiratory depression. Minimal cardiovascular effects.	None available
Meperidine (Demerol)	IM, IV	1-2 mg/kg (100 mg max)	2-4 hr	Although often combined with promethazine and chlorpromazine, not currently recommended for procedural sedation. Interacts unfavorably with numerous medications. Accumulation of metabolite may precipitate seizures.	Naloxone (Narcan), Nalmefene (Revex)
Methohexital (Brevital)	PR IM IV	25 mg/kg 10 mg/kg 0.75-1.0 mg/kg	45-90 min 45-90 min 8-10 min	Respiratory depression is more common following IV bolus administration than rectal dosing. Apnea may occur because of the relaxed head position, causing airway obstruction. Seizures have been reported; however, usually only in those patients with underlying seizure disorder.	None available

Continued

APPENDIX 8-1
Commonly used agents for analgesia and sedation in pediatric emergency medicine—cont'd

Agent	Route	Dose	Duration	Comments	Reversal agent
Midazolam (Versed)	PO, IN, PR IM IV	0.4-0.8 mg/kg 0.1-0.2 mg/kg 0.035-0.1 mg/kg (2 mg max/dose)	30-60 min 30-60 min 30-60 min	Intranasal administration is not always well tolerated and has been associated with paradoxical hyperactivity. Midazolam administered by any route can cause respiratory depression, particularly when combined with opioids. Sedation may become more pronounced when the painful procedure has been completed and the child is no longer being stimulated.	Flumazenil (Romazecon)
Morphine	IM, SQ, IV	0.1 mg/kg (2 mg max/dose)	1-2 hr	May cause respiratory depression, particularly when combined with benzodiazepines. Sedation may become more pronounced when the painful procedure has been completed and the child is no longer being stimulated.	Naloxone (Narcan), Nalmefene (Revex)
Propofol (Diprivan)	IV	50-200 μg/kg/min (a loading or bolus dose of 1mg/kg may be given as needed)	8-10 min	Excellent sedative with ultra-short half-life. Lower doses do not provide analgesia. Use of additional local anesthesia is recommended whenever possible. Higher doses produce respiratory depression, hypotension, and general anesthesia (induction dose for intubation 2-4 mg/kg).	None available

APPENDIX 8-2
Commonly used reversal and adjuvant agents in analgesia and sedation

Agent	Dose	Action	Comments
Atropine	0.01 mg/kg (0.3 mg max)	Antisecretory (anticholinergic)	Commonly used with ketamine. May produce tachycardia.
Flumazenil (Romazecon)	0.1 mg aliquots every 60 sec (Max initial dose 1 mg)	Reversal agent for benzodiazepines	Onset of action is 1-3 min. Duration of action may be shorter than benzodiazepine and therefore might require multiple doses. May precipitate seizures in those habituated.
Glycopyrrolate (Robinal)	0.01 mg/kg (0.2 mg max)	Antisecretory (anticholinergic)	Commonly used with ketamine. Produces less tachycardia than atropine.
Nalmefene (Revex)	0.25 μg/kg Repeated every 2-5 min to effect or 1.0 μg/kg max	Reversal agent for opioids	Onset of action is rapid. Duration of action (3-5 hr) is longer than naloxone but may still be shorter than opioid. May precipitate withdrawal in those habituated.
Naloxone (Narcan)	0.1 mg/kg (2.0 mg max)	Reversal agent for opioids	Onset of action is almost immediate. Duration of action may be shorter than opioid and therefore might require multiple doses. May precipitate withdrawal in those habituated.

CHAPTER 9

Local and Regional Anesthesia

Sean P. Kelly
Mark A. Hostetler

INTRODUCTION

Anesthesia allows physicians to perform otherwise painful procedures such as wound exploration, laceration repair, fracture reduction, incision and drainage, and foreign body removal with relative ease and patient comfort. The three types of local and regional anesthesia that are discussed in this chapter include commonly used specific nerve blocks, local infiltration, and regional field blocks.

INDICATIONS

- Local anesthesia is indicated for procedures such as wound explorations, wound debridements, laceration repairs, fracture reductions, incision and drainages, foreign body removals, paronychia drainages, nailbed injuries, and skin biopsies.
- Local wound infiltration is indicated for most uncomplicated wound explorations, laceration repairs, and skin biopsies.
- Field blocks are indicated for areas that are infected, or difficult or painful to infiltrate directly. They are also indicated if direct infiltration would distend the tissues and interfere with wound approximation.
- Peripheral nerve blocks are indicated for areas that are infected, or difficult or painful to inject directly. They are also indicated if direct infiltration would distend the tissues and interfere with wound approximation, and in situations when direct infiltration would require more needlesticks (painful) and higher total doses of anesthetic (increased potential toxicity) than a nerve block.

CONTRAINDICATIONS

- Local anesthetics are contraindicated in patients with known hypersensitivity.
- Allergic reactions to aminoester compounds (e.g., procaine, chlorprocaine, and tetracaine) are not uncommon.

- Allergic reactions to aminoamides (e.g., lidocaine, bupivicaine, mepivicaine, prilocaine, and etidocaine) are extremely rare. When allergic reactions to amides occur, they are usually attributable to the methyl-paraben preservative used in most multidose commercial preparations. Multidose vials are therefore contraindicated in patients with known sensitivity.
- No cross-reactivity occurs between esters and amides. A patient with sensitivity to esters can be given amides without increased risk of allergic reaction.
- Injecting anesthetic through infected tissue is contraindicated.
- Injecting anesthetic in the setting of profound anticoagulation or bleeding disorders is contraindicated.
- Epinephrine is contraindicated in areas where vasoconstriction could cause tissue ischemia and necrosis. It should not be used in the fingers, toes, penis, nose, or earlobes. It may also cause ischemia in avulsion flaps with poor blood supply. Practitioners should also remember that patients with known peripheral vascular disease can exhibit an exaggerated vasoconstrictor response.

SELECTING AN ANESTHETIC AGENT

- There are two major types of local anesthetics: aminoesters and aminoamides.
- Aminoesters include tetracaine, procaine, and chlorprocaine. They are primarily metabolized by the liver. Patients can have allergic reactions to the paraamino benzoic acid (PABA) nucleus.
- Aminoamides include lidocaine, bupivicaine, mepivicaine, prilocaine, and etidocaine. They are primarily metabolized in the serum. Allergic reactions to these compounds are extremely rare. When allergic reactions occur, they are usually attributable to the methyl-paraben preservative used in most multidose commercial preparations. Most single-dose preparations do not contain this preservative. Single-dose vials should therefore be used whenever possible.
- No cross-reactivity occurs between esters and amides, so a patient with sensitivity to esters can be given amides without increased risk of allergic reaction.
- An easy memory device to distinguish between the two types is that the aminoamides all have an "i" in the prefix, whereas the aminoesters do not.
- Most anesthetics have a vasodilatory effect.
- A vasoconstrictor, such as epinephrine (1/100,000 to 1/400,000), can be used to decrease bleeding, provide better wound visualization, reduce systemic absorption, and prolong the duration of action. Epinephrine is contraindicated, however, in areas where vasoconstriction might cause tissue ischemia or necrosis. It should not be used in the fingers, toes, penis, nose, or earlobes. It may also cause ischemia in avulsion flaps with poor blood supply. Practitioners should also remember that patients with known peripheral vascular disease can exhibit an exaggerated vasoconstrictor response (Box 9-1).
- Notable variability in onset and duration of action exists among agents. Practitioners should keep these differences in mind when selecting an

BOX 9-1 SELECTION OF LOCAL ANESTHETICS/EFFECTS

Lidocaine (Xylocaine) *without* epinephrine

Can cause vasodilation
Duration of 0.5 to 1 hour depending on site/vascularity
Use in contaminated wounds
Use in fingers, nose, penis, toes, and earlobes
Use if vascular disease is present or if patient is immunocompromised
Use for nerve blocks

Lidocaine (Xylocaine) *with* epinephrine

Causes vasoconstriction
Has longer duration
Use in highly vascular areas to improve visualization of field
Use in clean wounds
In general, do not use on fingers, nose, penis, toes, and earlobes

Bupivacaine (Marcaine)

Use for longer duration
Use for nerve blocks

From Pfenninger JL, Fowler GC: *Procedures for primary care physicians,* St Louis, 1994, Mosby.

TABLE 9-1
Commonly used local anesthetics in the office setting

Local anesthetic	Onset (min.)	Duration (hr.)	Concentration (%)	Maximum dose
Lidocaine (Xylocaine)	1	0.5-1	1	4.5 mg/kg not to exceed 300 mg (30 ml in adult)
Lidocaine w/epinephrine	1	2-6	1	7 mg/kg not to exceed 500 mg (50 ml in adult)
Bupivacaine	5	2-4	0.25	3 mg/kg not to exceed 175 mg (50 ml per average adult)
Bupivacaine w/epinephrine	5	3-7	0.25	3 mg/kg not to exceed 225 mg

From Pfenninger JL, Fowler GC: *Procedures for primary care physicians,* St Louis, 1994, Mosby.

agent and tailor the agents specifically to the individual patient and procedure (Table 9-1).

MECHANISM OF ACTION

Local anesthetics work by blocking sodium channels. They prevent sodium from entering nerve cells. The lack of ion movement prevents the formation of an action potential. Sensory nerve transmission to the central nervous system (CNS) is blocked, and anesthesia is achieved.

COMPLICATIONS, TOXICITY, AND DOSING

- *Local complications* include bleeding, infection, muscle inflammation, and neuropathy from direct injection of a nerve, and tissue ischemia from epinephrine injection into an end-organ area.
- *Systemic complications* may arise from inadvertent intravascular injection or from excessive extravascular infiltration. Systemic complications include excitability, apprehension, disorientation, parasthesias, a metallic taste in the mouth, tremors, nystagmus, seizures, and hypotension. In large doses, prilocaine and benzocaine have been reported to cause methemoglobinemia. Bupivicaine is not recommended for children less than 12 years old.
- The toxic dose of lidocaine, the most commonly used topical anesthetic, is 4.5 mg/kg.
- The toxic dose of lidocaine with epinephrine is 7 mg/kg because vasoconstriction limits systemic spread of local anesthetic.
- Remember that 1 ml of 1% lidocaine equals 10 mg of lidocaine, and 1 ml of 2% lidocaine equals 20 mg. The simplest way to remember this formula is to simply add a zero to the percent concentration (1% = 10 mg/ml, 10% = 100 mg/ml).
- In infants and small children, the blood–brain barrier is more permeable to anesthetic agents, resulting in relatively higher CNS concentrations. They are at higher risk than adults for toxic reactions to anesthetic agents; therefore dosing should not exceed 80% of the usual recommended maximum doses listed previously. (See Table 9-1 for maximum toxic doses of common anesthetics.)

TYPES OF LOCAL AND REGIONAL ANESTHESIA

- *Local infiltration* involves direct infiltration of anesthesia into the wound margins and is the most commonly used technique for wound anesthesia. Using this technique, injecting into the wound edge may minimize the pain of injection caused by injecting through intact, highly innervated skin. Local infiltration has several notable limitations and potential disadvantages. It may distort wound edges and make amlurate approximation more difficult. It also may spread infection through high-risk areas, such as abscesses or contaminated wounds. Also, some anatomic regions, such as the ear or the nailbed, are difficult or painful to infiltrate directly. Some wounds are so large that direct infiltration would require a significant amount of local anesthetic, which raises the risk of toxicity, particularly for children. In such cases, field or peripheral nerve blocks may be preferred.
- *Field block* involves infiltration of anesthetic into the soft tissue in a field pattern around the wound, instead of injecting into the wound itself. Also called "parallel margin infiltration," this technique blocks nerves proximal to the injured area. Advantages of the field block are that it lowers the risk of spreading infection through a contaminated wound, it will not distort the wound edges, and it can be used in difficult-to-infiltrate areas such as the nose and ear.

- *Peripheral nerve block* involves injection of anesthetic proximally around the nerve(s) supplying sensation to the injured area. One advantage of the nerve block is that it produces a large field of anesthesia with a relatively small amount of anesthetic, thereby reducing risk of toxicity. Similar to the field block, it does not distort the wound edges. It is also recommended over local infiltration in highly contaminated wounds.

TECHNIQUES USED TO MINIMIZE PAIN OF INJECTION

1. Use the smallest size needle possible for each procedure. For peripheral nerve blocks, a 25- to 27-gauge needle is usually appropriate. For local infiltration or field blocks, a 27- to 30-gauge needle is usually appropriate.
2. Topical anesthetics, which are acidic, may be buffered with bicarbonate to make the pH more neutral and ease the pain of injection. To do this, add 1 ml of sodium bicarbonate (1 mg/1 ml solution) to 10 ml of lidocaine to create an anesthetic with physiologic pH. Converting to a more physiologic pH also increases the anesthetic's potency.
3. Remember to inject slowly because most of the pain of injection is associated with rapidity of tissue distortion.
4. Proceed from an anesthetized to an unanesthetized area.
5. Allow sufficient time for onset of anesthesia before beginning the procedure.

NECESSARY EQUIPMENT

- Buffer solution (sodium bicarbonate 1 mg/1 ml solution) (+/–)
- Local anesthetic (1% lidocaine)
- Needle (25- to 30-gauge, 0.5- to 1.5-inch)
- Needle (18-gauge) to draw up solution (+/–)
- Povidine-iodine solution 10%, or other antiseptic solution
- Sterile gauze
- Syringe (5-10 ml)
- Vasoconstrictor, if not contraindicated (epinephrine 1/100,000) (+/–)

LOCAL INFILTRATION

1. Obtain informed consent before procedure. Discuss the risks and benefits of the procedure with the patient and/or the family.
2. Assess local and distal sensory function, motor function, perfusion status, and associated injuries before procedure.
3. Document all findings, particularly if a sensory motor deficit is present before procedure.
4. Prepare the skin around the injured area with 10% povidine-iodine solution or

another antiseptic solution. Avoid application to the wound itself, however, because most antiseptics are toxic to tissues.

5. Select a topical anesthetic. See the Selection of an Anesthetic Agent section for further discussion.
6. Do not use epinephrine on fingers, nose, penis, toes, or ears.
7. Wipe the top of the anesthetic bottle with an alcohol swab. Using an 18-gauge needle, draw up an appropriate amount of local anesthetic; 10 ml is usually adequate for most procedures described in this text. See the Toxicity and Dosing section for further discussion of dosing.
8. If lidocaine is not buffered, add 1 ml of sodium bicarbonate (1 mg/1 ml solution) to 10 ml of lidocaine to create an anesthetic with physiologic pH. This will decrease the pain of injection and increase the anesthetic's potency.
9. Discard the 18-gauge needle into an appropriate container. Do not recap needles.
10. Screw an appropriately sized needle onto the syringe. A 27- to 30-gauge, 0.5- to 1.0-inch needle is appropriate for most procedures described in this text.
11. Inject into the dermal layer, through the wound margins, as shown in Fig. 9-1. Subcutaneous injection may also be used, depending on the depth of the wound.
12. Before infiltration, aspirate back on the syringe to avoid intravascular injection of anesthetic.
13. Inject slowly and proceed from anesthetized to unanesthetized areas to reduce pain. See the Minimizing Pain of Injection section for further discussion.
14. Some blanching of the anesthetized area is to be expected; however, rapid blanching, cooling, or pain in the injured area, or distal to it, may signify intraarterial injection of anesthetic. If this occurs, immediately stop the injection, reassess the patient, reposition the needle, and aspirate again before reinjecting. Also, if any systemic symptoms of anesthetic toxicity occur, immediately stop the injection and reassess the patient. See the Toxicity and Dosing section for further discussion.

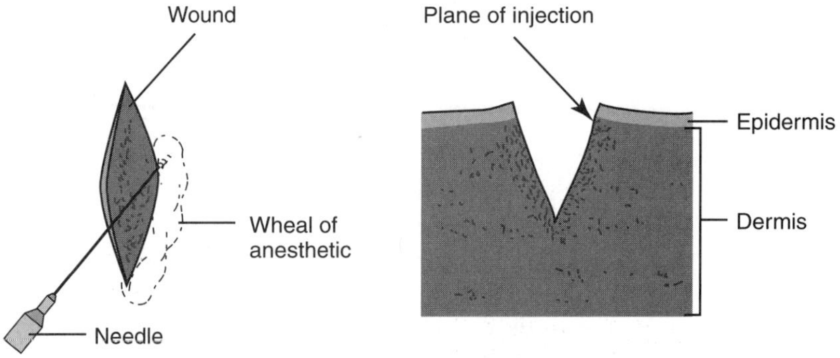

FIG. 9-1. Local infiltration technique.

15. Allow sufficient time for onset of anesthesia before starting the procedure.
16. Ensure complete anesthesia by checking for sensation to pain around entire wound before starting the procedure.

FIELD BLOCK

1. Obtain informed consent before procedure. Discuss the risks and benefits of the procedure with the patient and/or the family.
2. Assess local and distal sensory function, motor function, perfusion status, and associated injuries before procedure.
3. Document all findings, particularly if a sensory motor deficit is present before procedure.
4. Prepare the skin around the injured area with 10% povidine-iodine solution or another antiseptic solution. Avoid application to the wound itself, however, because most antiseptics are toxic to tissues.
5. Select a topical anesthetic. See the Selection of an Anesthetic Agent section for further discussion.
6. Do not use epinephrine on fingers, nose, penis, ears, or toes.
7. Wipe the top of the anesthetic bottle with an alcohol swab. Using an 18-gauge needle, draw up an appropriate amount of local anesthetic; 10 ml is usually adequate for most procedures described in this text. See the Toxicity and Dosing section for further discussion of dosing.
8. If lidocaine is not buffered, add 1 ml of sodium bicarbonate (1 mg/1 ml solution) to 10 ml of lidocaine to create an anesthetic with physiologic pH. This will decrease the pain of injection and increase the anesthetic's potency.
9. Discard the 18-gauge needle into an appropriate container. Do not recap needles.
10. Select an appropriately sized needle for the procedure. A 25- to 30-gauge, 0.5- to 1.5-inch needle is appropriate for most procedures described in this text.
11. Inject into the intact skin in a field around the injured area (Fig. 9-2). Do not inject into the wound itself. Depending on the depth of the wound, injections may need to be dermal or subcutaneous. Fig. 9-3 illustrates a field block around the ear.
12. Before infiltration, aspirate back on the syringe to avoid intravascular injection of anesthetic.
13. Inject slowly and proceed from anesthetized to unanesthetized areas to reduce pain. See the Minimizing Pain of Injection section for further discussion.
14. Some blanching of the anesthetized area is to be expected; however, rapid blanching, cooling, or pain in the injured area, or distal to it, may signify intraarterial injection of anesthetic. If this occurs, immediately stop the injection, reassess the patient, reposition the needle, and aspirate again before reinjecting. Also, if any systemic symptoms of anesthetic toxicity occur, immediately stop the injection and reassess the patient. See the Toxicity and Dosing section for further discussion.

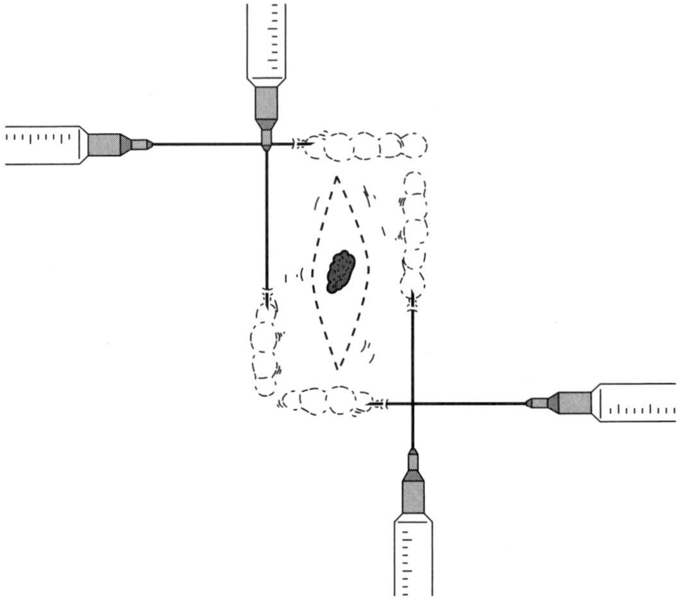

FIG. 9-2. Basic field block technique.

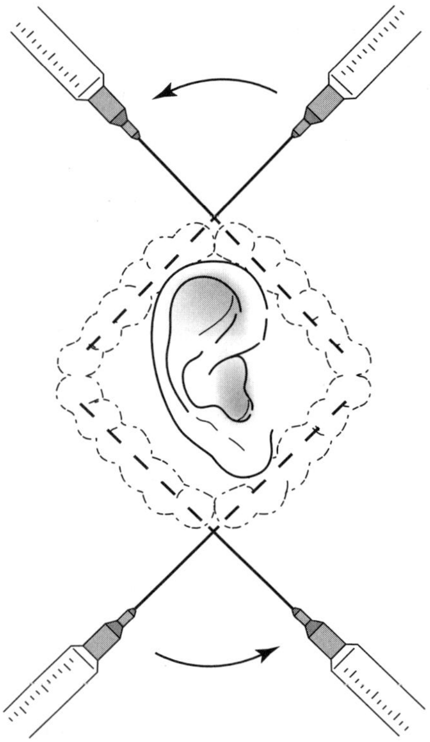

FIG. 9-3. Field block of the ear.

15. Allow sufficient time for onset of anesthesia before starting the procedure.
16. Ensure complete anesthesia by checking for sensation to pain around entire wound before starting the procedure.

NERVE BLOCK

1. Obtain informed consent before procedure. Discuss the risks and benefits of the procedure with the patient and/or the family.
2. Assess local and distal sensory function, motor function, perfusion status, and associated injuries before procedure.
3. Document all findings, particularly if a sensory motor deficit is present before procedure.
4. Identify the appropriate nerve(s) that provides sensation to the injured area(s). Determine the site of injection for the peripheral nerve block to be performed. See the following section for a description of several common nerve blocks.
5. Prepare the skin around the injured area with 10% povidine-iodine solution or another antiseptic solution. Avoid application to the wound itself, however, because most antiseptics are toxic to tissues.
6. Select a topical anesthetic. See the Selection of an Anesthetic Agent section for further discussion.
7. Do not use epinephrine on fingers, nose, penis, ears, or toes.
8. Wipe the top of the anesthetic bottle with an alcohol swab. Using an 18-gauge needle, draw up an appropriate amount of local anesthetic; 10 ml is usually adequate for most procedures described in this text. See the Toxicity and Dosing section for further discussion of dosing.
9. If lidocaine is not buffered, add 1 ml of sodium bicarbonate (1 mg/1 ml solution) to 10 ml of lidocaine to create an anesthetic with physiologic pH. This will decrease the pain of injection and increase the anesthetic's potency.
10. Discard the 18-gauge needle into an appropriate container. Do not recap needles.
11. Screw an appropriately sized needle onto the syringe. A 25- to 27-gauge, 0.5- to 1.5-inch needle is appropriate for most procedures described in this text.
12. Insert the needle into the appropriate site. See following section for descriptions of some of the most commonly used peripheral nerve blocks.
13. The patient may feel paresthesias, signifying mechanical stimulation of the nerve by the needle. If this occurs, withdraw the needle 1 to 2 mm to avoid intraneural injection. Note that, with young children, it may be difficult to distinguish the pain of the needlestick from paresthesias.
14. Before injecting, aspirate back on the syringe to ensure that you are not in a vascular space to avoid intravascular injection of anesthetic.
15. Inject anesthetic slowly. Most nerve blocks described in this text require only 1 to 2 mm of anesthetic to achieve full effect.
16. Some blanching of the anesthetized area is to be expected; however, rapid blanching, cooling, or pain in the injured area, or distal to it, may signify

intraarterial injection of anesthetic. If this occurs, immediately stop the injection, reassess the patient, reposition the needle, and aspirate again before reinjecting. Also, if any systemic symptoms of anesthetic toxicity occur, immediately stop the injection and reassess the patient. See the Toxicity and Dosing section for further discussion.

17. Allow sufficient time for onset of anesthesia before starting the procedure. It may take 15 minutes to attain complete anesthesia.
18. Ensure complete anesthesia by checking for sensation to pain around entire wound before starting the procedure.

COMMON NERVE BLOCKS

Forehead Block (Supraorbital and Supratrochlear Nerve Blocks)

Anatomy

- The supraorbital and supratrochlear nerves emerge from the superior orbital ridge and supply sensation to the forehead and anterior scalp, as shown in Fig. 9-4.

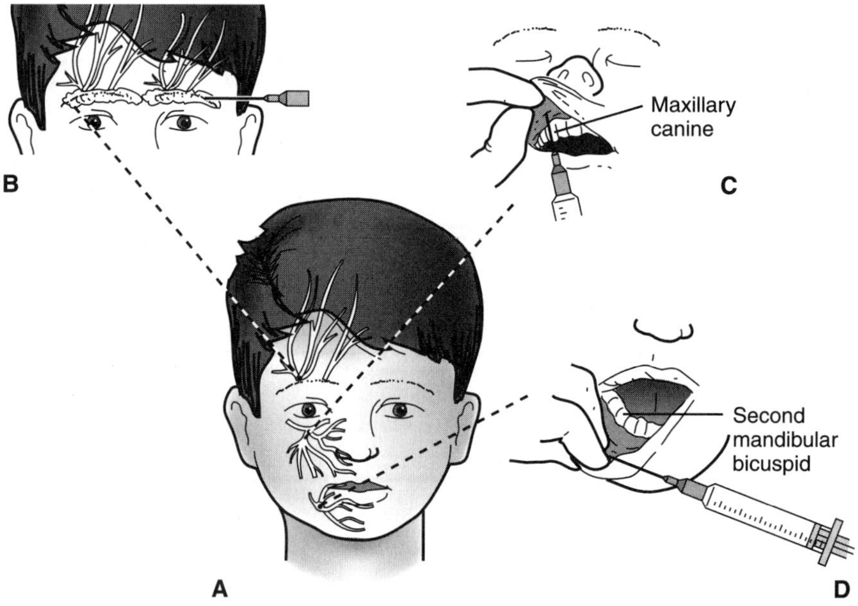

FIG. 9-4. Locations and approaches to common facial nerve blocks. **A,** Sensory distribution of supraorbital, supratrochlear, infraorbital, and mental nerves. **B,** Horizontal approach for supraorbital and supratrochlear nerve forehead block. **C,** Intraoral insertion point for infraorbital nerve block. **D,** Intraoral insertion point for mental nerve block.

Procedure

- Follow the basic nerve block procedure described previously, using 1% lidocaine with epinephrine. Make sure to prepare the skin, and always aspirate before injection, as instructed previously.
- In order to block all branches of both nerves, inject the anesthetic subcutaneously, just superficial to bone, in a line of anesthesia running horizontally across the supraorbital ridge, as shown in Figs. 9-4 and 9-5. This line can be extended bilaterally to anesthetize the entire forehead.

Infraorbital Nerve Block

Anatomy

- The infraorbital nerve emerges from the infraorbital foramen, inferior to a notch in the infraorbital ridge and superior to the first premolar (Fig. 9-4). It supplies sensation to the face, as shown in Fig. 9-6.

Procedure

- Follow the basic nerve block procedure described previously, using 1% lidocaine with epinephrine. Make sure to prepare the skin, and always aspirate before injection, as instructed previously.
- There are two techniques: extraoral and intraoral. Both are equally efficacious. The intraoral technique may be easier and less painful.
- To perform the intraoral infraorbital nerve block, introduce a 27-gauge, 1.5-inch needle into the gingival-buccal margin superior to the maxillary canine tooth.

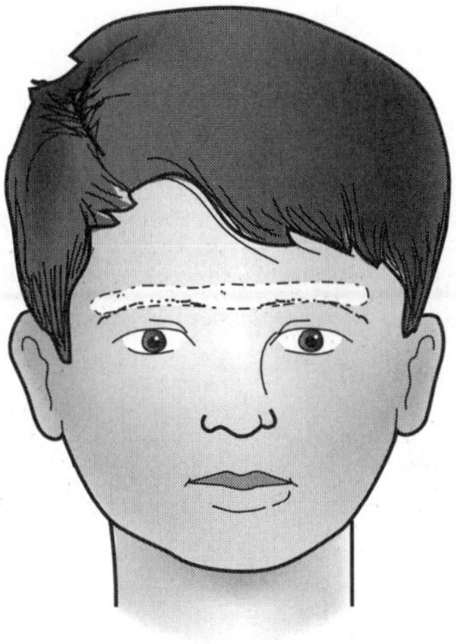

FIG. 9-5. Horizontal approach for supraorbital and supratrochlear nerve forehead block.

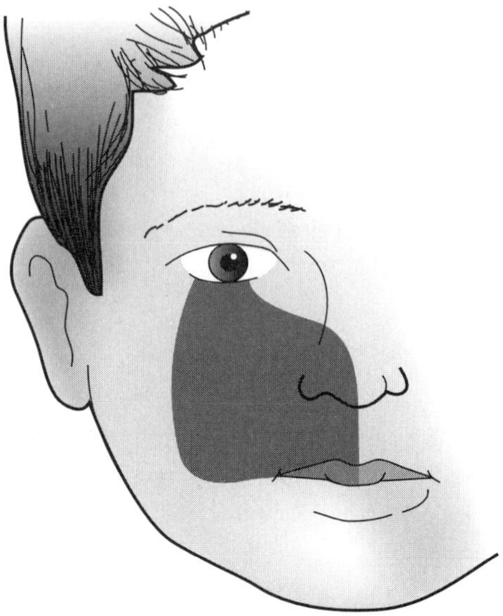

FIG. 9-6. Sensory distribution of the infraorbital nerve.

Advance it under the skin to the infraorbital foramen. Inject approximately 1 ml of anesthetic subcutaneously, as shown in Fig. 9-4.

- To perform the extraoral infraorbital nerve block, infiltrate approximately 1 ml of anesthetic directly into the subcutaneous tissue over the infraorbital foramen.

Mental Nerve Block

Anatomy

- The mental nerve is a branch of the inferior alveolar nerve. It runs through the mental foramen (Fig. 9-7, *A*) and supplies sensation to the lower lip, as shown in Fig. 9-7, *B*. The mental foramen lies below the second premolar at the level of the inferior sulcus.

Procedure

- Follow the basic nerve block procedure described previously, using 1% lidocaine with epinephrine. Make sure to prepare the skin, and always aspirate before injection, as instructed previously.
- There are two techniques: extraoral and intraoral. They are equally as effective, but the intraoral technique is recommended because it is easier and less painful.
- To perform the extraoral mental nerve block, infiltrate approximately 1 to 2 ml of 1% lidocaine with epinephrine directly into the subcutaneous tissue over the mental foramen.

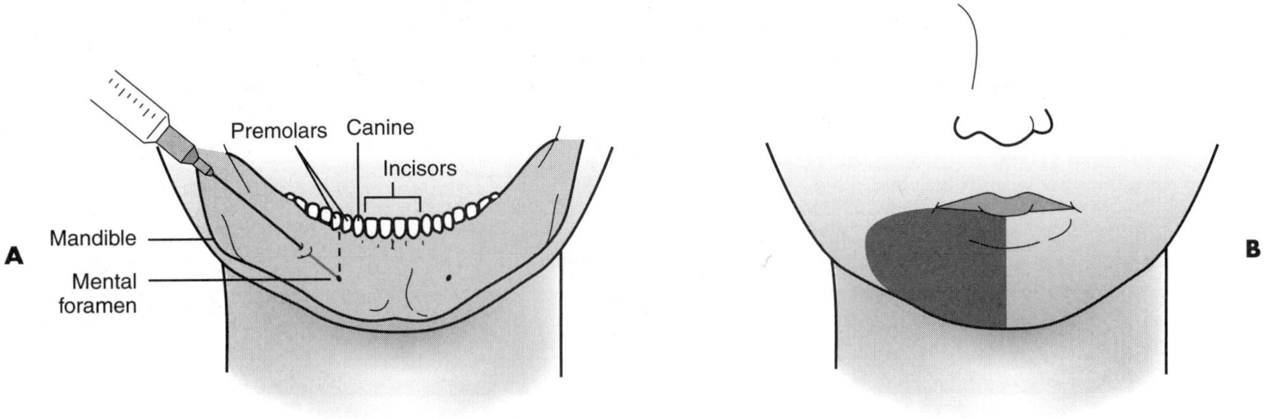

FIG. 9-7. A, Location of the mental foramen directly inferior to the second premolar. **B,** Sensory distribution of the mental nerve.

- To perform the intraoral mental nerve block, introduce a 27-gauge, 1.5-inch needle into the gingival-bumlal margin inferior to the second premolar. Advance it to the mental foramen. Inject approximately 1 to 2 ml of 1% lidocaine with epinephrine subcutaneously, as shown in Fig. 9-8.

Digital Nerve Block of the Finger

Anatomy

- Four digital nerves supply sensation to the finger, arising from branches of the median, ulnar, and radial nerves (Fig. 9-9).
- Two dorsal digital nerves run dorsally along each side of the phalynx.
- Two plantar digital nerves run ventrally along each side of the phalynx.

Procedure

- Follow the basic nerve block procedure described previously, using 1% lidocaine *without* epinephrine. Make sure to prepare the skin, and always aspirate before injection, as instructed previously.
- Dorsal or palmar approaches can be used. The dorsal approach is preferred because palmar skin is more sensitive to the needlestick.
- Digital blocks can be performed distally or proximally (Fig. 9-10). The proximal approach is also known as the metacarpal block.

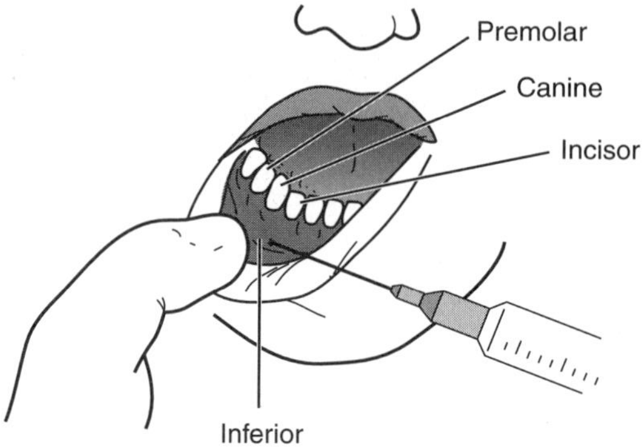

FIG. 9-8. Illustration of the intraoral approach to the mental nerve block.

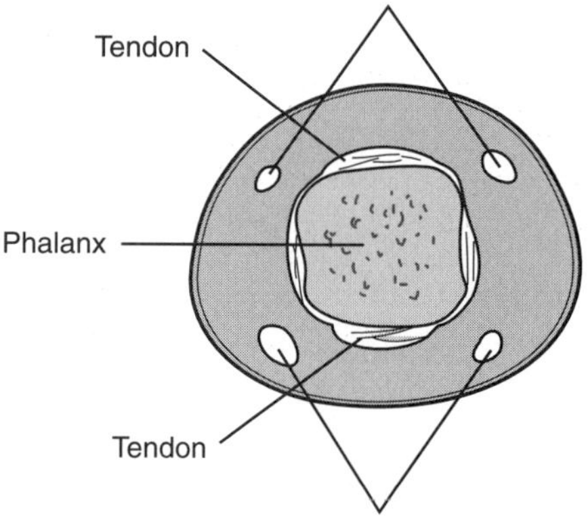

FIG. 9-9. Basic anatomy of the four digital nerves.

Procedure—proximal digital block (metacarpal block)

1. To perform the proximal digital block, also known as the metacarpal block, follow the basic nerve block procedure described previously, using 1% lidocaine *without* epinephrine. Make sure to prepare the skin, and always aspirate before injection, as instructed previously.
2. Raise a wheal of anesthetic in the skin between the metacarpal bones on either side of the affected digit, approximately 1 to 2 cm proximal to the web space at the level of the metacarpal heads (Fig. 9-11).
3. Insert a 25-gauge needle through the anesthetized skin on one side.
4. Advance the needle until it rests just underneath the skin on the palmar aspect.

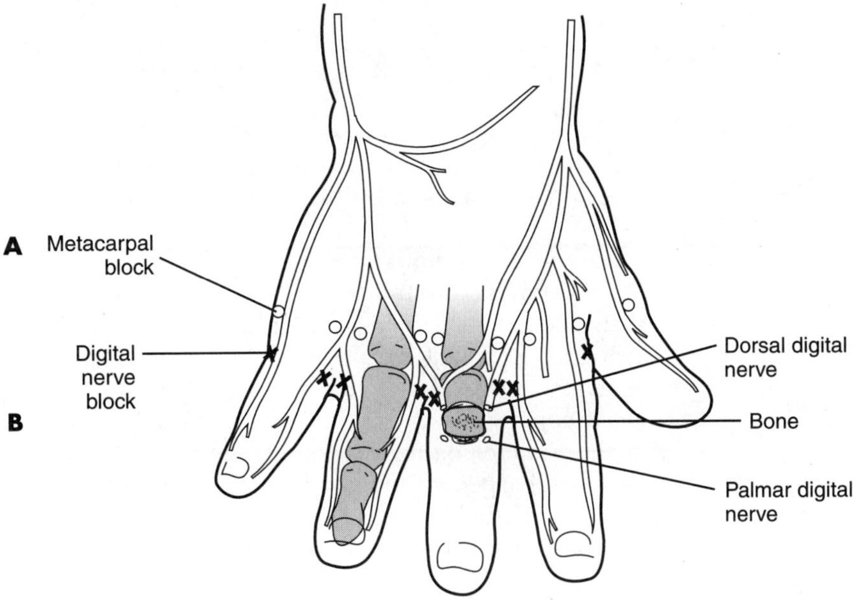

FIG. 9-10. Diagrammatic illustration of the two common approaches to digital nerve blocks. **A,** Proximal metacarpal block. **B,** Distal digital nerve block.

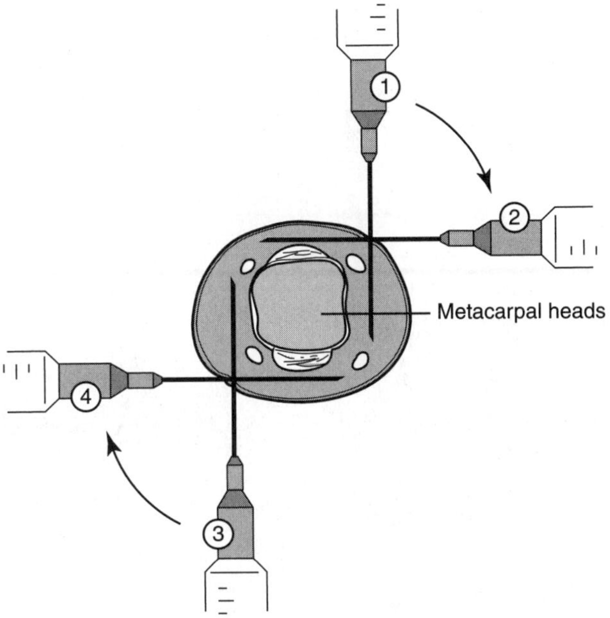

FIG. 9-11. Metacarpal ring block. Four-step process provides for anesthesia around all four sides of the digit with two needlesticks.

5. Inject approximately 2 to 3 ml of anesthetic, while slowly withdrawing the needle.
6. The common digital nerve lies closer to the palmar side, so most of the anesthetic should be deposited there.
7. Repeat the procedure on the other side of the affected digit.

Procedure—distal digital block

1. To perform the distal digital block, insert the needle into the dorsal webspace distal to the metacarpal-pharyngeal joint (Fig. 9-12, *A*).
2. Advance the needle in a palmar direction, next to the phalynx of the affected finger.
3. Inject approximately 1 ml of lidocaine *without* epinephrine at the palmar aspect of the phalynx, partially withdraw the needle, and inject approximately 1 ml at the dorsal aspect of the phalynx (Fig. 9-12, *B*).
4. Without removing the needle from the skin, redirect the needle across the dorsal surface of the digit and inject anesthetic along the back of the finger.
5. Then insert the needle on the other side of the affected digit, through the anesthetized skin, and repeat the procedure to anesthetize the palmar and dorsal digital nerves on the other side (Fig. 9-10).

A

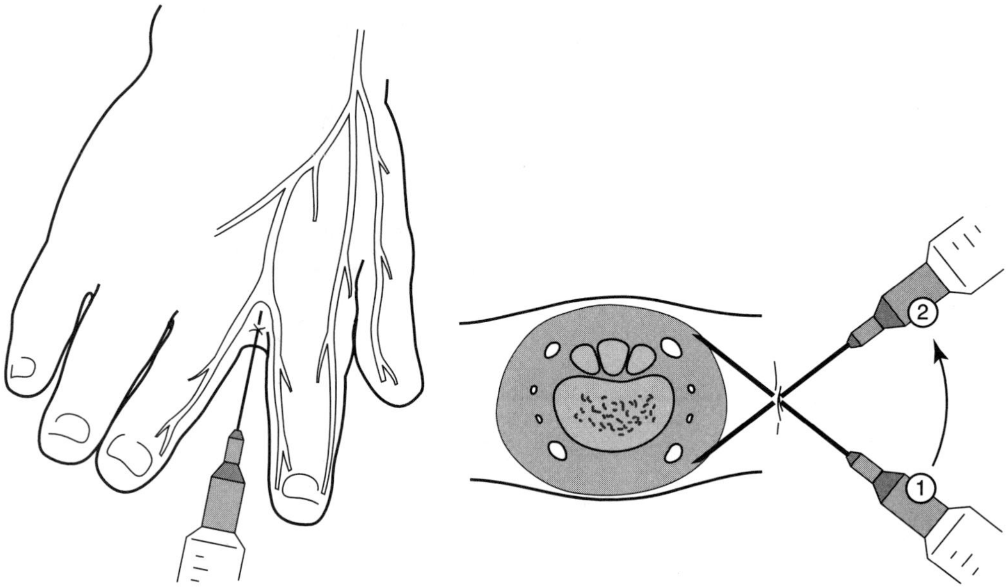

B

FIG. 9-12. Distal digital nerve block. **A,** Insertion into the webspace. **B,** Manipulation of needle to provide anesthesia of palmar and dorsal branches on the same side of the finger using one needlestick.

Digital Nerve Block of the Toe

Anatomy

- Four digital nerves supply sensation to the toe similar to the fingers (Fig. 9-9).
- Two dorsal digital nerves run dorsally along each side of the toe.
- Two palmar digital nerves run ventrally along each side of the toe.

Procedure—digital nerve block of the toe

1. Follow the basic nerve block procedure described previously, using 1% lidocaine *without* epinephrine. Make sure to prepare the skin, and always aspirate before injection, as instructed previously.
2. Dorsal or plantar approaches can be used, but the plantar skin is more sensitive to the needlestick, so the dorsal approach is preferred.
3. Digital block of the toe is similar to digital block of the finger; however, because the toes are narrower than the fingers, it is possible to anesthetize both sides of the phalynx with one midline needlestick.
4. Insert the 25- to 27-gauge needle into the skin, midline at the base of the injured toe, as shown in Fig. 9-13.
5. Advance the needle toward the plantar surface on one side of the bone, passing as close as possible to the bone.
6. Inject approximately 1 to 2 ml of anesthetic as the needle is withdrawn toward the dorsal surface.
7. Without removing the needle from the skin, redirect it toward the other side of the injured toe.
8. Repeat the same procedure to complete the block (Fig. 9-12).

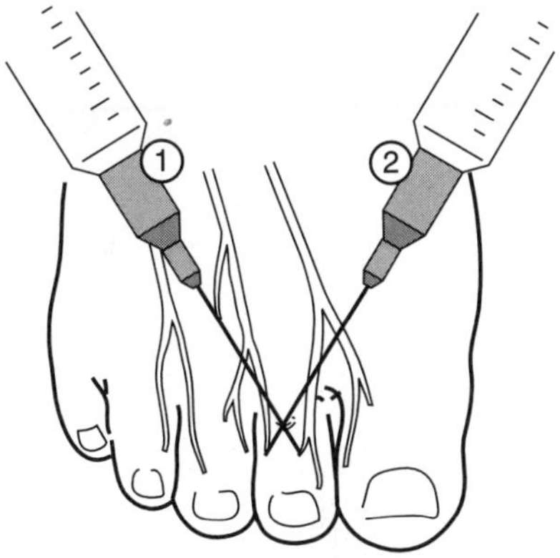

FIG. 9-13. Digital nerve block of toe.

Procedure—digital nerve block of the first toe

1. Follow the basic nerve block procedure described previously, using 1% lidocaine *without* epinephrine. Make sure to prepare the skin, and always aspirate before injection, as instructed previously.
2. Digital block of the first toe requires a circumferential ring of anesthetic. The technique is similar to the digital block of the finger, except a line of anesthetic is deposited on the plantar side of the toe in addition to the other sides (Fig. 9-14).
3. Insert a 25- to 27-gauge, 1-inch needle dorsally into the skin at the base of the first toe, just medial to the proximal phalynx.
4. Advance the needle perpendicularly toward the plantar surface. Inject approximately 1 to 2 ml of anesthetic as the needle is withdrawn.
5. Without removing the needle from the skin, redirect the needle across the dorsal surface of the digit and inject anesthetic along the back of the great toe.
6. Then insert the needle on the lateral side of the great toe, through the anesthetized skin, and again advance the needle perpendicularly toward the plantar surface.
7. Inject approximately 1 to 2 ml of anesthetic as the needle is withdrawn.
8. Then insert the needle into the medial side of the base of the great toe, under the anesthetized plantar skin.
9. Advance the needle in a medial-to-lateral direction. Inject approximately 1 to 2 ml of anesthetic to complete the circumferential digital block of the great toe (Fig. 9-14).

Wrist Block

The wrist block is a combination of the *median, ulnar,* and *radial nerve blocks* discussed as follows. It is used to achieve complete anesthesia of the hand.

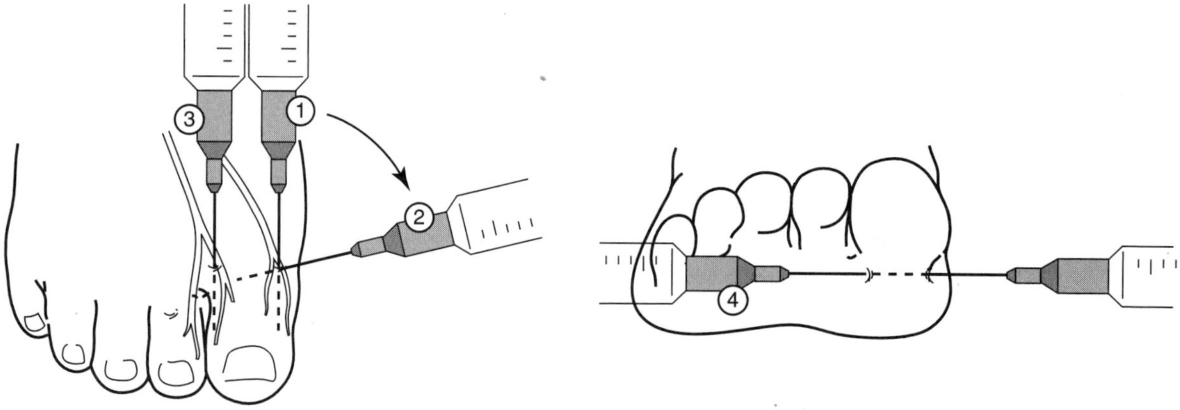

FIG. 9-14. Ring block of great toe. Requires three needlesticks but provides excellent anesthesia of an otherwise difficult-to-anesthetize area.

Median Nerve Block

Anatomy

- The median nerve supplies sensation to parts of the palm, thumb, and index and middle fingers, as shown in Fig. 9-15. It runs between the palmaris longus and the flexor carpi radialis tendons beneath the flexor retinaculum in the wrist (Fig. 9-16).

Procedure

1. Follow the basic nerve block procedure described previously, using 1% lidocaine *without* epinephrine. Make sure to prepare the skin, and always aspirate before injection, as instructed previously.
2. Locate the palmaris longus and flexor carpi radialis tendons by having the patient make a fist and flex the wrist against resistance. The point of insertion is between these two tendons (just radial to the palmaris longus tendon), at the proximal wrist crease (Fig. 9-17).
3. Insert a 25- to 27-gauge, 0.5-inch needle perpendicular to the skin. Advance the needle approximately 0.5 cm. A "pop" may be felt as the needle goes through the flexor retinaculum.
4. The patient may feel paresthesias, signifying mechanical stimulation of the nerve by the needle. If this occurs, withdraw the needle 1 to 2 mm to avoid intraneural injection. Note that, with young children, it may be difficult to distinguish the pain of the needlestick from paresthesias.
5. Parasthesias indicate close proximity to the nerve. If parasthesias are elicited, inject approximately 2 to 3 ml of local anesthetic. If parasthesias are not elicited, inject approximately 3 to 5 ml of local anesthetic.

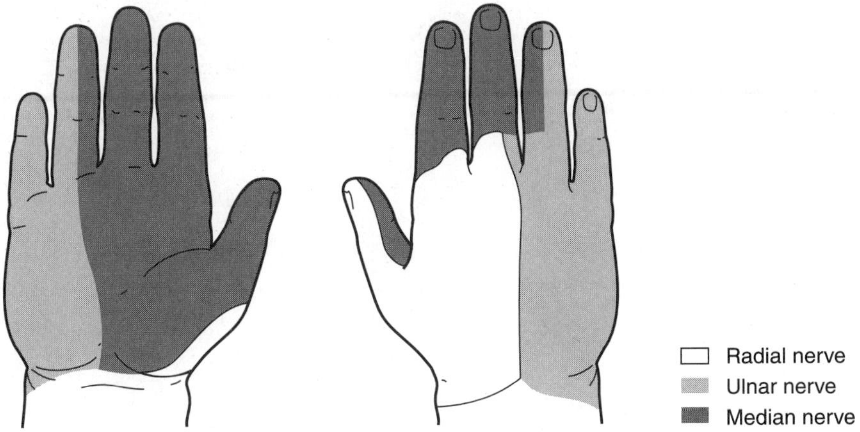

FIG. 9-15. Sensory distribution of the radial, ulnar, and median nerves.

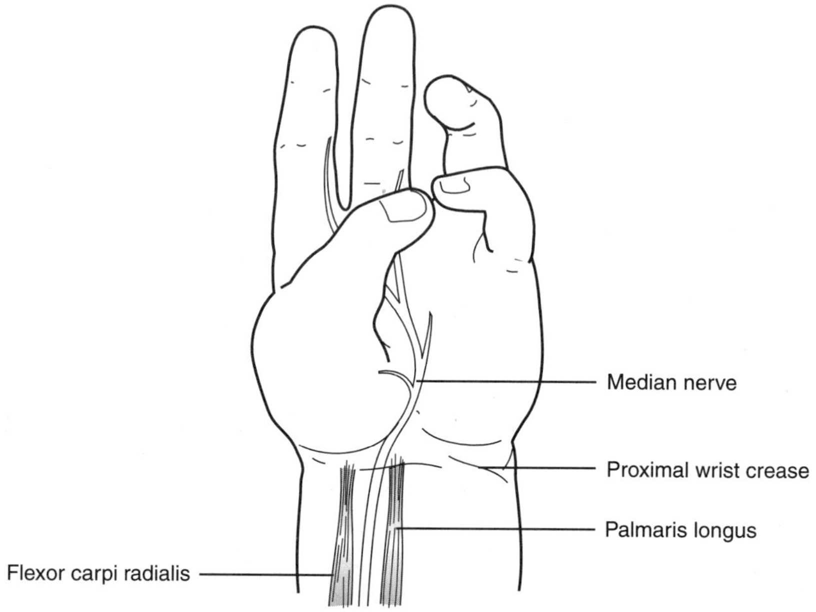

FIG. 9-16. Anatomy of the wrist, illustrating the location of the median nerve between the flexor carpi radialis and palmaris longus tendons.

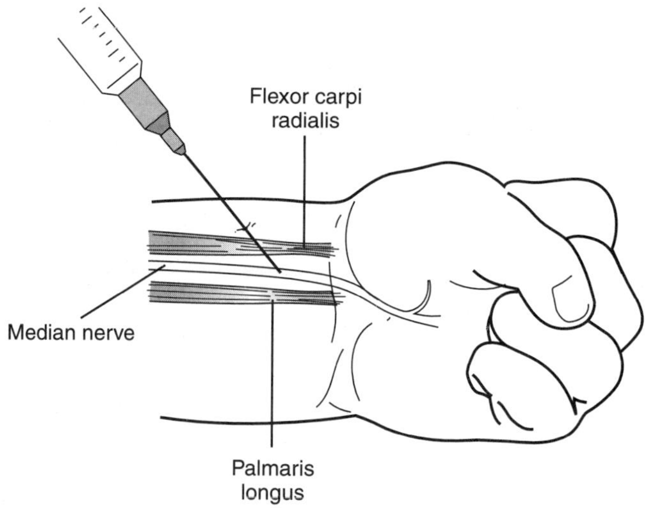

FIG. 9-17. Illustration of the insertion point for the median nerve block at the wrist.

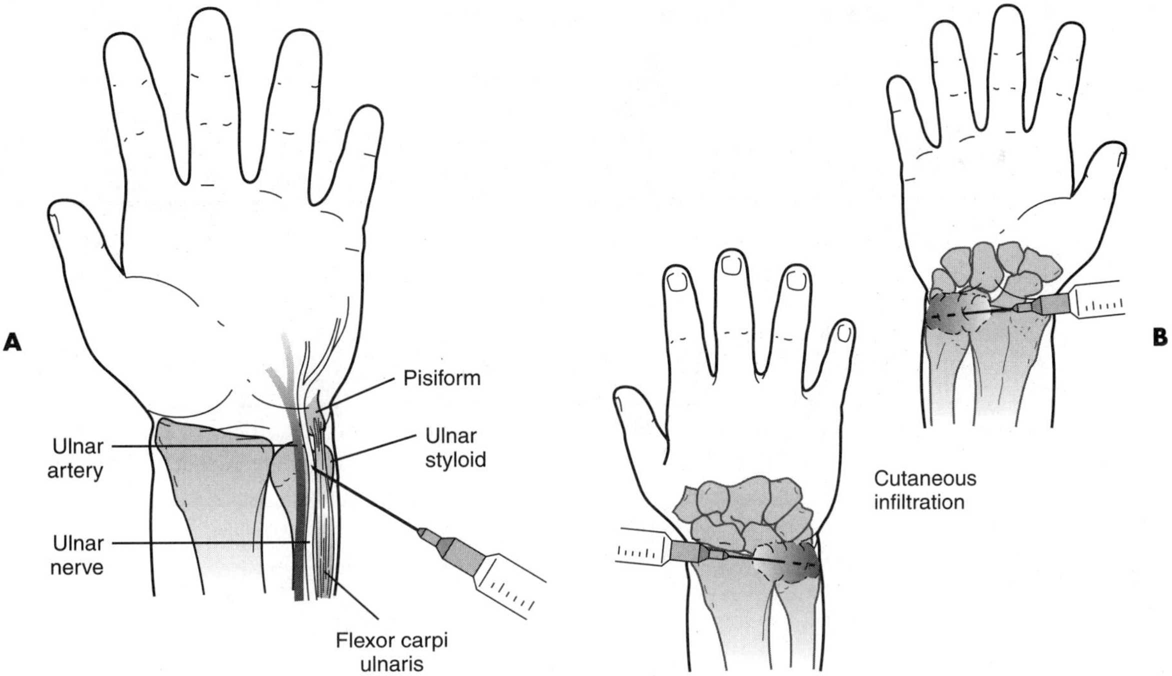

FIG. 9-18. A, Anatomy of the wrist, illustrating the location of the ulnar nerve between the flexor carpi ulnaris and the ulnar artery, with an insertion point at the level of the ulnar styloid. **B,** Illustration of wheal infiltration for ulnar nerve block at the wrist.

Ulnar Nerve Block

Anatomy

- The ulnar nerve supplies sensation to the ulnar side of the hand, as shown in Fig. 9-15.
- At the elbow, the ulnar nerve runs between the olecrenon and the medial epicondyle.
- At the wrist, the ulnar nerve runs beneath the flexor retinaculum, just radial to the flexor carpi ulnaris tendon, in close proximity to the ulnar artery (Fig. 9-18, *A*); however, approximately 5 cm proximal to the wrist, the ulnar nerve gives off a palmar branch that crosses the wrist superficial to the flexor retinaculum and a dorsal cutaneous branch that runs superficially on the dorsal aspect of the wrist.
- In order to perform a complete ulnar block at the wrist, anesthetic must be deposited deep to the flexor retinaculum, near the ulnar artery, as well as superficially on the ventral and dorsal aspects of the ulnar wrist.
- Therefore it is safer and easier to perform the ulnar nerve block at the elbow, rather than the wrist.

Procedure—ulnar nerve block at the wrist

1. Follow the basic nerve block procedure described previously, using 1% lidocaine *without* epinephrine. Make sure to prepare the skin, and always aspirate before injection, as instructed previously.
2. Raise a skin wheal of anesthetic from the ventral aspect of the wrist, at the ulnar styloid, around to the dorsal aspect, as shown in Fig. 9-19, *B*.
3. Locate the flexor carpi ulnaris tendon by having the patient make a fist and flex the wrist against resistance, and feeling for the tendon's insertion on the pisiform bone over the ulnar styloid.
4. Insert a 25- to 27-gauge, 0.5-inch needle perpendicular to the skin just radial to the flexor carpi ulnaris tendon, at the proximal wrist crease.
5. Advance the needle approximately 0.5 cm. A "pop" may be felt as the needle goes through the flexor retinaculum.
6. The patient may feel paresthesias, signifying mechanical stimulation of the nerve by the needle. If this occurs, withdraw the needle 1 to 2 mm to avoid intraneural injection. Note that, with young children, it may be difficult to distinguish the pain of the needlestick from paresthesias.
7. Parasthesias indicate close proximity to the nerve. If parasthesias are elicited, inject approximately 2 to 3 ml of local anesthetic. If parasthesias are not elicited, inject approximately 3 to 5 ml of local anesthetic.

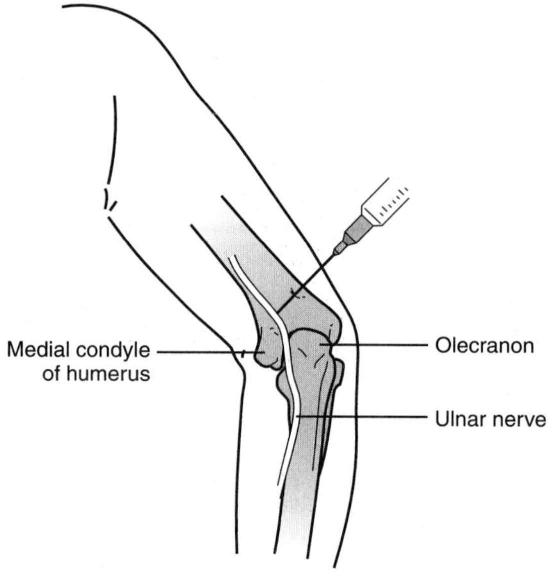

FIG. 9-19. Anatomy of the elbow, illustrating the location of the ulnar nerve and insertion point into the groove between the olecranon and the medial epicondyle of the elbow.

Procedure—ulnar nerve block at the elbow

1. Follow the basic nerve block procedure described previously, using 1% lidocaine *without* epinephrine. Make sure to prepare the skin, and always aspirate before injection, as instructed previously.
2. Palpate the ulnar nerve in the groove between the olecranon and the medial epicondyle of the elbow.
3. Flex the elbow to 90 degrees.
4. Injecting proximal to the groove reduces the risk of nerve injury, so the point of insertion is 1 to 2 cm distal and parallel to the ulnar nerve as it runs through the groove (Fig. 9-19).
5. Insert a 25-gauge, 0.5-inch needle perpendicular to the skin. Advance the needle approximately 0.5 cm.
6. The patient may feel paresthesias, signifying mechanical stimulation of the nerve by the needle. If this occurs, withdraw the needle 1 to 2 mm to avoid intraneural injection. Note that, with young children, it may be difficult to distinguish the pain of the needlestick from paresthesias.
7. Parasthesias indicate close proximity to the nerve. If parasthesias are elicited, inject approximately 2 to 3 ml of local anesthetic. If parasthesias are not elicited, inject approximately 3 to 5 ml of local anesthetic.

Radial Nerve Block

Anatomy

- The radial nerve supplies sensation to parts of the hand, thumb, and index and middle fingers, as shown in Fig. 9-15.
- The radial nerve splits into several peripheral branches proximal to the wrist. One of the major branches runs just radial to the flexor carpi radialis tendon, near the radial artery. The other branches run cutaneously around the dorsal and ventral aspects of the radial side of the wrist.

Procedure

1. Follow the basic nerve block procedure described previously, using 1% lidocaine *without* epinephrine. Make sure to prepare the skin, and always aspirate before injection, as instructed previously.
2. Locate the flexor carpi radialis tendon by having the patient make a fist and flex the wrist against resistance.
3. Deposit a line of local anesthetic subcutaneously at the level of the proximal wrist crease, superficial to the flexor carpi radialis (Fig. 9-20, *A*).
4. Extend this line from the ventral aspect of the wrist, around the radial styloid, to the dorsal aspect of the wrist, into the "snuff box," as shown in Fig. 9-20, *B*.
5. This may require as much as 8 ml of total anesthetic. If more than one needlestick is needed, it is best to inject through anesthetized skin whenever possible.
6. Locate the radial artery.
7. Insert a 25- to 27-gauge, 0.5-inch needle perpendicular to the skin just radial to the radial artery, at the level of the proximal wrist crease (Fig. 9-20).

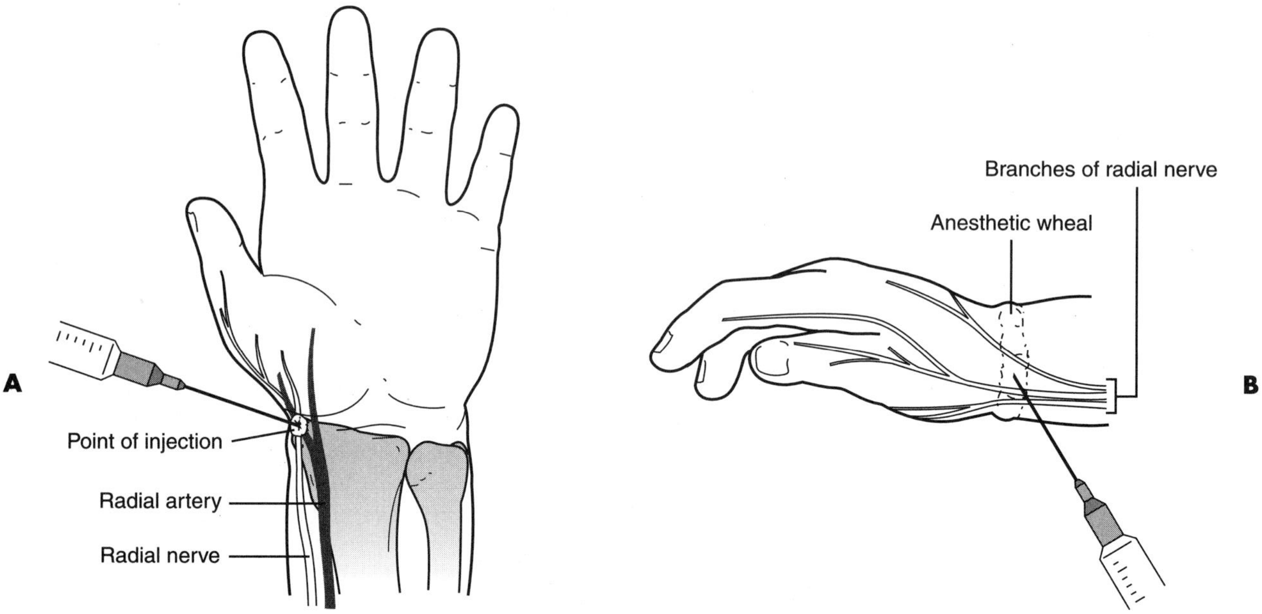

FIG. 9-20. A, Anatomy of the wrist, indicating the location of the radial nerve and artery at the level of the wrist. **B,** Illustration of wheal infiltration for radial nerve block at the wrist.

8. Advance the needle approximately 0.5 cm.
9. The patient may feel paresthesias, signifying mechanical stimulation of the nerve by the needle. If this occurs, withdraw the needle 1 to 2 mm to avoid intraneural injection. Note that, with young children, it may be difficult to distinguish the pain of the needlestick from paresthesias.
10. Parasthesias indicate close proximity to the nerve. If parasthesias are elicited, inject approximately 2 to 3 ml of local anesthetic. If parasthesias are not elicited, inject approximately 3 to 5 ml of local anesthetic.

Ankle Block

Anatomy

- The posterior tibial, sural, deep peroneal, superficial peroneal, and saphenous nerves supply sensation to the foot, as shown in Fig. 9-21.
- A true ankle block involves regional nerve blocks of all of these nerves.
- Posterior tibial nerve blocks and sural nerve blocks are the most commonly used lower extremity blocks. Together, they are called a *posterior ankle block*. They are used because the posterior tibial and sural nerves supply sensation to the sole of the foot. This area can be painful to infiltrate with local anesthesia because of dense innervation. It can also be difficult to infiltrate because of highly septated subcutaneous tissue. For these reasons, regional nerve blocks are recommended over local infiltration.

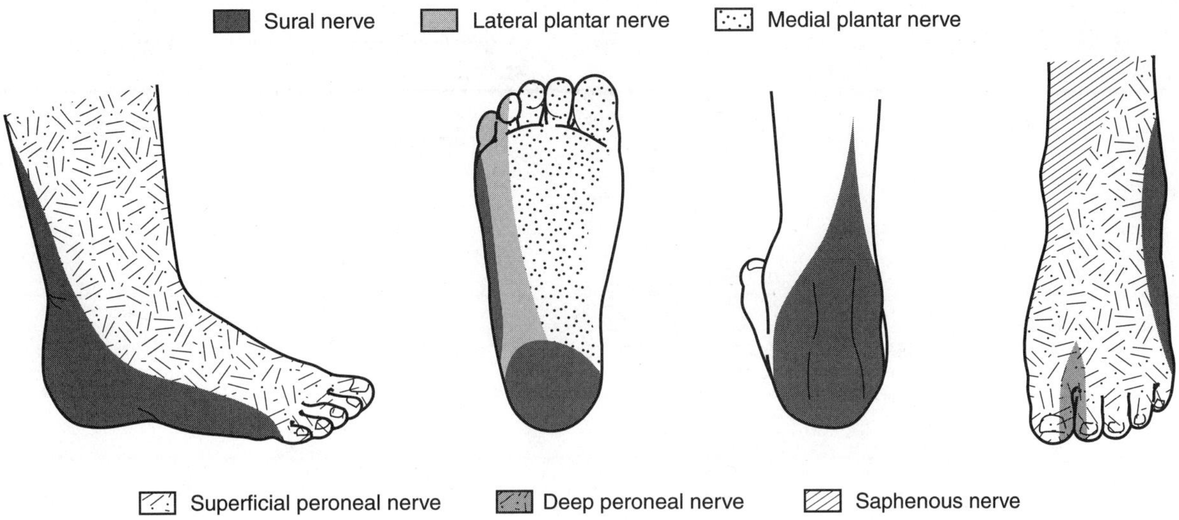

FIG. 9-21. Sensory innervation of the foot. The posterior tibial nerve branches to become the medial and lateral plantar branches.

- The saphenous and superficial peroneal nerves supply sensation to the dorsal aspect of the foot, as shown in Fig. 9-21. These areas are easily and effectively infiltrated with local anesthetic. Therefore local infiltration is used more commonly than nerve blocks.

Posterior Tibial Nerve Block

Anatomy

- The posterior tibial nerve supplies sensation to the foot, as shown in Fig. 9-21.
- At the ankle, the posterior tibial nerve runs behind the medial malleolus, between the posterior tibial artery and the Achilles tendon.

Procedure

1. Follow the basic nerve block procedure described previously, using 1% lidocaine *without* epinephrine. Make sure to prepare the skin, and always aspirate before injection, as instructed previously.
2. Place the patient in a prone position, with the foot partially dorsiflexed and extended off the end of the stretcher.
3. Palpate the posterior tibial artery behind the medial malleolus.
4. Insert a 25-gauge, 1.0- to 1.5-inch needle perpendicular to the skin, just posterior to the artery (Fig. 9-22).
5. Advance the needle until it rests approximately 1 mm superficial to the tibia.

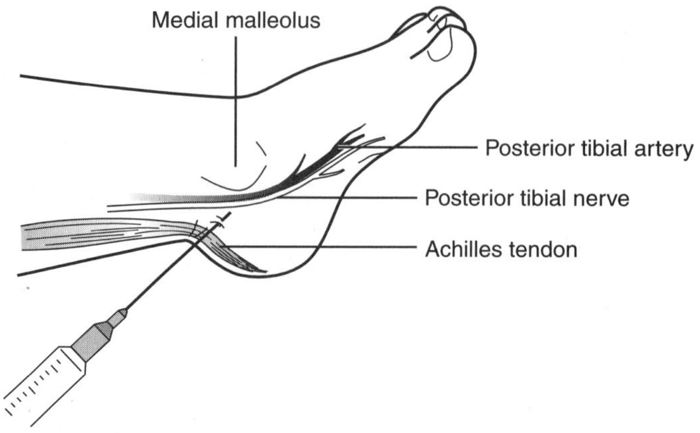

FIG. 9-22. Anatomy of the ankle, illustrating the location for the posterior tibial nerve and insertion point behind the medial malleolus, between the posterior tibial artery and the Achilles tendon.

6. The patient may feel paresthesias, signifying mechanical stimulation of the nerve by the needle. If this occurs, withdraw the needle 1 to 2 mm to avoid intraneural injection. Note that, with young children, it may be difficult to distinguish the pain of the needlestick from paresthesias.
7. Parasthesias indicate close proximity to the nerve. If parasthesias are elicited, inject approximately 5 ml of local anesthetic. If parasthesias are not elicited, inject approximately 10 ml of local anesthetic.

Sural Nerve Block

Anatomy

- The sural nerve supplies sensation to the foot, as shown in Fig. 9-21.
- At the ankle, the sural nerve runs behind the lateral malleolus, between the lateral malleolus and the Achilles tendon.

Procedure

1. Follow the basic nerve block procedure described previously, using 1% lidocaine *without* epinephrine. Make sure to prepare the skin, and always aspirate before injection, as instructed previously.
2. Place the patient in a prone position, with the foot partially dorsiflexed and extended off the end of the stretcher.
3. Insert a 25- to 27-gauge, 1.0- to 1.5-inch needle, perpendicular to the skin, just lateral to the Achilles tendon, approximately 1 cm above the level of the lateral malleolus (Fig. 9-23).
4. Advance the needle in the subcutaneous space toward the lateral malleolus, until the needle strikes the malleolus.
5. Inject the anesthetic as the needle is slowly withdrawn.

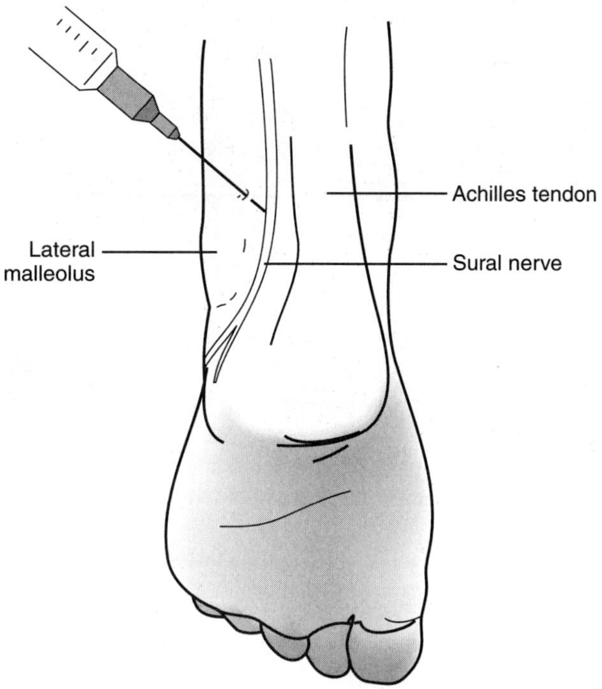

FIG. 9-23. Anatomy of the ankle, illustrating the location for the sural nerve and insertion point behind the lateral malleolus, between the lateral malleolus and the Achilles tendon.

6. The patient may feel paresthesias, signifying mechanical stimulation of the nerve by the needle. If this occurs, withdraw the needle 1 to 2 mm more, to avoid intraneural injection. Note that, with young children, it may be difficult to distinguish the pain of the needlestick from paresthesias.
7. Parasthesias indicate close proximity to the nerve. If parasthesias are elicited, inject approximately 5 ml of local anesthetic. If no parasthesias are elicited, inject approximately 10 ml total of local anesthetic into the space between the lateral malleolus and the Achilles tendon.

Deep Peroneal Nerve Block

Anatomy

- The deep peroneal nerve supplies sensation to the foot, as shown in Fig. 9-21.
- At the ankle, the deep peroneal nerve runs through the dorsum of the foot deep to the hallicus longus tendon.

Procedure

1. Follow the basic nerve block procedure described previously, using 1% lidocaine *without* epinephrine. Make sure to prepare the skin, and always aspirate before injection, as instructed previously.

2. Place the patient in a supine position.
3. Identify the hallicus longus tendon by having the patient dorsiflex the big toe.
4. The needle insertion point is on the dorsum of the ankle, approximately 1 cm above the level of the malleoli, just medial to the hallicus longus tendon.
5. Raise a superficial skin wheal of anesthetic at this spot.
6. Insert a 25- to 27-gauge, 1.0- to 1.5-inch needle, perpendicular to the skin (Fig. 9-24).
7. Direct the needle at a 30-degree angle laterally, aiming beneath the hallicus longus tendon.
8. Advance the needle approximately 1 cm, until it reaches the tibia.
9. Inject the anesthetic as the needle is slowly withdrawn.

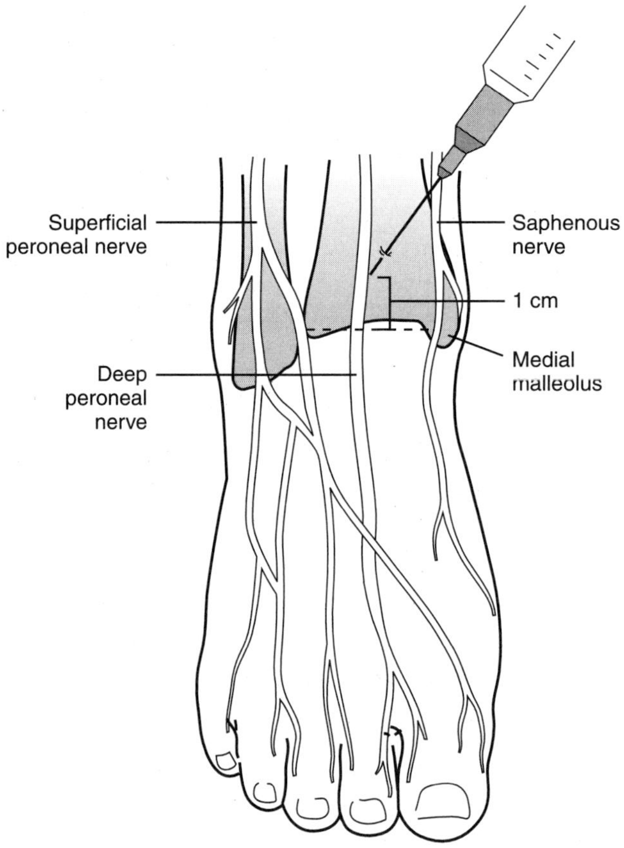

FIG. 9-24. Anatomy of the ankle, illustrating the locations of the saphenous, deep peroneal, and superficial peroneal nerves.

10. The patient may feel paresthesias, signifying mechanical stimulation of the nerve by the needle. If this occurs, withdraw the needle 1 to 2 mm more, to avoid intraneural injection. Note that, with young children, it may be difficult to distinguish the pain of the needlestick from paresthesias.
11. Parasthesias indicate close proximity to the nerve. If parasthesias are elicited, inject approximately 2 to 3 ml of local anesthetic. If no parasthesias are elicited, inject approximately 3 to 5 ml total of local anesthetic into the space between the lateral malleolus and the Achilles tendon.

Superficial Peroneal and Saphenous Nerve Blocks

Anatomy

- The superficial peroneal and saphenous nerves supply sensation to the foot, as shown in Fig. 9-21.
- At the ankle, the superficial peroneal nerve runs in the subcutaneous space along the dorsum of the foot. The saphenous nerve runs in the subcutaneous space along the dorsal medial aspect of the ankle.

Procedure

1. Follow the basic nerve block procedure described previously, using 1% lidocaine *without* epinephrine. Make sure to prepare the skin, and always aspirate before injection, as instructed previously.
2. Place the patient in a supine position.
3. Identify the hallicus longus tendon by having the patient dorsiflex the big toe.
4. Use a 25- to 27-gauge, 1-inch needle to infiltrate a line of subcutaneous anesthetic from the hallicus longus to the lateral malleolus. This blocks the superficial peroneal nerve and may require 5 to 10 ml of local anesthetic.
5. Without withdrawing the needle, redirect and extend the line from the hallicus longus medially to the medial malleolus. Another 5 to 10 ml is deposited to block the saphenous nerve.
6. The patient may feel paresthesias, signifying mechanical stimulation of the nerve by the needle. If this occurs, withdraw the needle 1 to 2 mm more, to avoid intraneural injection. Note that, with young children, it may be difficult to distinguish the pain of the needlestick from paresthesias.

AFTERCARE INSTRUCTIONS

- Keep the affected area clean and dry.
- The anesthetized area may look blanched and be numb for several minutes to hours after the procedure, but this is normal.
- Avoid exposure to extreme heat or cold or any possible trauma to the affected areas because the child will not regain full sensation for several minutes to hours, depending on the agent used.
- Complications from properly administered local and regional anesthesia are extremely rare, but they can happen.

- Return to your doctor or go to the emergency room if the child develops any of the following:
  - Weakness, numbness, or tingling in the affected areas
  - Redness, swelling, or drainage from the affected areas
  - Red streaks from the affected areas
  - Fevers, chills, nausea, vomiting, or swollen glands
  - Metallic taste in the mouth, agitation, tremors, or seizures

MODIFICATIONS FOR SITUATIONS OF LIMITED RESOURCES OR KNOWN SENSITIVITY TO LOCAL ANESTHETICS

- Ice is perhaps the cheapest and most effective anesthetic.
- Allergies to local anesthetics are rare. Patients can have allergic reactions to esters, but allergic reactions to amides are almost nonexistent. When sensitivity occurs, it is usually attributable to the preservative used in most multidose commercial preparations. Single-dose preparations do not contain this preservative; therefore single-dose vials should be used whenever possible. See the Selection of Anesthetic Agent section for further discussion.
- If a true drug allergy exists, or if no local anesthetic is available, several alternatives may be used.
  - A cooling agent such as ethyl chloride or ice may be applied topically.
  - Use normal saline in place of anesthetic.
  - Use diphenhydramine in place of local anesthetic. To obtain the appropriate concentration, mix 1 ml of 50 mg/ml diphenhydramine with 4 ml of normal saline.

CHAPTER 10

Surgical Procedures

Andrew K. McVie
Steven J. White

WOUND CLOSURE

Background

- Traumatic lacerations account for a large number of pediatric emergency department and urgent care visits.
- Physicians caring for these children must consider cosmetic results, pain, time, expense, complications, and follow-up associated with different wound closure techniques.

Indications

- Hemostasis
- Improve the cosmetic appearance of a wound
- Facilitate wound healing
- Reduce the chance of wound infection

Contraindications

- Deep puncture wounds
- Heavily contaminated wounds or wounds unable to be thoroughly cleaned
- Wounds beyond 24 hours after injury
- Bite (human, dog, cat)*

Wound Preparation

- Wound care should always precede laceration closure.
- Proper wound care includes a focused history and physical examination.

*Often, the location of these wounds demands closure for cosmetic reasons. Consultation with a specialist is sometimes required. The high rates of infection associated with these injuries mandate antibiotics and close follow-up.

- History should include indicators of past wound healing, bleeding, and potential for infection, along with documentation of tetanus status.
- A careful physical examination includes a detailed neurovascular exam (before anesthesia), adequate anesthesia, and a thorough wound exploration for identification of damage to underlying vessels, tendons, nerves, and muscles, and removal of foreign bodies if identified.
- The wound should undergo copious irrigation before closure and debridement of devitalized tissue as indicated.
- Wound irrigation technique deserves special mention as it can significantly reduce the chance of wound infection. "The solution to pollution is dilution."
- High-pressure irrigation can be accomplished by using a pulsatile high-pressure flow system such as that attained by using water-pik-type devices or a syringe-pressure irrigation system using a 20-ml syringe and 18-gauge intravenous catheter. A good rule of thumb for irrigation volume is to use 50 ml of irrigant (sterile water or saline) per centimeter of laceration per number of hours elapsed since original injury.
- Once the wound has been properly prepared, closure may be accomplished by using sutures, staples, tissue adhesive, or wound-closure tape.

METHOD 1: SUTURING

Background

- Suturing remains the time-honored method of primary wound closure.

Indications

- Complex laceration requiring meticulous closure
- High-tension wound, particularly over a joint
- Deep wounds requiring multilayer closure

Contraindications

- A history of significant keloid scarring should prompt consideration of alternate closure methods or specialist referral because sutures incite the greatest tissue reactivity.

Suturing Materials

- Sutures can be classified as absorbable versus nonabsorbable, and natural versus synthetic.
- For cutaneous closure of traumatic lacerations, synthetic monofilament sutures are generally preferred (Table 10-1).
- Suture needles are composed of an eye, a body, and a point (Fig. 10-1).

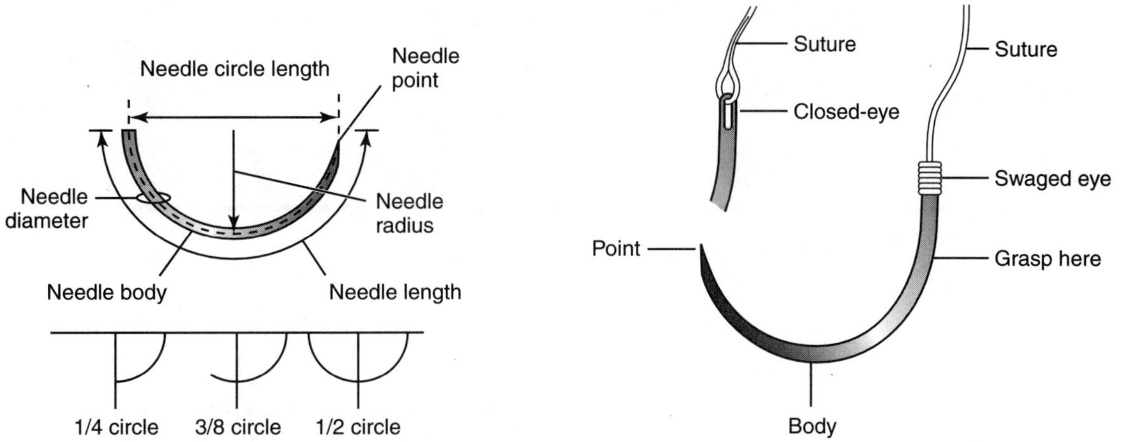

FIG. 10-1. Anatomy of a surgical needle.

TABLE 10-1
Recommendations for suture by location

Location	Suture material	Suture removal
Scalp	Deep sutures: Generally not indicated	
	Superficial sutures: 3-0 to 5-0 synthetic, nonabsorbable (nylon, ethylon, prolene)	5-10 days
Face	Deep sutures: 5-0 or 6-0 synthetic, absorbable (dexon, vicryl)	
	Superficial sutures: 6-0 synthetic nonabsorbable or 6-0 fast-absorbing gut	3-5 days
Oral cavity	Deep sutures: Generally not indicated	
	Superficial sutures: 4-0 or 5-0 synthetic, absorbable	
Extremity	Deep sutures: 3-0 or 4-0 synthetic, absorbable	
Trunk/Back	Superficial sutures: 4-0 or 5-0 synthetic, nonabsorbable	7-10 days 10-14 days if sutures cross a joint
Hand/Foot	Deep sutures: Generally not indicated	
	Superficial sutures: 4-0 or 5-0 synthetic nonabsorbable	7-10 days 10-14 days if sutures cross a joint

- The eye of the needle attaches to the suture. Closed and French-eyed needles require threading of the suture. In general, only swaggered-eye needles, in which the needle is molded around the suture, are available in most acute care settings.
- The body of a needle has varying degrees of curvature to facilitate the passage of the needle through tissue (Fig. 10-2).

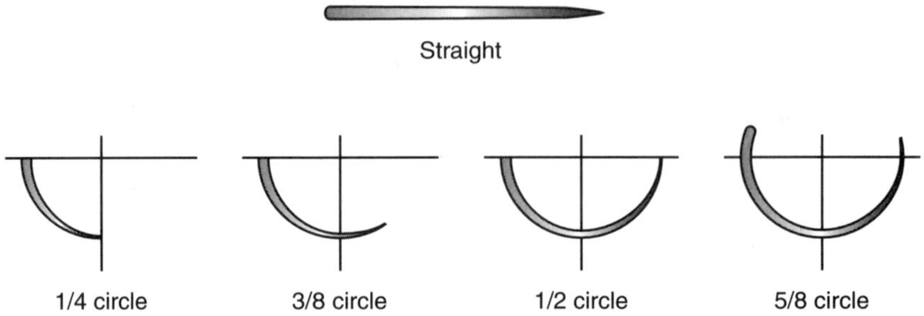

FIG. 10-2. Needle body shapes.

- The point of a cutting needle assists the easy passage of the needle through tough skin. The cutting edge of a conventional cutting needle is along the inner surface of the curvature. The cutting edge of a reverse-cutting needle is along the outer surface of the curvature. A reverse-cutting needle minimizes trauma to the inner path of the suture, thus reducing the incidence of the suture pulling through the wound.
- Tapered-point needles reduce tissue trauma and are useful for piercing low-tension tissue. Tapered-point needles are used in bowel anastamosis.
- Blunt-point needles are used for repair of parenchymal tissue such as liver and kidney (Fig. 10-3).
- In general, reverse-cutting, three-eighths-inch, swaggered-eyed needles are appropriate for most cutaneous closures. Pictures on the suture package may aid in the selection of the appropriate needle.

Contents of a Standard Suture Tray

- ABS towels
- Adson, serrated, 4.75″
- Cotton-tipped applicators, 6″
- Fenestrated drape
- Gauze sponges, 4 × 4″, 2 × 2″
- Iris scissors, straight, 4.5″
- Mosquito, curved, 5″
- Needles: 27-gauge × 1.25″, 25-gauge × 5/8″, 18-gauge × 1.5″
- Syringe, 10 ml
- Webster needle holder, 6″
- Medicine cups, 2 oz.

Types of Suture Material

Absorbable

Absorbable natural

- Collagen strands derived from serosa of beef intestine or submucosa of sheep intestine. Digested by proteolytic enzymes.

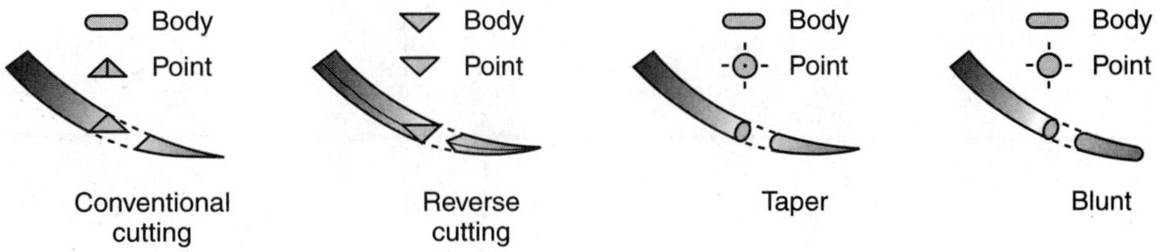

FIG. 10-3. Needle points.

- Plain gut
- Fast-absorbing gut: Plain gut heat-treated to accelerate absorption
- Chromic gut: Plain gut treated with chromic salt solution to resist proteolytic enzymes

Absorbable synthetic
- Synthetic polymers developed for more predictable rates of absorption and less tissue reaction
- Polyglycolic acid (Dexon)
- Polygalactin 910 (Vicryl)

Nonabsorbable

Nonabsorbable natural
- Silk: Historically associated with higher rates of reactivity and infection
- Metal: Stainless steel used in orthopedic and neurosurgical procedures

Nonabsorbable synthetic
- Nylon: Low tissue reactivity, commonly used in cutaneous procedures
- Polyester: Used in vessel anastamosis
- Polypropylene (e.g., Prolene): Used in cutaneous closures

Suturing Technique

- Although each wound requires an individualized approach, several fundamental goals should guide every closure.
- Acceptable methods for suturing commonly encountered wounds are depicted in Figs. 10-4 through 10-9 and include the following:
  — Skin edge eversion.
  — Skin/superficial sutures should achieve "approximation without strangulation."
  — Minimize tension on skin wound edges.
  — Minimize number of sutures.
  — Deep sutures aid greatly in minimizing tension on skin sutures.

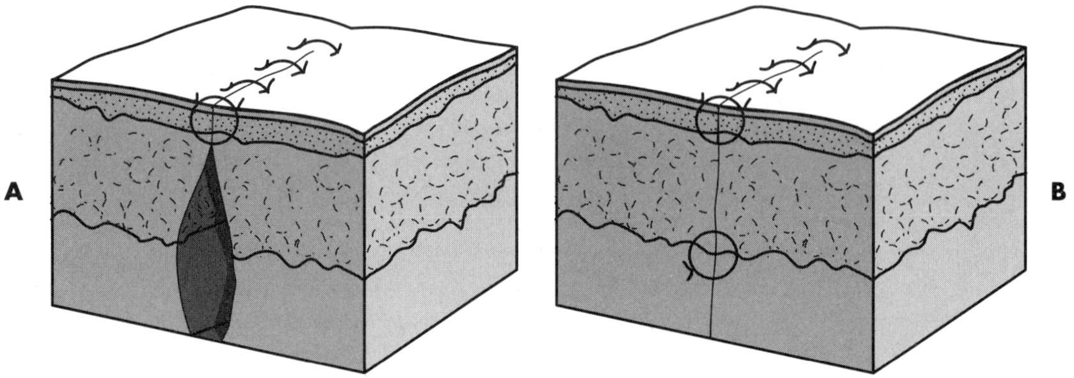

FIG. 10-4. A, Improper and **B,** proper wound closure.

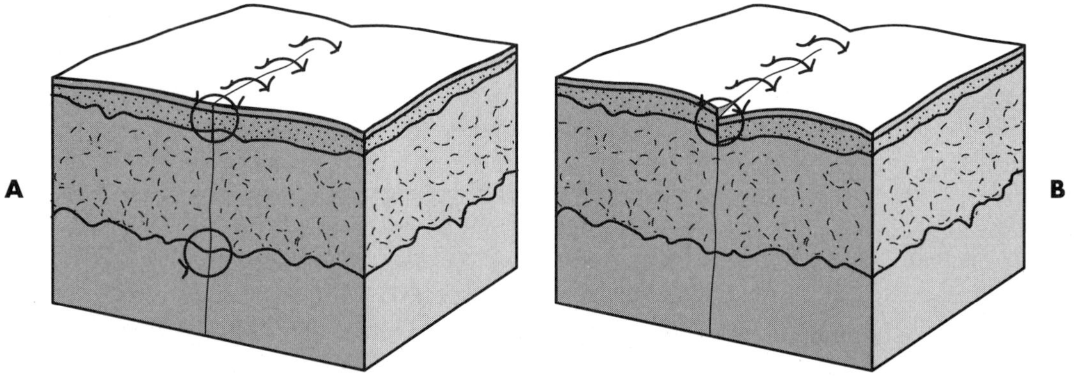

FIG. 10-5. A, Proper tissue apposition and **B,** improper tissue apposition and inappropriate excess tightness.

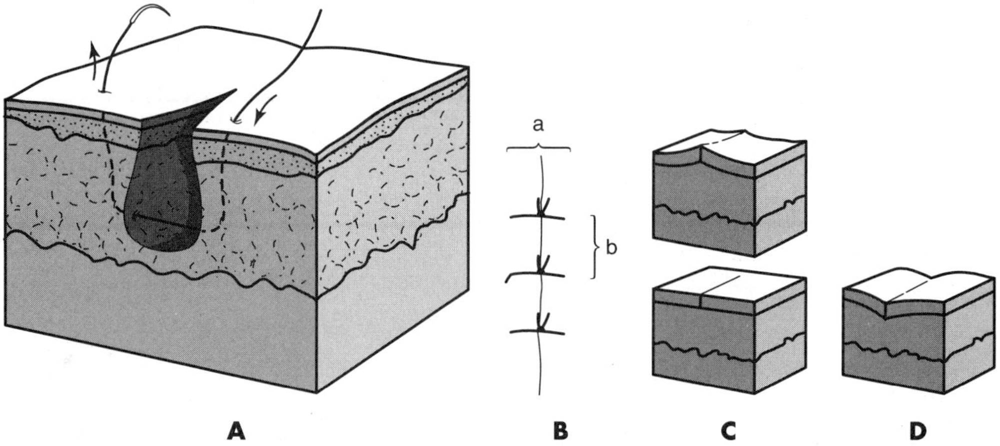

FIG. 10-6. Simple, interrupted dermal suture. **A,** Proper depth; **B,** Proper spacing (a = b); **C,** Proper final appearance (everted or flat); **D,** Improper final appearance (inverted).

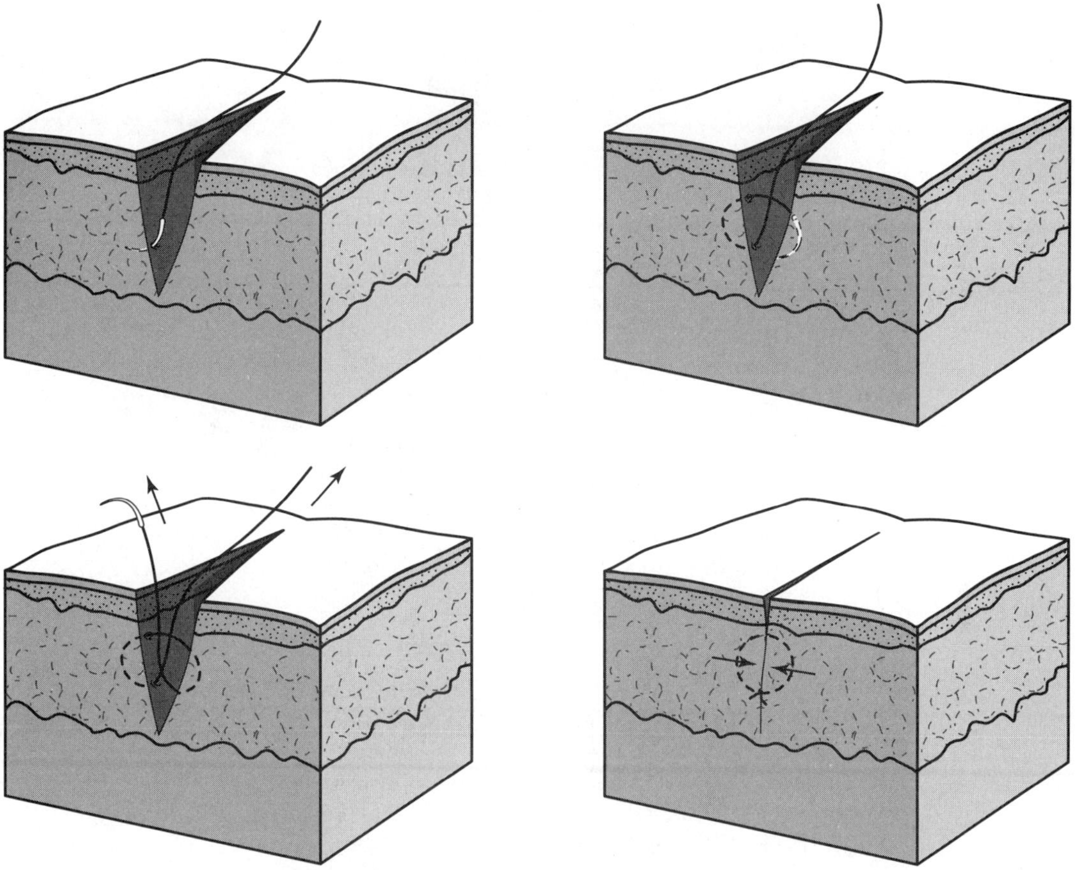

FIG. 10-7. Simple, interrupted inverted knot suture.

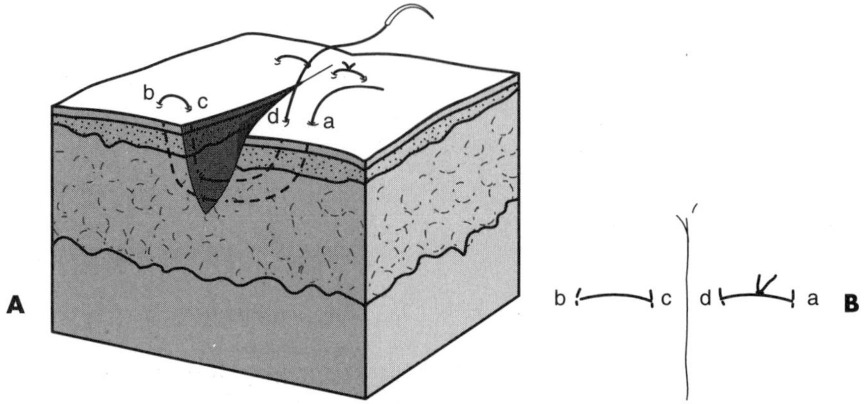

FIG. 10-8. Vertical mattress suture. **A,** Cross section; **B** Overhead view. Begin at *a* and go under skin to *b.* Come out, go in at *c,* and exit at *d.*

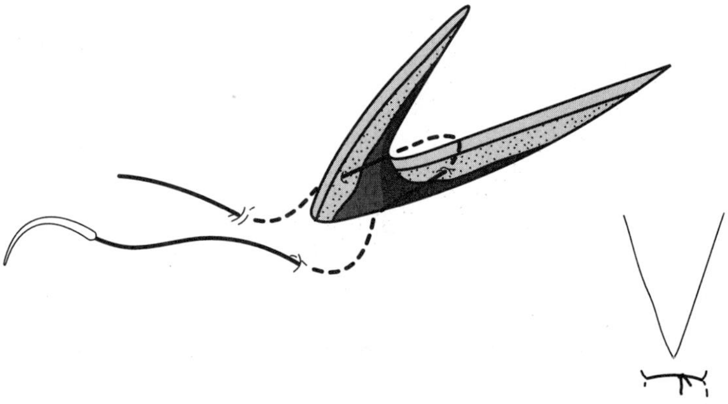

FIG. 10-9. Three-point or half-buried mattress incision, also known as the "corner stitch."

Discharge Instructions

- Keep the wound clean and dry.
- Wash the wound gently with antibacterial soap and pat dry.
- Apply antibiotic ointment to the wound twice per day.
- Cover wound with a nonadherent dressing for the first 24 hours.
- Return as instructed for suture removal.
- Return for signs or symptoms of infection, such as fever, redness of the wound, drainage from the wound, increasing pain at the site of injury, or increased swelling at the site of infection.

METHOD 2: STAPLES

Background

- Staples offer an alternative to sutures for superficial, linear tissue approximation on the scalp, trunk, and upper and lower extremities.
- Deep sutures are sometimes required for wound closure before cutaneous closure with staples.
- Staples are unacceptable for closure of wounds on the face, neck, hands, or feet.
- Ideally, an assistant everts the skin edges with forceps before staple placement.

Indications

- Simple linear lacerations requiring superficial closure

Advantages

- Less tissue reactivity than sutures
- Less costly than sutures
- Shorter application time compared with sutures

Contraindications

- Lacerations of the face, neck, hands, and feet
- Need for subsequent computed tomography (CT) or magnetic resonance imaging (MRI) scan. Metal staples interfere with both CT and MRI.

Equipment

- Forceps, two pairs
- Stapler
- Staple removal or suture kit (kits contain items useful for removing misplaced staples)

Procedure

1. After appropriate wound care, have an assistant evert the wound edges with forceps.
2. Hold the stapler in contact with the skin.
3. Squeeze the lever, dispensing a staple.
4. Center the staples on the laceration. Staples should not be flush with the skin, but instead should have several millimeters between the staple bar and the skin.

Discharge Instructions

- Discharge instructions are identical to instructions for sutured wounds.
- The interval before staple removal is based on the location of the wound and is identical to the recommended interval for suture removal.

METHOD 3: TISSUE ADHESIVE

Background

- Tissue adhesives (octylcyanoacrylate, N-2-butylcyanoacrylate) have been heralded as alternatives to sutures for repair of small, superficial lacerations under minimal tensile stress.
- The liquid monomer cyanoacrylates polymerize when exposed to the basic environment provided by skin and tissue moisture.
- The polymerization reaction is exothermic. Patients may complain of a burning sensation in an inadequately dried wound as a result of excess polymerization.

Indications

- Superficial linear laceration with minimal skin tension

Advantages

- Less tissue reactivity than sutures or staples
- Shorter application time compared with sutures or staples
- Anesthesia not required for adhesive application, however, may be necessary for proper wound irrigation and exploration
- Follow-up for removal unnecessary

Disadvantages

- The adhesive material is significantly more expensive than suture material.

Contraindications

- High-tension wounds, particularly wounds across joints
- Excessively moist areas such as the axilla or groin
- Mucous membranes or wounds close to the eye

Equipment

- Forceps (special forceps are often sold with the tissue adhesive)
- Tissue adhesive

Procedure

1. After appropriate wound care, pat skin dry. (Proper hemostasis ensures that the skin remains dry during adhesive application.)
2. Break the ampule, allowing tissue adhesive to form on the applicator tip, or draw the adhesive into a syringe equipped with a 25-gauge needle.
3. An assistant apposes and everts the skin edges with forceps.
4. Apply the tissue adhesive parallel to the wound and allow it to dry. Wound edges should be supported for at least 1 minute while the glue dries.
5. Apply three or four layers of adhesive and allow it to dry between each layer.

Discharge Instructions

- Minimize exposure to water. Avoid swimming, and showers preferred over bathing. Blot dry after showers.
- Do not apply antibiotic ointment to wound. Antibiotic ointment acts as a solvent and weakens the tissue adhesive bond.
- Return for signs or symptoms of infection, such as fever, redness, drainage, increasing pain, or swelling at the site.

METHOD 4: WOUND CLOSURE TAPE

Background

- Wound-closure tapes (e.g., Steri-Strips, Cover-Strips, Shur-Strips, Clearon, Curi-Strip, Cicagraf, and Suture Strip) are readily available in most emergency rooms for closing simple, superficial lacerations with minimal tension or for reinforcing suture-closure repairs.

Indications

- Low-tension superficial lacerations
- Reinforcement of sutured wounds or after suture removal for additional protection against wound dehiscence

Advantages

- Less tissue reactivity than sutures or staples
- Less costly than sutures or staples
- Shorter application time compared with sutures or staples
- Anesthesia not required for adhesive application, however, may be necessary for proper wound irrigation and exploration.
- Follow-up for removal unnecessary

Contraindications

- High-tension laceration
- Wound requiring deep closure
- Excessively moist areas such as the axilla or groin
- Allergy or hypersensitivity to tincture of benzoin or mastisol

Equipment

- Scissors
- Tincture of benzoin or mastisol
- Two pairs of forceps
- Wound tape

Procedure

1. After appropriate wound care, blot wound dry. (Proper hemostasis ensures that the skin remains dry during tape application.)
2. Apply tincture of benzoin or mastisol to the skin that will anchor the tape.
3. Have an assistant evert the skin edges with forceps.
4. Apply tape perpendicular to the wound axis.

Discharge Instructions

- Leave taped wounds open—no occlusive dressing or adhesive bandages. The resulting moisture facilitates dehiscence.
- Clean the wound with a moist washcloth.
- Trim curled tape edges.
- Return if the tape is removed.
- Return if the wound remains open.
- Return for signs or symptoms of infection, such as fever, ill-appearing, redness of the wound, drainage from the wound, increasing pain at the site of injury, or increased swelling at the site of infection.

INCISION AND DRAINAGE

Background

- Soft tissue and superficial skin abscesses are a common pediatric problem.
- Antibiotics are ineffective at relieving the symptoms or eradicating the bacteria of a soft tissue abscess.
- The treatment of choice for superficial abscesses is incision and drainage.
- Simple incision and drainage can be accomplished in an office or emergency room.
- Doctors who care for children should be familiar with the basic technique of

incision and drainage, as well as more location-specific techniques involving paronychia and felons.

Indications

- Well-localized collection of pus as evidenced by visualization of purulent material superficially below the epidermis or fluctuance
- Induration alone is generally not an indication. In questionable cases, syringe aspiration can be performed with an 18-gauge needle after local anesthesia to ensure that pus is present.

Contraindications

- Soft tissue hematoma
- Ill-defined collection of pus. Incision and drainage of an immature abscess or cellulitis may spread the infection into different tissue planes and can potentially result in bacteremia.
- A kerion is sometimes mistaken for a scalp abscess. Kerions respond to oral antibiotics, steroids, and antifungal medications. Incision and drainage is not indicated.
- Inability to provide adequate anesthesia
- Clinical uncertainty of surrounding anatomy, especially neurovascular structure. Special attention is required in the axilla, neck, groin, hand, foot, and posterior knee/popliteal region.
- Cosmetic considerations such as the face deserve consultation.
- If osteomyelitis is suspected, radiographs should be obtained, and parenteral antibiotics should be given in consultation with a specialist.

Equipment

Contents of a standard suture tray and accessories used for incision and drainage

- ABS towels
- Adson, serrated, 4.75″
- Cotton-tipped applicators, 6″
- Fenestrated drape
- Gauze sponges, 4 × 4″, 2 × 2″
- Iris scissors, straight, 4.5″
- Medicine cups, 2 oz.
- Mosquito, curved, 5″
- Needles: 27-gauge × 1.25″, 25-gauge × 5/8″, 18-gauge × 1.5″
- Syringe, 10 ml
- Webster needle holder, 6″

Procedure

1. Consider oral or parental analgesics (narcotic) and anxiolytics (benzodiazepines) to aid in patient comfort.

2. Consider regional nerve blocks as appropriate, particularly for facial, hand, or finger abscesses.
3. Gently scrub the area with betadine-soaked gauze.
4. Using a 25-gauge needle, infiltrate the dome of the abscess with lidocaine; to avoid injecting lidocaine into the abscess cavity, insert the needle parallel to the skin (not perpendicular). If the needle is positioned correctly, the skin overlying the abscess should blanch.
5. At this point, the skin is adequately anesthetized, but patients may still experience significant discomfort caused by the deeper innervation of the abscess cavity. Regional blocks or conscious sedation can greatly aid patient comfort.
6. Using a No. 11 or 15 scalpel, puncture the abscess and extend a linear incision parallel to the natural skin folds (Fig. 10-10).
7. Express the pus with gentle pressure at the edges of the abscess cavity.
8. Using cotton swabs or gauze-wrapped hemostats, open loculations and explore the depth of the abscess; never explore an abscess cavity with a finger because the nidus of the abscess may be a sharp, foreign body.
9. Gently irrigate the exposed abscess cavity with normal saline.
10. Loosely pack the cavity with 0.25″ or 0.5″ packing gauze (plain or iodoform). Document the approximate length of packing gauze used. If more than one piece of packing gauze is used, document the number and ensure that one end of each piece exits the abscess cavity.
11. Dress the packed wound with several layers of gauze pads to aid absorption of draining material.

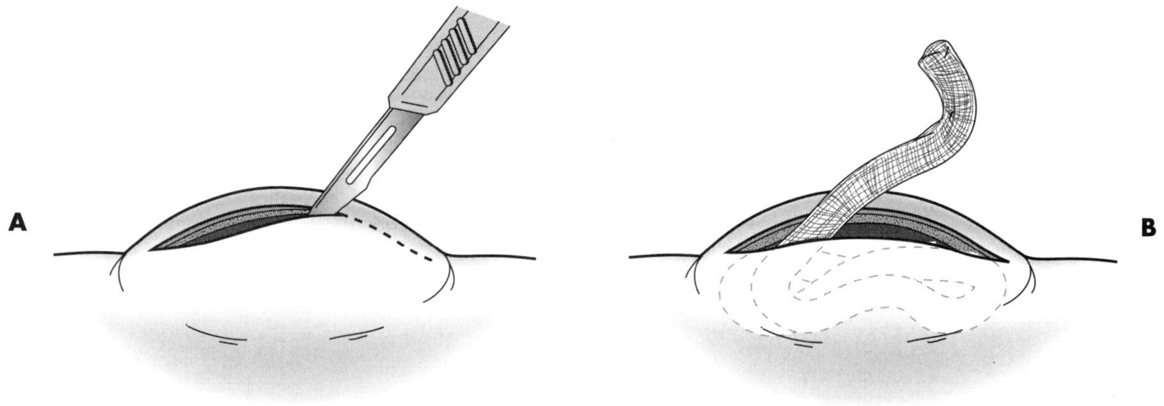

FIG. 10-10. Incision and drainage of an abscess. **A,** Prepare and drape the area. After appropriate anesthesia, make an incision the length of the abscess. **B,** After allowing the abscess to drain, loosely pack the abscess cavity to prevent premature closure and recurrence.

Follow-up

- Patients with co-morbid illness (particularly immunosupression), those who are cosmetically sensitive (face), or those who have functionally crucial wounds (hands) should be followed closely by the same physician.
- Keep affected area clean and dry.
- Follow up in 24 to 48 hours for wound check, packing removal, and possible repacking.

Repacking

Procedure

1. Offer patients anesthesia as appropriate. Anesthesia may not always be required, but patient comfort may be enhanced with oral narcotics and benzodiazepines. Occasionally, parenteral analgesia may be required to facilitate repacking of abscess cavities. Local anesthetic infiltration is of limited usefulness.
2. Moisten the packing with normal saline before removal. Some analgesia may be provided by using 4% lidocaine solution applied to the packing material, several minutes before removal. Do not exceed 0.1 ml/kg.
3. Gently remove the packing.
4. Repack the abscess cavity as necessary. The goal of repacking an abscess cavity is to provide continued drainage and to prevent premature closure of the opened abscess, resulting in reaccumulation of pus.

Other considerations

- Compliant patients with adequately draining, well-granulated abscess cavities can be managed with dressing changes and irrigation two to four times per day.
- Patients can irrigate at home by gently holding the cavity open under running water from a faucet or shower.
- Abscesses that must be repacked should be followed up in 24 to 48 hours.
- Patients should be followed until the wound has healed.

PARONYCHIA

Background

- Paronychia refers to an infection of the tissues surrounding the fingernail.
- An acute paronychia can be cellulitis, an abscess, or both.
- Treatment of acute paronychia cellulitis is warm soaks or warm compresses eight times per day and a short course of oral antistaphylococcal antibiotics.
- Treatment of an acute paronychia abscess requires incision and drainage; treatment of a mixed paronychia (cellulitis and abscess) requires both antibiotic therapy and drainage.
- As with abscess in general, an invasive drainage procedure should not be performed unless the practitioner can localize a discrete area of pus.

- Clinical uncertainty should prompt more conservative treatment with warm compresses, oral antibiotics, and close follow-up.
- Chronic paronychia should be referred to a dermatologist.

Indications

- A well-defined area of pus surrounding the fingernail causing symptoms

Contraindications

- Ill-defined collection of pus. Incision and drainage of an immature abscess or cellulitis can potentially spread the infection into different tissue planes and result in bacteremia.
- Subungual pus requires removal of the proximal nail to ensure adequate drainage.
- Inability to provide adequate anesthesia
- Clinical uncertainty of surrounding anatomy, especially neurovascular structures
- Tenosynovitis of the phalanges should be treated with intravenous antibiotics and consultation with a hand surgeon.

Equipment

- ABS towels
- Fenestrated drape
- Gauze sponges, 4 × 4″, 2 × 2″
- Iris scissors, straight, 4.5″
- Needle: 18-gauge, 1.5″

Procedure

1. Consider oral or parental analgesia (narcotics) and anxiolytics (benzodiazepines) to aid in patient comfort.
2. Consider digital blocks as appropriate.
3. Soak the eponychium in warm water for 10 minutes.
4. Gently scrub the area with betadine-soaked gauze.
5. Advance the scissors parallel to the nail.
6. Insert the scissors into the potential space between the nail and the eponychium.
7. Lift the eponychium and open the scissors while providing counterpressure on the abscess (Fig. 10-11). Alternatively, an 18-gauge needle can be used in place of scissors. As the eponychium is lifted, a small incision can be made with the cutting edge of the needle to facilitate drainage.
8. Loosely pack the abscess cavity as necessary. Larger abscesses benefit from continued drainage, whereas small abscesses do not require packing.
9. Dress the wound with antibiotic ointment or prescribe a short course of oral antistaphylococcal antibiotics and apply a dry dressing.

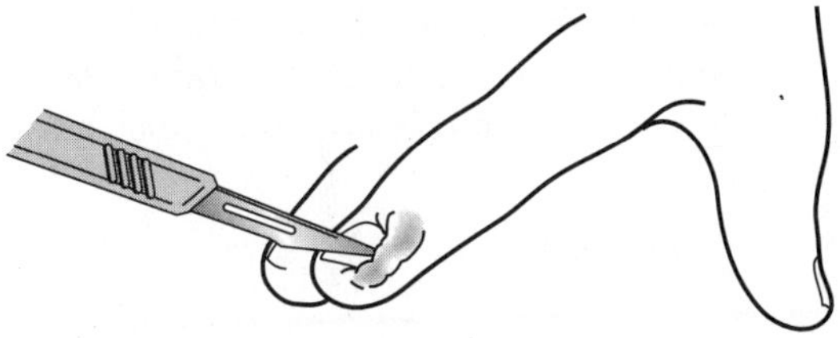

FIG. 10-11. Drainage of a paronychia.

Follow-up

- Keep the wound clean and dry
- Remove any packing after 24 hours. Soak in warm water before removing packing.
- Soak in warm water and gently massage the wound four to eight times per day.
- Keep the wound covered in antibiotic ointment or take oral antibiotics as prescribed.
- Return for wound check in 24 to 48 hours.

FELON

Background

- Felon refers to an infection of the distal dorsal pad of the finger. Localizing an abscess can be difficult but remains essential before beginning any invasive procedure.
- Patients sometimes relate a history of minor trauma days to weeks earlier; thus differentiating a felon from osteomyelitis can be difficult.
- A complete history should include documenting right or left hand dominance and occupation.
- Radiographs before incision may identify a retained foreign body or osteomyelitis.
- Care should be taken to avoid flexor tendons and digital nerves and arteries.
- Consultation with a hand surgeon may be appropriate.

Indications

- A well-defined abscess on the dorsal tip of the finger

Contraindications

- Inability to localize pus
- Involvement of the radial aspect of the dorsal surface of the second phalanx or

the ulnar aspect of the dorsal surface of the first or fifth phalanx; injury to the digital nerve and resulting numbness can impair pinch.
- Inability to provide adequate anesthesia

Equipment

- Betadine
- Curved hemostat
- Gauze pads, 4 × 4″
- Lidocaine
- Normal saline
- Penrose drain
- Scalpel
- Syringe/needle

Procedure

1. Consider oral or parental analgesia (narcotics) and anxiolysis (benzodiazepines) to aid in patient comfort.
2. Consider digital blocks as appropriate.
3. Clean the digit with betadine-soaked gauze.
4. Make an incision at the lateral edge of the distal phalanx at the junction of the dorsal and volar skin. The incision should stop 5 mm short of the interphalangeal crease, extending to or past the crease risks tendon or joint involvement (Fig. 10-12).
5. Loculations should be broken with curved forceps.
6. If drainage is inadequate, then a similar incision should be made on the other side of the finger. Once the loculations have been broken, a penrose drain can be passed through the finger to ensure continued drainage.

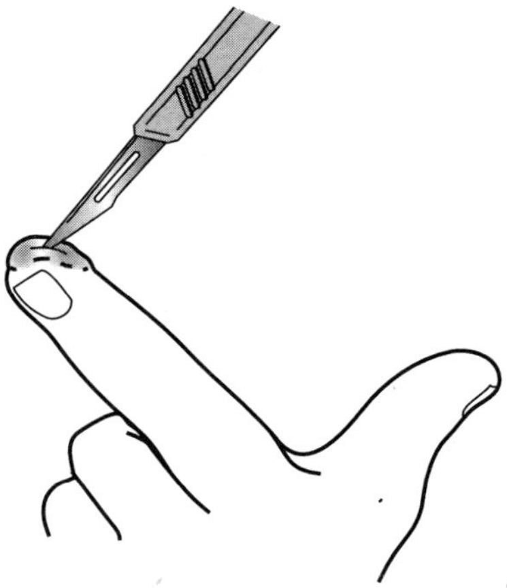

FIG. 10-12. Drainage of a felon.

7. Dress the wound.
8. Prescribe at least 7 days of broad-spectrum antibiotics.
9. Prescribe narcotic pain medicine as necessary.

Follow-up

- Keep the wound clean and dry.
- Return in 24 to 48 hours for wound check.
- Take antibiotics as prescribed.

SUGGESTED READINGS

Bresnahan KA, Howell JM, Wizorek J: Comparison of tensile strength of cyanoacrylate tissue adhesive closure of lacerations versus suture closure, *Ann Emerg Med* 26:575, 1995.

Bruns TB et al: A new tissue adhesive for laceration repair in children, *J Pediatr* 132: 1067, 1998.

Harwood-Nuss AL et al: *The clinical practice of emergency medicine,* ed 2, Philadelphia, 1996, Lippincott-Raven.

Hollander JE, Singer AJ: Laceration management, *Ann Emerg Med* 34:356, 1999.

Kanegaye JT et al: Comparison of skin stapling devices and standard sutures for pediatric scalp lacerations: a randomized study of cost and time benefits, *J Pediatr* 130:808, 1997.

Liebelt EL: Current concepts in laceration repair, *Curr Opin Pediatr* 9:459, 1997.

Mayhew HE, Rodgers LA: *Basic procedures in family practice,* Bethany, CT, 1984, Fleschner Publishing.

Noeller T, Cydulka R: Laceration repair techniques, *Emerg Med Rep* 17:207, 1996.

Osmond MH: Pediatric wound management: the role of tissue adhesives, *Pediatr Emerg Care* 15:137, 1999.

Osmond MH, Klassen TP, Quinn JV: Economic comparison of a tissue adhesive and suturing in the repair of pediatric facial lacerations, *J Pediatr* 126:892, 1995.

Osmond MH et al: A randomized clinical trial comparing butylcyanoacrylate with octylcyanoacrylate in the management of selected pediatric facial lacerations, *Acad Emerg Med* 6:171, 1999.

Pfenninger JL, Fowler GC: *Procedures for primary care physicians,* St Louis, 1994, Mosby.

Roberts JR, Hedges JR: *Clinical procedures in emergency medicine,* ed 3, Philadelphia, 1998, WB Saunders.

Saxena AK, Willital GH: Octylcyanoacrylate tissue adhesive in the repair of pediatric extremity lacerations, *Am Surg* 65:470, 1999.

Simon RR, Brenner BE: *Emergency procedures and techniques,* ed 3, Baltimore, 1994, Williams & Wilkins.

Simon HK et al: Long-term appearance of lacerations repaired using a tissue adhesive, *Pediatrics* 99:193, 1997.

Singer A, Hollander J, Quinn JV: Evaluation and management of traumatic lacerations, *N Engl J Med* 337:1142, 1997.

CHAPTER 11

Orthopedic Procedures

Mark A. Hostetler
David S. Weisman

INTRODUCTION

- Extremity injuries are a common reason for children presenting to the emergency department or doctor's office.
- Children present with unique types of fractures because of the presence of growth centers and the unusual flexibility of their skeletal system. Basic bone anatomy and terminology are illustrated in Fig. 11-1.
- Unique pediatric fractures are illustrated in Figs. 11-2 and 11-3.
- A bowing or plastic deformity involves bending of the bones without a fracture line. This occurs most often after a fall onto an outstretched arm and appears as though the forearm is bent or bowed (Fig. 11-2).
- Torus or buckle fractures are seen as a buckling of the cortex of the bone, without a complete break in the cortical line (Fig. 11-2).
- Greenstick fractures have a complete break in one side of the cortex of the bone, while the other side remains intact. Radiographs resemble a combination of bending and breaking similar to that seen when attempting to break a twig that is still green (Fig. 11-2).
- Fractures involving the growth center (physis) are classified according to the Salter-Harris classification system (Fig. 11-3).
- Growth plates close at variable ages depending on which bones are involved. Box 11-1 lists the age of appearance of ossification centers of the elbow. When in doubt, comparison views of the uninvolved extremity are often helpful.
- Caution should be used when diagnosing strains or sprains in young children. Epiphyseal plates are weaker than the ligaments or capsule supporting joints and, therefore, fail first when forces are applied.
- Point tenderness and swelling along an epiphysis, even in the absence of radiographic abnormality, should be considered a Salter-Harris Type I fracture.
- Joint dislocations are also rare in children; instead, a fracture will similarly occur along the growth plate.

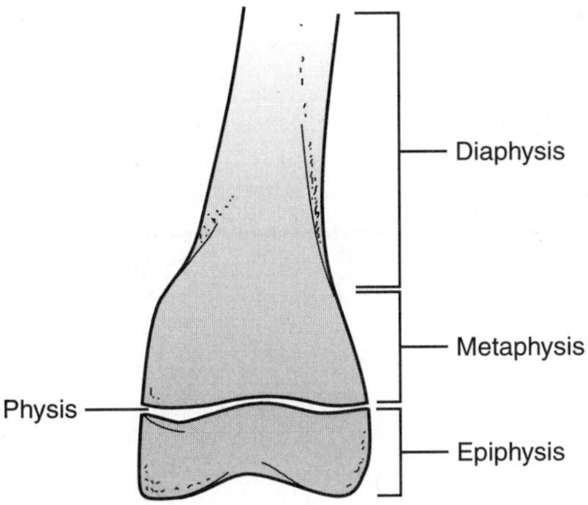

FIG. 11-1. Basic bone anatomy.

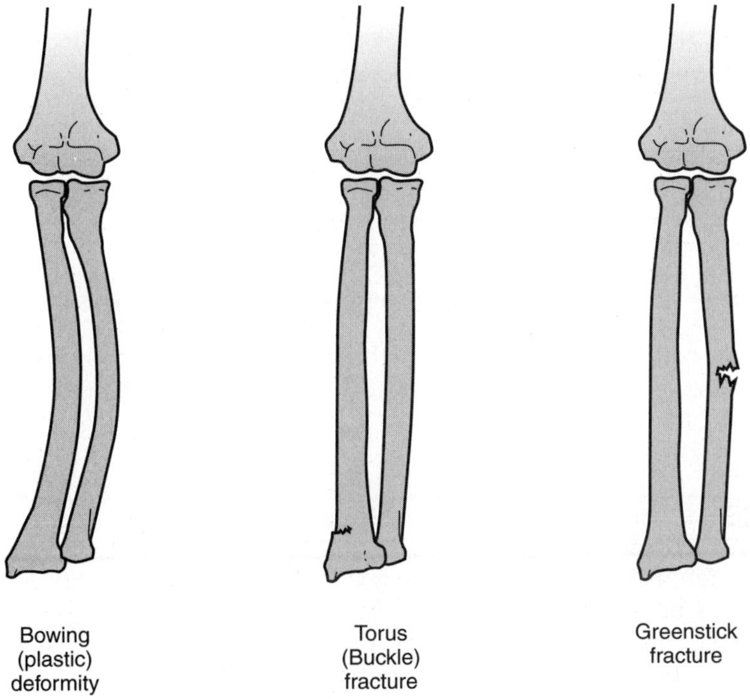

FIG. 11-2. Unique pediatric fractures.

PHYSICAL EXAMINATION

- The presentations of some children may be dramatic, with significant swelling and deformity of an extremity; however, don't forget to examine the rest of the patient. Always begin by assessing the ABCs and ensuring that no other life-threatening or limb-threatening emergencies are present.
- A complete examination requires a thorough neurovascular evaluation.

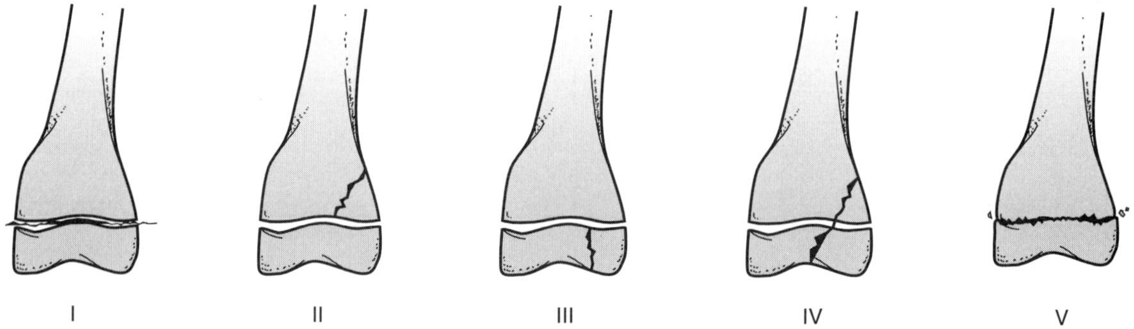

FIG. 11-3. Salter-Harris classification of epiphyseal fractures.

BOX 11-1 AGE OF APPEARANCE OF OSSIFICATION CENTERS OF THE ELBOW (CRITOE)

Capitellum (1 yr)
Radial head (3 yrs)
Internal (medial) epicondyle (5 yrs)
Trochlea (7 yrs)
Olecranon (9 yrs)
External (lateral) epicondyle (11 yrs)

- If a full-thickness wound communicates with the fracture, there is a high risk of patients developing osteomyelitis. All such wounds require thorough irrigation, debridement, and antibiotics.

COMPARTMENT SYNDROME

- Compartment syndrome may occur in several anatomical areas but most notably occurs in the forearm and lower leg.
- Compartment syndrome occurs when the swelling within a confined muscle compartment exceeds its capacity, and the pressure begins to occlude vascular structures and compress nerves.
- Commonly, five "Ps" are associated with compartment syndrome: pain, paresthesia, pallor, paralysis, and pulselessness.
- The earliest finding is pain that is worsened by passive movement of the muscles within that compartment and rest pain out of proportion to what might normally be expected.
- The muscles and soft tissues are typically firm to the touch, with significant swelling and tenderness.

- The last finding to occur is pulselessness. The presence of a pulse does not rule out compartment syndrome, however.
- Compartment syndrome is a true orthopedic emergency.
- The initial treatment is release of constricting bandages and evaluation. If this does not improve symptoms, surgical evaluation is necessary to determine if fasciotomy is necessary to return blood flow.

EXTREMITY IMMOBILIZATION

- To minimize pain and further injury, always immobilize the joints above and below the site of injury.
- Leave the fingers and toes accessible for monitoring neurovascular status.
- If tenting of the skin or vascular compromise is present, the fracture should be reduced before splinting.
- Open wounds should be covered with a sterile, moist, nonadherent dressing before splinting.
- Care should be taken when applying splinting materials because those that are applied too tightly may cause pain, swelling, and neurovascular compromise.

Indications

- Liberal use of splints is highly recommended because some childhood fractures are not apparent on initial radiographic evaluation.
- Even if no fracture is subsequently found, splints can hasten the recovery of ligamentous injuries.

Reasons for Referral to a Specialist

- In general, all children diagnosed with an extremity fracture should be referred to an orthopedic surgeon.
- Children with simple, uncomplicated fractures may be splinted and referred for follow-up within the week.
- Children with an open fracture, a significantly angulated fracture, or one that has neurovascular compromise should be referred emergently to an orthopedic surgeon.

Nursing Skills and Procedures

- An assistant who is trained in the application of splints can be very helpful.
- Assistants should support the extremity both above and below the fracture site to provide adequate stability and to reduce pain.
- As the splint is being applied, the hand should remain flat to prevent indentations in the casting material, which can cause dimpling and potential areas of excess pressure.

Supplies and Equipment

- ACE bandages
- Disposable gloves
- Heavy-duty scissors
- Padding material (Webril)
- Plaster or fiberglass splinting material
- Water bucket

Posterior Mold (Posterior Splint)

- The basic splint is called a posterior mold and may be used in a variety of ways for short or long splinting of the arm or leg.
- Splints are commonly used to prevent motion and swelling at a fracture or dislocation site. They are used as the initial treatment when the swelling, or the potential for swelling, is too great for a circumferential cast.
- The materials are sized to the involved extremity so that the splint is long enough to completely extend from the joint above to the joint below.

Procedure

- Fashion a splint in one of two basic ways (Fig. 11-4): The first way is to apply circumferential padding material over the involved extremity and then apply the

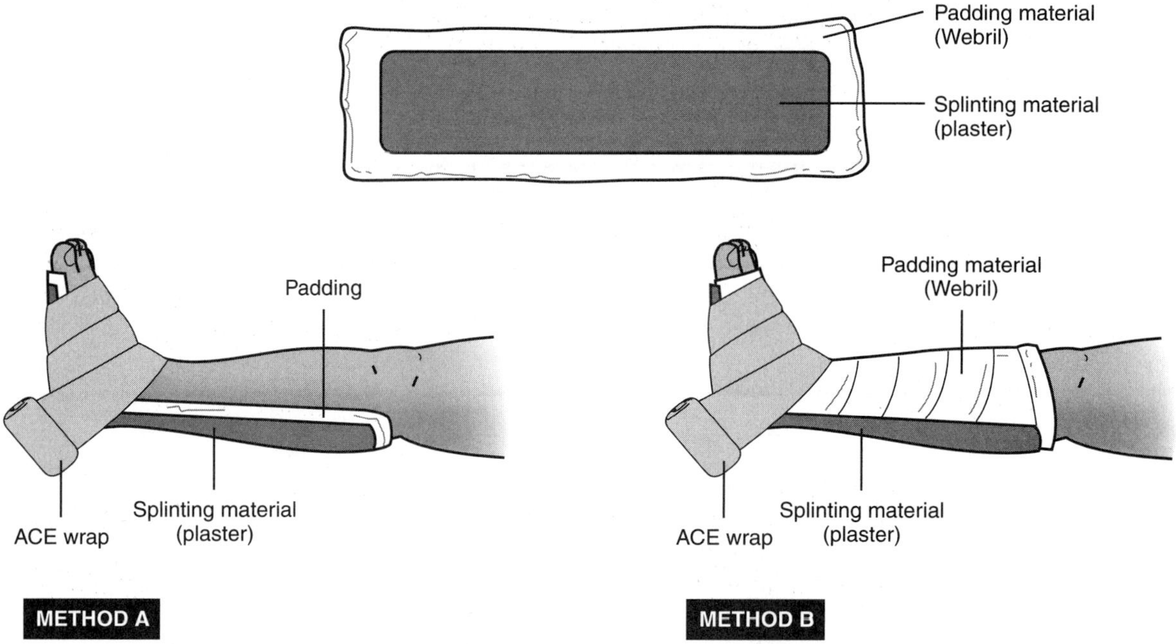

FIG. 11-4. Methods of applying posterior molds.

splinting material (plaster) over the posterior aspect. The other method is to lay out the padding in a long strip of the desired length, apply the wet plaster to the padding, and then apply the combined unit all at once to the extremity. The basics of both application techniques are the same.

1. Measure out one length of material needed by unrolling it onto the patient's unaffected extremity, using it as a template to estimate size. A minimum of four layers of padding material are required.
2. Using the template, size the casting materials. The padding material should be slightly wider than the splinting material to ensure that all areas receive adequate padding and to prevent excess contact with and pressure on the skin. The splinting material, however, should be just slightly longer when rolled out because it will shrink slightly as it dries.
3. Determine the appropriate number of layers of splinting material depending on patient size and the extremity involved. Usually, 8 to 12 layers are adequate, with lower extremities and larger patients requiring more layers.
4. Submerge the casting material in room temperature water before applying so that it is completely saturated.
5. Wring excess water out of the material by squeezing the material between the fingers until all of the air bubbles come out. Place the casting material on top of the padding.
6. Apply the entire unit (padding plus plaster) to the patient, with the padding side toward the patient along the posterior surface of the involved extremity.
7. Hold the padding and plaster in place using an ACE wrap. Hold the extremity in the neutral position until the casting material has completely hardened.
8. As the cast hardens, it gives off heat; do not use warm water because it increases the amount of heat generated by the casting material and can actually burn the patient. In addition, do not place the drying splint onto plastic-covered pillows because this may also intensify the heat and cause unintended burns.

POSTERIOR MOLD VARIATIONS

Sugar Tong (Fig. 11-5)

- This type of splint is commonly used for nondisplaced torus or buckle fractures involving the wrist or forearm.
- Sugar tong splints offer reasonable immobilization for minor fractures but may be inadequate for complete fractures.

Double Sugar Tong (Fig. 11-5)

- This type of splint is commonly used for true complete fractures involving the wrist or forearm and offers excellent immobilization of the entire forearm, elbow, and wrist.

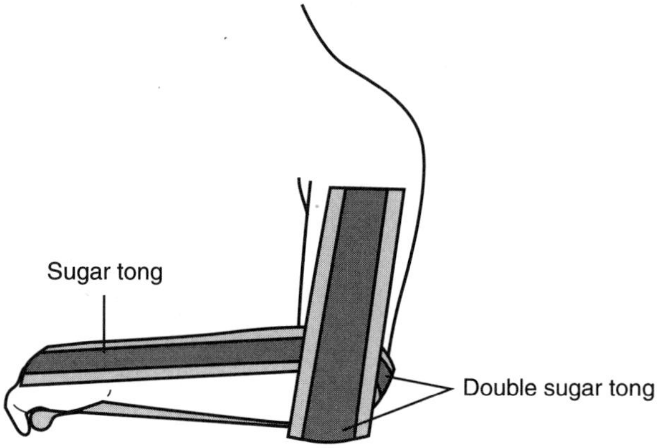

FIG. 11-5. Arm splints.

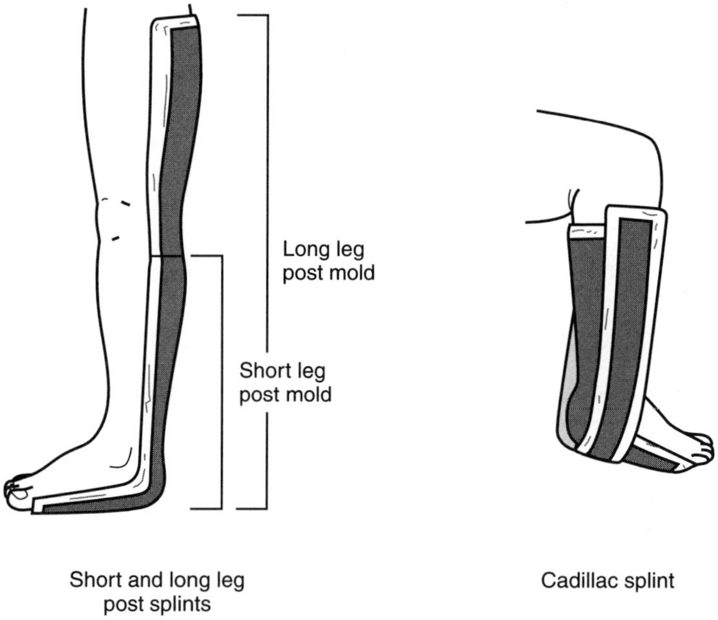

FIG. 11-6. Leg splints.

Short Leg Posterior Mold (Fig. 11-6)

- This type of splint is commonly used for mild injuries involving the ankle or foot.
- This splint is adequate for patients who require only to limit movement from a comfort standpoint. If a true fracture or any question of stability is present, a Cadillac splint is preferred.

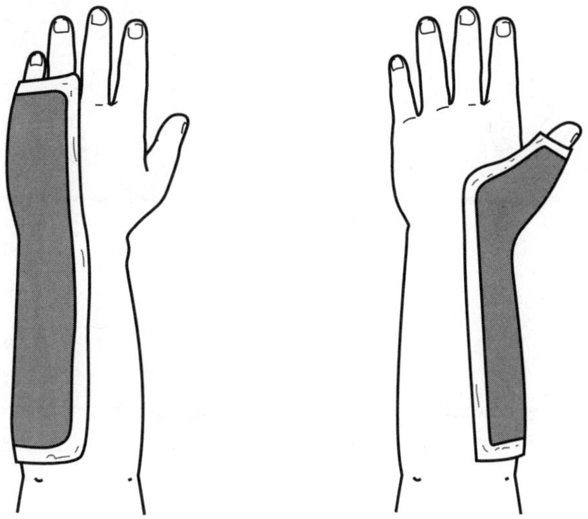

FIG. 11-7. Short arm splints.

Cadillac (Fig. 11-6)

- This type of splint is preferred for most ankle injuries because it offers significantly more support. It provides limitation of flexion and extension as well as lateral movement.

Thumb Spica (Fig. 11-7)

- This type of splint is commonly used for navicular or thumb fractures and extends along the radial aspect of the forearm.
- Fig. 11-8 demonstrates the safe position for splinting that involves the hand.

Ulnar Gutter (Fig. 11-7)

- This type of splint is commonly used for various fractures involving the hand and extends along the ulnar aspect of the forearm.
- Fig. 11-8 demonstrates the safe position for splinting that involves the hand.

Prefabricated Support Devices (Incomplete Immobilization)

ACE wrap

- An ACE (all cotton elastic) wrap is an effective treatment for control of swelling in both the acute and nonacute setting.
- Although commonly used for sprains, the ACE wrap provides no support to the joint. It functions merely as a compressive dressing to limit the amount of space available for swelling.

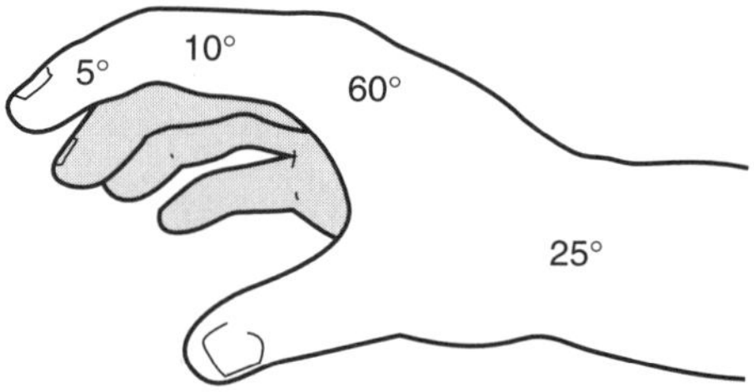

FIG. 11-8. Safe hand position for splinting.

- The wrap should not be stretched to the point that it is transparent, and it should be applied from the distal to the proximal part of the extremity in order to aid in return of edema fluid to the central circulation. For example, an ACE wrap applied to the knee only may trap fluid distally and cause the foot to swell.
- Similar to any circumferential compressive dressing, if the swelling exceeds the capacity of the extremity to compensate, then pain will occur and the dressing should be loosened or removed.
- The ACE wrap is also an effective method of holding dressings, splints, or ice bags in place.

Air bladder splints (air cast)

- These splints are most commonly used for ankle sprains. They typically function to reduce medial and lateral motion of the ankle.
- They are applied as a stirrup, with a medial and lateral plastic support with an underlying air bladder to conform to ankle anatomy.
- These splints permit full flexion and extension of the ankle.
- Air bladder splints are not indicated for anterior and posterior injuries (Achilles tendonitis, overuse syndrome), but they are indicated for medial and lateral injuries (ankle sprains).
- Instructions for application are included in the packaging materials.

Wrist splints

- These splints consist of a sleeve, usually with Velcro straps for tightening and a metal "spoon" to place in the palm to immobilize the wrist.
- They are indicated for treatment of wrist sprains, overuse syndrome, and postcasting fracture care.
- The straps should not be applied too tightly because the splint is intended only to resist wrist motion, not to completely immobilize the joint.

Clavicle straps

- A figure-of-eight strapping system was originally indicated for treating clavicle fractures in children.
- These complex and often uncomfortable straps have now been replaced by the use of simple arm slings.
- Slings with swath attachments that encircle the waist and include an attachment for the sling to the swath are also available.

Knee immobilizer

- Knee immobilizers consist of a long sleeve with Velcro straps that are placed over the leg and centered on the knee joint. Metal slats are located posteriorly to immobilize the knee.
- They are indicated for the transport or initial treatment of soft tissue knee injuries when immobilization is intended to be short term.
- The straps should not be applied too tightly because the splint is used only to resist knee motion, not to completely immobilize the joint.

SPINE IMMOBILIZATION

- Spinal cord injuries in children are uncommon but devastating.
- It is important to remember that children with a loss of consciousness or a high mechanism of injury (e.g., motor vehicle crash or fall from a height greater than 10 to 20 feet) should be considered to have a cervical spine injury until proven otherwise.
- Spinal injuries should also be considered when children have any neurologic complaints consistent with a spinal cord injury.
- A thorough neurovascular examination includes mental status, sensation, motor function, reflexes, and a rectal examination.

Anatomy

- The cervical spine in children differs from adults because of a higher fulcrum of flexion (C2-3) and more ligamentous laxity. Younger children tend to involve the upper cervical spine, whereas spinal injuries tend to be lower in older children and adults.
- Evaluation of the spine should include three to five views of the spine. The most important view is the lateral radiograph as approximately 90% of injuries are noted in this area.
- Radiographic analysis should include evaluation of the curvature of the spine, prevertebral soft tissue, predental space, odontoid, individual vertebrae, disc spaces, neural arches, and spinous processes.
- Other radiographic views include an anteroposterior (AP) view, open mouth odontoid, and oblique views. Unfortunately, the open mouth odontoid view is often difficult to obtain in young children; therefore in order to assess the odontoid and lateral masses, a computed tomography (CT) scan may be necessary.

Indications

- All patients with a potential spine injury should be immobilized.
- There are no set guidelines regarding who needs radiographic clearance of a spinal injury, but radiographic studies should be liberally ordered for children with an appropriate mechanism of injury who have neck pain, are preverbal, or have neurologic deficits.

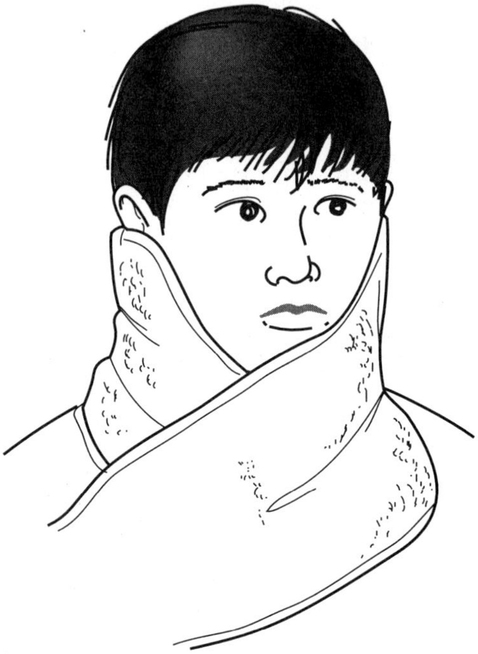

FIG. 11-9. Towel wrap for cervical spine immobilization.

Supplies and Equipment

- Age-appropriate and size-appropriate backboard immobilization
- Age-appropriate and size-appropriate cervical immobilization (collar, sandbags, towel rolls)
- Padding

Nursing Skills and Procedures

- Padding: The backboard should be padded whenever possible to prevent pain and the potential for pressure sore necrosis.
- Reassurance: Lying fully immobilized on a backboard is a terrifying experience for most children, and they often require a lot of handholding and reassurance.
- Vomiting: Patients who are fully immobilized on their backs should not be left alone. If children were to have unrecognized vomiting, they could very easily aspirate.

Procedure

1. Keep the patient immobilized as a single unit. Immobilization of the neck can often be created with something as simple as a towel roll placed around the neck like a thick scarf (Fig. 11-9), or with towel rolls taped at the sides of the head, pending the availability of a rigid cervical collar.

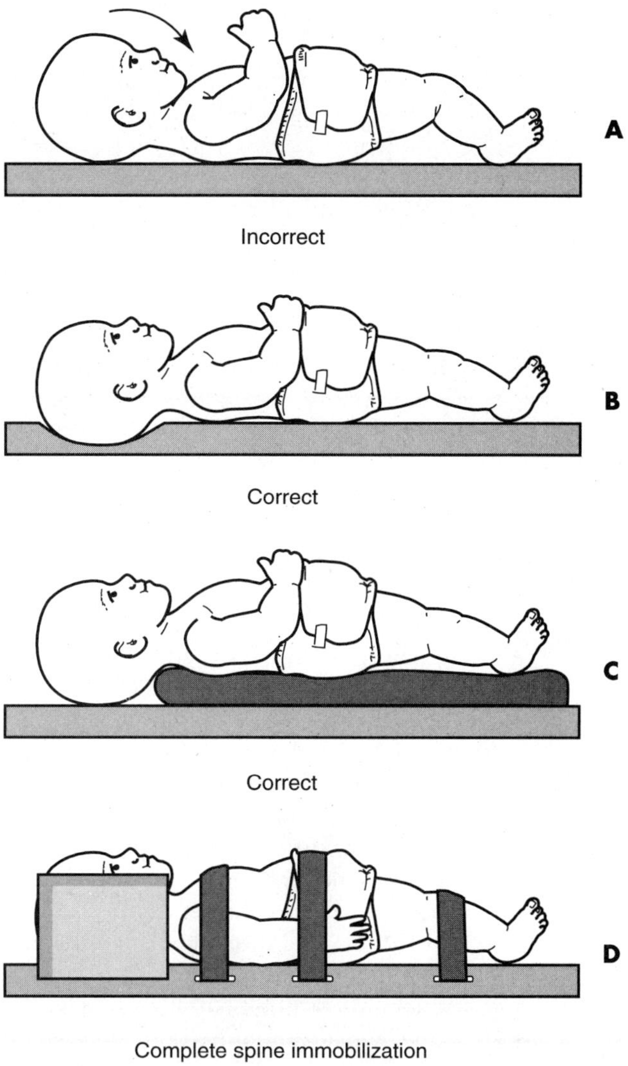

FIG. 11-10. Pediatric spine immobilization. **A,** Inadvertant neck flexion caused by child's relatively large occiput. **B,** Modified pediatric backboard with scooped-out area for head. **C,** Additional padding used on a standard backboard. **D,** Complete spinal immobilization.

2. For transport purposes, place children on a rigid backboard with sandbags or rolled towels placed at either side of the head and taped in place. This positioning prevents side bending, rotation, and flexion of the neck.
3. Modify the backboard for transporting children (Fig. 11-10). The size of children's heads is proportionately larger than that of adults when compared to the body. Placing children on a standard backboard causes their necks to flex because of this increased head-body proportion. A pediatric backboard requires a cutout for the head (occiput) to allow it to extend to a neutral position.

If none is available, a pad may alternatively be placed under the body to modify positioning.

4. Remove children from the board as soon as initial clinical and radiographic evaluation is completed. A 6-hour maximum is allowed on the backboard. Skin breakdown can occur with longer times on the board.
5. A thoracic or lumbar injury is unusual in children but more common in adolescents and teenagers. The evaluation and treatment is similar for these injuries.

Reasons for Referral to a Specialist

- Any children with abnormal radiographs, neurologic deficit consistent with a spinal cord injury, or significant neck pain even with normal radiographs should be referred to a spine specialist.

JOINT REDUCTIONS

Nursemaid's Elbow

- Nursemaid's elbow is a common injury in toddlers and young preschool children; however, it may occur in children up to the age of 10.
- Typically, a history of a longitudinal force being applied to the extended elbow (such as when a child's arm is pulled forcefully) is reported. The classic example is when the child's arm is pulled by a caregiver going up a curb or set of stairs, hence the term "nursemaid's elbow."
- Another common mechanism of injury is when older family members swing children around by their wrists when playing.
- Immediately after the forceful pull, children refuse to move the elbow and hold it limp at their side, flexed at the elbow and slightly pronated.
- There should be no swelling or tenderness on palpation. Pain occurs only with movement, most notably with supination.
- If the mechanism and the examination are consistent with the diagnosis, then no radiographs are needed and reduction can proceed.
- A fall onto an outstretched arm does not cause nursemaid's elbow; it causes supracondylar fractures. Similarly, blunt trauma to the arm does not result in nursemaid's elbow.
- If any question exists, a radiograph should be obtained first to rule out fracture.

Anatomy

- Nursemaid's elbow is often inappropriately described as a radial head subluxation; however, there is no abnormal movement of the radial head out of the joint.
- Nursemaid's elbow occurs as a result of natural laxity within a young child's elbow combined with the normal redundancy of the annular ligament surrounding the radial head.
- A longitudinal force applied to the arm can distract the elbow joint, allowing

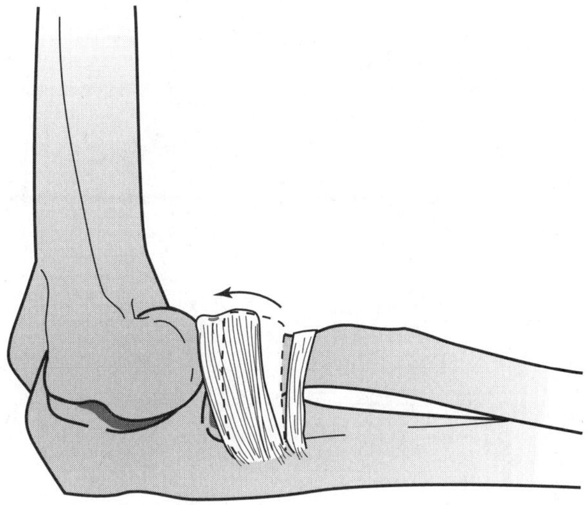

FIG. 11-11. Anatomical representation of nursemaid's elbow. The annular ligament slips or is torn out of place, becoming wedged between radial head and capitellum.

the redundant portion of the annular ligament to fall into the joint and become entrapped when the longitudinal force is removed and the joint closes (Fig. 11-11).

Indications

- Reduction is indicated when the diagnosis of nursemaid's elbow is strongly suspected based on history and physical findings, and when fracture or injury to neurovascular structures can be reasonably excluded on clinical examination.

Contraindications and reasons for referral to a specialist

- The manipulation of the extremity necessary for reduction involves the application of force and torque to the elbow joint. Such maneuvers are, therefore, contraindicated in any situation in which a fracture of the bones of the arm or forearm is strongly suspected.
- If successful reduction cannot be accomplished after one or two attempts, radiographs should be obtained to ensure that another injury is not present.
- Referral to a pediatric orthopedic specialist should occur whenever a fracture is identified or when reduction of the injury is unsuccessful.

Procedure

1. Use one of two methods for reduction: hyperpronation or supination-flexion. The supination-flexion method has historically been the standard; however, the hyperpronation method may be more successful.
2. Perform the hyperpronation maneuver with children's arms left pronated at their side. Grab the wrist with one arm, position your thumb over the radial head, and with one swift motion provide a firm twist at the wrist, causing hyperpronation. A "click" should be simultaneously felt under the thumb on

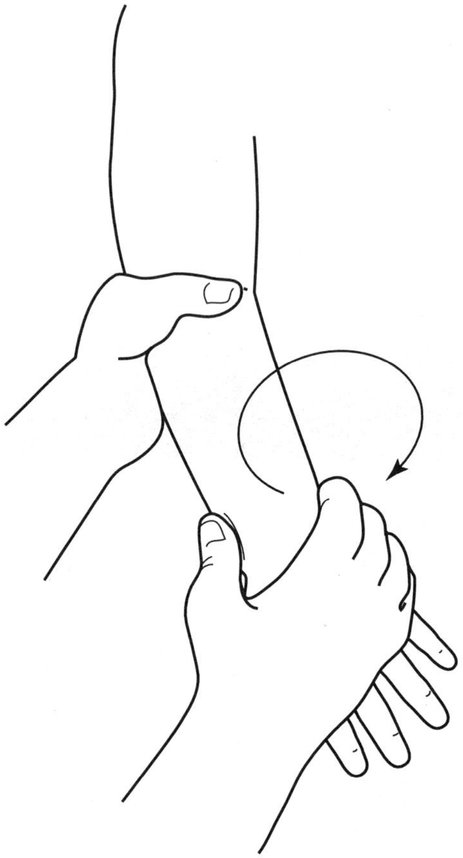

FIG. 11-12. Hyperpronation method. With one thumb placed over radial head, practitioner performs one swift and forceful hyperpronation of wrist and hand.

the other hand. Using this maneuver, there is no need to flex children's arms at the elbow (Fig. 11-12).

3. The child should begin using the arm normally within 10 to 15 minutes following the procedure.
4. Perform the supination-flexion procedure using stepwise supination of the forearm and flexion of the elbow, with the thumb placed over the radial head while flexing the elbow. A "click" should be felt under the thumb as the annular ligament snaps back into place (Fig. 11-13). A "click" may be palpated during either maneuver, but the definitive test is verification that patients begin using the arm normally within 10 to 15 minutes after the procedure. If either maneuver doesn't work, the other may be tried.

What the patient and family should know

- The family should understand that this common injury may occur again with similar pulling motions. The family, therefore, needs to avoid lifting children by the hand or wrist.

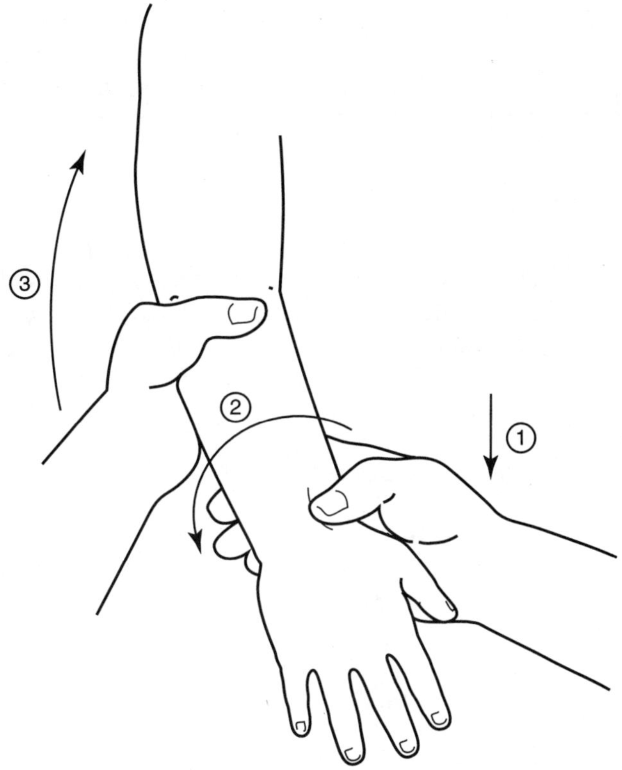

FIG. 11-13. Supination/flexion method. Following three steps are done in rapid succession: (1) With one thumb applying pressure over radial head, apply longitudinal traction by pulling at wrist. (2) Supinate forearm fully by twisting wrist outward. (3) Flex elbow fully while continuing to press on radial head.

- If this injury becomes a recurrent problem, parents can be instructed on how to perform the reduction at home themselves.

Shoulder Dislocation

Anatomy

- History and physical examination is necessary to establish the diagnosis of shoulder dislocation and to evaluate for neurovascular injury before reduction.
- Document any decreased sensation, especially in the distribution of the axillary nerve.
- Radiographs of the shoulder should include both anteroposterior and lateral views (axillary or scapular Y view). This process establishes if any fractures are present and demonstrates the direction of the dislocation.

- More than 90% of shoulder dislocations are anterior (humerus in front of glenoid).
- The type of dislocation determines the reduction maneuver used.
- These procedures are generally most successful when good relaxation has been obtained. Often, the use of a benzodiazepine alone is sufficient; however, many patients benefit from the addition of an analgesic such as fentanyl or morphine sulfate.

Indications

- All dislocations require reduction.

Contraindications and reasons for referral to a specialist

- All patients with shoulder dislocations should be referred to an orthopedic surgeon.
- If reduction attempts are unsuccessful, or there is open injury or evidence of neurovascular compromise, patients should be referred emergently.
- Otherwise, if the reduction is successful, patients may be immobilized (shoulder immobilizer or sling and swath) and sent for follow-up referral within the week.

Procedure

- The traction-countertraction method is perhaps the most common reduction maneuver described. Using this technique, have one practitioner wrap a sheet around the patient's chest and pull (countertraction), while the other practitioner holds the patient's arm abducted and externally rotated, applying continuous longitudinal traction until the shoulder relocates with a "clunk" (Fig. 11-14). A considerable amount of force may be required, especially in the large or muscular adolescent.

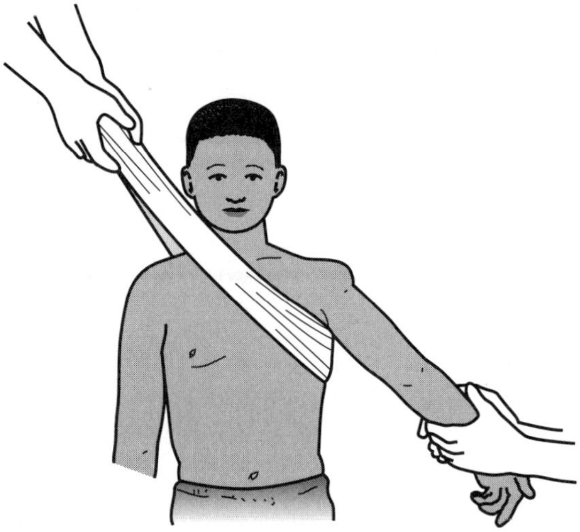

FIG. 11-14. Traction-countertraction method of shoulder reduction.

- Another technique is to have patients reduce the dislocation themselves by placing their hand on their forehead and progressively walking their hand over their head. This technique is known as the "greaser" technique because of the appearance of the hand sliding over the top of the head (Fig. 11-15). This technique is often successful but requires a significant amount of cooperation from children.
- One of the techniques believed to be the least painful, and perhaps most physiologic, is the Stimson technique (Fig. 11-16). Using this technique, patients lie on their stomach with their arm hanging over the side of the bed. The shoulder is allowed to reduce itself using the weight of gravity or can be augmented by hanging weights from the arm. This technique has the added advantage of being able to be done at home. Instead of weights, patients can hold onto a bag of IV fluid, a can of food, or any other similar type of object.
- Once the shoulder has been reduced, place patients into some type of immobilization (shoulder immobilizer or sling and swath) and obtain a repeat neurovascular examination and confirmatory radiograph.

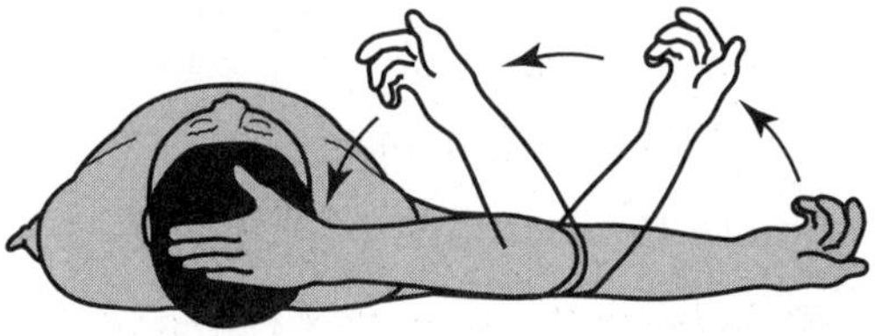

FIG. 11-15. "Greaser" method of shoulder reduction.

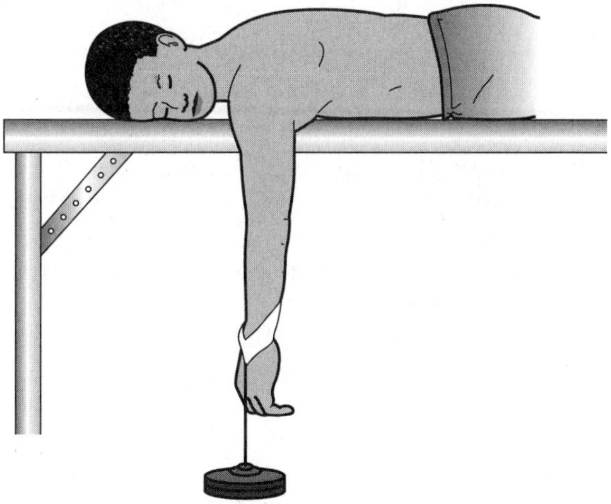

FIG. 11-16. Stimson technique.

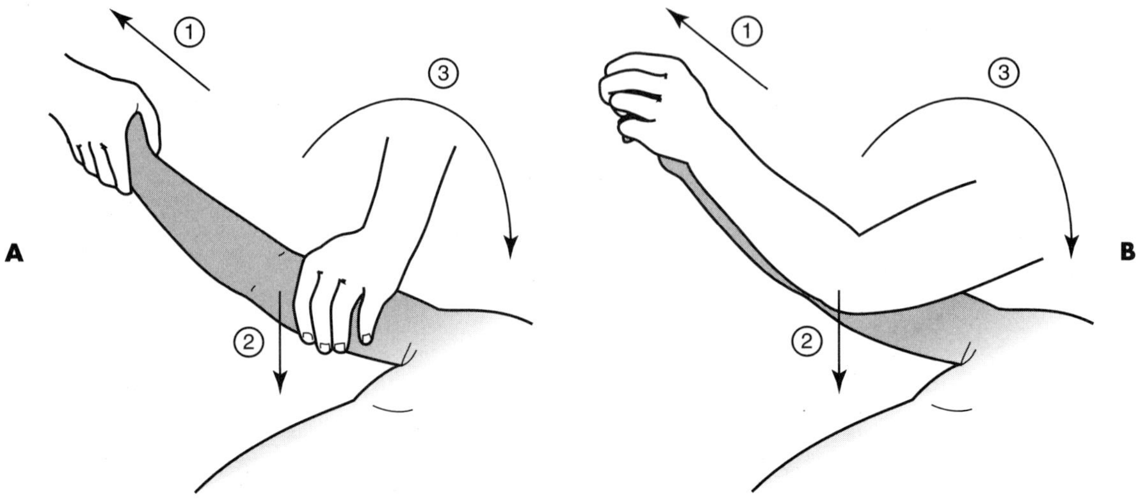

FIG. 11-17. Elbow dislocation reduction techniques. Method A: (1) Apply longitudinal traction. (2) Apply downward (posterior) force at distal humerus. (3) Flex at elbow. Method B: All three steps can be accomplished simultaneously by using your elbow as a fulcrum and grasping patient's hand. (1) Extending your wrist results in a longitudinal traction. (2) Your elbow exerts a simultaneous posterior force at the distal humerus. (3) Flexing your elbow also causes the patient's elbow to flex and reduction of the olecranon back into anatomical position.

Elbow Dislocation

Anatomy

- The evaluation is similar to that of a shoulder dislocation.
- Elbow dislocations are usually posterior (olecranon behind humerus).

Procedure

1. Apply a longitudinal force to the arm, exert a posteriorly directed force to the distal humerus, and flex the elbow to 90 degrees (Fig. 11-17, *A*). A palpable "clunk" follows the reduction.
2. One of the easiest ways to reduce the elbow and ensure proper positioning is to use your elbow as the fulcrum to provide the force necessary to reduce the joint. Grasp the patient's hands with your opposite hand, interlacing the fingers, and place your elbow into their antecubital fossa.
3. Tighten your fingers and pull up on the wrist to produce a fulcrum with your elbow, causing the end of the humerus to remain stationary while exerting significant force on the forearm, flexing at the forearm and allowing the olecranon to be reduced back into its proper position (Fig. 11-17, *B*).
4. If the reduction cannot be obtained or maintained, or if an associated fracture occurs, request an orthopaedic consult to assess the obstructing structure.
5. After reduction, take the elbow through a gentle range of motion to assess stability; however, these dislocations are often unstable.
6. Immobilize the elbow initially with a posterior splint at 90 degrees and a sling.

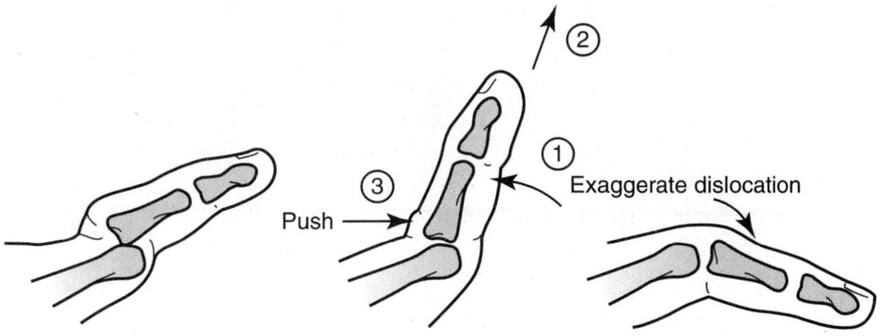

FIG. 11-18. Reduction of finger dislocation.

7. Postreduction films should be obtained to ensure that the joint has been reduced and remains in good position after splinting.

Contraindications and reason for referral to a specialist

- All patients with elbow dislocations should be referred to an orthopedic surgeon.
- If reduction attempts are unsuccessful, or there is open injury or evidence of neurovascular compromise, patients should be referred emergently.
- Otherwise, if the reduction is successful, patients may be immobilized (posterior long arm splint or double sugar tong with the elbow at 90 degrees and a sling) and sent for follow-up referral within the week.

Finger

Anatomy

- Finger dislocations can be at the proximal interphalangeal (IP) joint or less commonly at the distal IP joint. They may also be volar (anterior) or more commonly dorsal (posterior) dislocations. Dorsal dislocations at the proximal IP joint produce a characteristic prominence of the middle phalanx. Anterior dislocations do not have a characteristic appearance and can more easily be missed.
- The evaluation requires a thorough history, physical examination, and radiographs.
- On examination, these patients have tenderness over the joint and inability to fully extend the finger.
- All patients suspected of a dislocation should have radiographs taken to confirm the diagnosis and to evaluate for associated fractures.

Procedure

1. Use a digital block to control pain during the maneuver, if needed.
2. Apply traction in a direction that exaggerates the deformity. First, exaggerate the deformity, applying longitudinal traction in the same direction, and then push the dislocated segment back into a neutral anatomical position (Fig. 11-18).

3. After reduction, test the joint for ligamentous stability.
4. Apply a finger splint with the finger in full extension. Anterior dislocations invariably involve tendon damage.
5. If the reduction cannot be obtained, request an orthopaedic consult to assess the obstructing structure (volar plate or fracture segment).

Contraindications and reason for referral to a specialist

- In general, all patients with dislocations should be referred to an orthopedic surgeon.
- If reduction attempts are unsuccessful, or if there is open injury or evidence of neurovascular compromise, patients should be referred emergently.
- Otherwise, if the reduction is successful, patients may be immobilized (posterior splint in extension) and sent for follow-up referral within the week.

Hip Dislocation

Anatomy

- The evaluation is similar to that of a shoulder dislocation.
- Hip dislocations are usually posterior (femoral head behind the acetabulum).

Procedure

1. Reduction of the hip joint requires at least two practitioners and a certain amount of brute strength in order to lift and manipulate the entire leg.
2. Apply a longitudinal force to the leg, exert a posteriorly directed force to the proximal femur so that it can come back over the acetabulum, and then apply

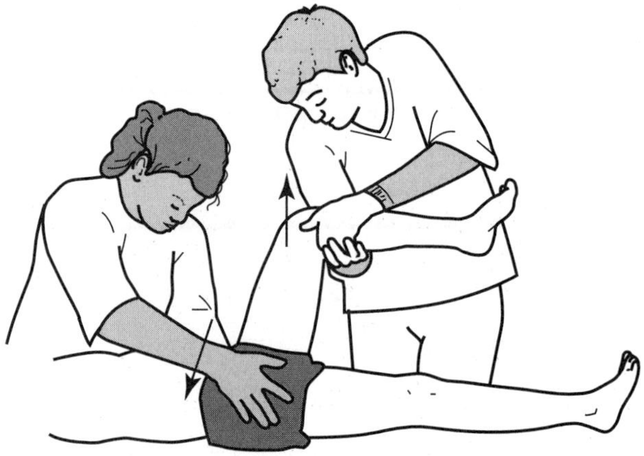

FIG. 11-19. Reduction of hip dislocation.

an upward pull back up into the acetabulum (Fig. 11-19). These movements are all done while a second person applies a downward force to keep the pelvis stable. A palpable "clunk" signifies reduction.

3. After reduction, take the hip through a gentle range of motion to assess stability.

Contraindications and reason for referral to a specialist

- All patients with hip dislocations should be referred to an orthopedic surgeon.
- If reduction attempts are unsuccessful, or there is open injury or evidence of neurovascular compromise, patients should be referred emergently.

Knee Dislocation

Anatomy

- The evaluation is similar to that of a shoulder dislocation.
- Radiographs should be obtained to verify that the knee (not just the patella) is truly dislocated because true tibiofemoral dislocations require emergent evaluation to rule out vascular injury.

Procedure

1. A great deal of force is required to dislocate the knee, and in doing so most, if not all, of the supporting joint capsule is usually torn; therefore reduction is usually surprisingly easy.
2. Apply a longitudinal force to the leg while returning the tibiofemoral joint to a neutral anatomical position. A palpable "clunk" occurs with the reduction. Neurovascular compromise is a chief concern, and detailed serial examinations should be documented.
3. After reduction, apply a long leg posterior splint.
4. True tibiofemoral knee dislocations require imaging and assessment of vascular structures.

Contraindications and reason for referral to a specialist

- All patients with knee dislocations should be referred emergently to an orthopedic surgeon.

Patella

Anatomy

- The patella dislocates out of the femoral groove, displacing laterally. Patients with patellar dislocation present with the knee flexed and the patella sitting laterally.
- If the patella dislocated and spontaneously reduced before examination, the knee will be mildly swollen and tender over the medial side of the patella.
- Patellar dislocation is one of the few cases in which reduction may be performed

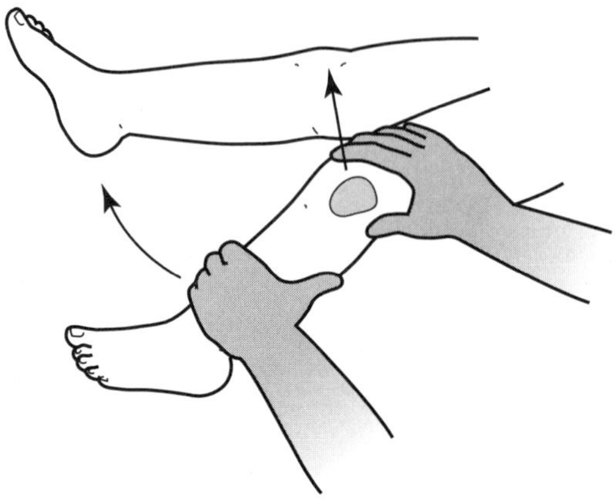

FIG. 11-20. Reduction of patella dislocation.

without first obtaining a radiograph, as long as the practitioner is sure that no other injuries are present.
- If there is any question, complete radiographs of the knee should be obtained.

Procedure

Reduction of the patella is easily done and gives immediate relief of pain. Patients frequently have an "apprehension sign" in that they are intensely fearful of any movement of the leg.

1. First, gain their trust and let them know what is going on.
2. Second, let them know that the reduction will not hurt and they will have immediate relief.
3. When ready, count to three and let patients know exactly when the reduction is commencing.
4. Perform the simultaneous and swift movement of extending the knee with one hand placed under the lower leg while at the same time moving the patella medially with the other (Fig. 11-20). Perform the two motions rapidly and simultaneously, not slowly. Once reduced, flex and extend the knee to assess stability and verify that the quadricep mechanism is functioning normally (knee extension).
5. If the reduction cannot be obtained or maintained, or if an associated fracture occurs, request an orthopaedic consult to assess the obstructing structure.
6. Place the knee into a knee immobilizer.

Contraindications and reason for referral to a specialist

- In general, all patients with dislocations should be referred to an orthopedic surgeon.
- If reduction attempts are unsuccessful, or there is open injury or evidence of neurovascular compromise, patients should be referred emergently.

- Otherwise, if the reduction is successful, patients may be immobilized (knee immobilizer in extension) and sent for follow-up referral within the week. Crutches are usually not necessary.

Ankle Dislocation

Anatomy

- The evaluation is similar to that of other dislocations, and radiographs are always necessary.

Procedure

- Most ankle dislocations also involve fractures and are associated with a significant force that results in instability and severe damage to the joint capsule. Generally, that process also makes ankles relatively easy to reduce.
- The reduction maneuver varies slightly depending on the location; however, it basically involves applying a longitudinal force to the foot and gentle movement of the foot and ankle back into a neutral anatomical position. A palpable "clunk" signifies reduction.
- Initial immobilization is with a posterior mold or cadillac splint. A cadillac splint is preferred.

Contraindications and reason for referral to a specialist

- All patients with ankle dislocations should be referred to an orthopedic surgeon.
- If reduction attempts are unsuccessful, or there is open injury or evidence of neurovascular compromise, patients should be referred emergently.

JOINT ASPIRATIONS AND INJECTIONS

- The most important factor in aspirating or injecting any joint is the ability to locate and recognize the anatomical landmarks that signify entry into the joint.
- Fluoroscopy may be used for difficult cases.
- Topical anesthesia such as eutectic mixture of local anesthetic (EMLA) cream may be used.
- Generally, lidocaine injection is avoided because this increases the number of injections necessary without any significant analgesia. If lidocaine is used, it should not contain epinephrine.
- If steroids are injected, patients should be warned of skin lightening and sun sensitivity that may occur in that area.
- Table 11-1 lists drug dosages for injection therapy, and Table 11-2 lists the differential considerations for synovial fluid analysis.

Equipment

- Needle, 18- to 22-gauge
- Sterile draping

TABLE 11-1
Drug dosages for joint injections

Joint	Lidocaine 1% (ml)	Methylprednisolone acetate (mg)
Shoulder	5-7	20-40
Elbow	3-5	10-20
Wrist	1-2	10-40
Hip	5	40-80
Knee	5	20-80
Ankle	3-5	20-40
Finger/Toe	0.5-1.0	4-10

TABLE 11-2
Synovial fluid analysis

	Normal	Gout	Pseudogout	Inflammatory arthritis*	Septic
Appearance	Clear	Turbid	Turbid	Turbid	Purulent
WBCs/mm^3	<200	2,000-50,000	2,000-50,000	2,000-50,000	>50,000
% PMNs	<25%	>75%	>75%	50-75%	>75%
Glucose	90-100	80-100	80-100	70-80	<50
Crystals	None	Negative birefringence	Positive birefringence	None	None

*Rheumatoid arthritis, psoriatic arthritis, Reiter's disease

- Sterile skin preparation
- Sterile specimen container (for aspiration)
- Syringe, 10 ml

Shoulder (Fig. 11-21)

- The shoulder joint is most easily and safely approached posteriorly. This is typically performed in the seated position.
- Palpate the posterior lateral edge of the acromion.
- Internally and externally rotate the shoulder to palpate the humeral head in the joint.
- Palpate the coracoid anteriorly.
- Move 5 to 10 mm inferiorly from the acromion and 5 to 10 mm medially.
- Place the thumb of the noninjecting hand at this point.
- Place the index finger of the noninjecting hand on the coracoid.
- Place the needle at the point of the thumb and direct it toward the index finger. If bone is encountered, range the shoulder joint. If the needle moves, it is in the humerus; if not, it is in the glenoid.
- The joint capsule is generally no deeper than 2 cm. It will be more superficial if distended by an effusion.
- If the needle is too superior, enter the subacromial space. If too medial, the suprascapular nerve is near, sitting in its notch. If too inferior, the brachial plexus is nearby. Too lateral, and the needle is on the humeral head.

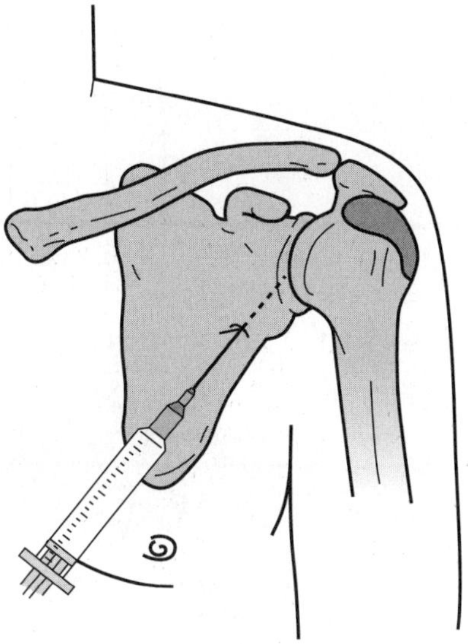

FIG. 11-21. Intraarticular shoulder joint injection/aspiration.

Elbow (Fig. 11-22)

- Viewed from the lateral aspect are three palpable bony landmarks: the lateral humeral epicondyle, the radial head, and the olecranon.
- With the elbow flexed to 90 degrees, these three landmarks form a triangle, in the center of which is the joint.
- If the needle is too proximal, the humerus is encountered; if too distal, the radial head is found. If the needle is too anterior, the neurovascular structures are at risk; and if too posterior, the ulna will be encountered.
- The joint capsule should be no more than 1 cm deep, although this may be altered by soft tissue swelling.

Knee (Fig. 11-23)

- At the superior lateral aspect of the patella, when viewed laterally, is an interval immediately anterior to the lateral femoral condyle. Both the condyle and the patella are palpable at this level, and this interval gives entry to the joint.
- If the needle is too proximal, the suprapatella bursa or quadriceps is present; if too distal, the interval becomes extremely narrow. If the needle is too anterior, the patella or prepatella bursa is encountered; if too posterior, the lateral femoral condyle is present.
- The joint is usually approximately 1 cm deep.
- If soft tissue swelling obscures bony landmarks, an alternative approach may be used. Flex the knee 30 to 45 degrees. Palpate the patella tendon. On either side there is a soft spot above the palpable tibial plateau. Through this soft spot approximately 2 cm is the knee joint. This entry is not recommended for

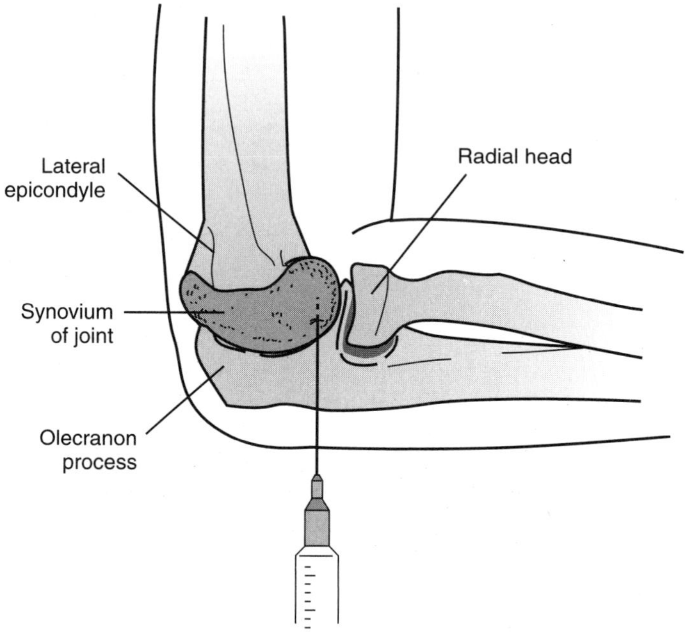

FIG. 11-22. Intraarticular elbow joint injection/aspiration.

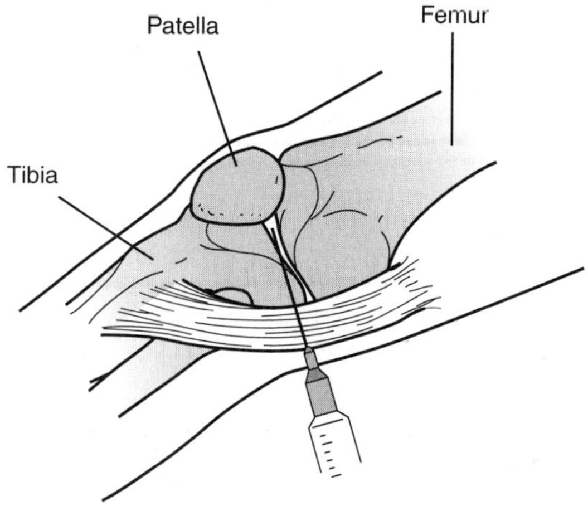

FIG. 11-23. Intraarticular knee joint injection/aspiration.

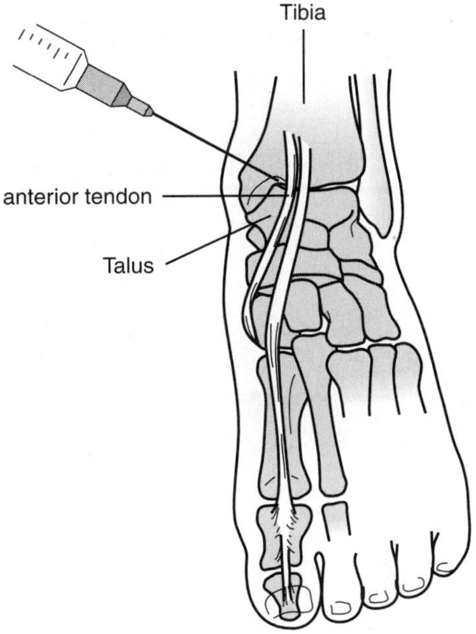

FIG. 11-24. Intraarticular ankle joint injection/aspiration.

injections of steroids because the fat pad is located here and the steroids may cause atrophy.

Ankle (Fig. 11-24)

- The ankle is most easily approached anteriorly.
- The tendon of the tibialis anterior is palpated as it crosses the ankle joint medially.
- With the foot in slight plantar flexion, place the needle lateral to the tendon.
- If bone is encountered, the ankle is dorsiflexed and plantar flexed. If the needle moves, it is in the talus; if not, it is in the tibia.
- If the needle is too medial, the interval narrows, making it more difficult to enter the joint. If the needle is too lateral, the neurovascular structures are at risk.
- The joint should be no more than 2 cm deep.

Toe (Fig. 11-25)

- The interphalangeal and the metatarsal phalangeal joints should be entered straight laterally to avoid neurovascular and tendinous structures.
- The joint is palpated and entered.
- If bone is encountered, redirect the needle.
- The joint should be no more than 1 cm deep.

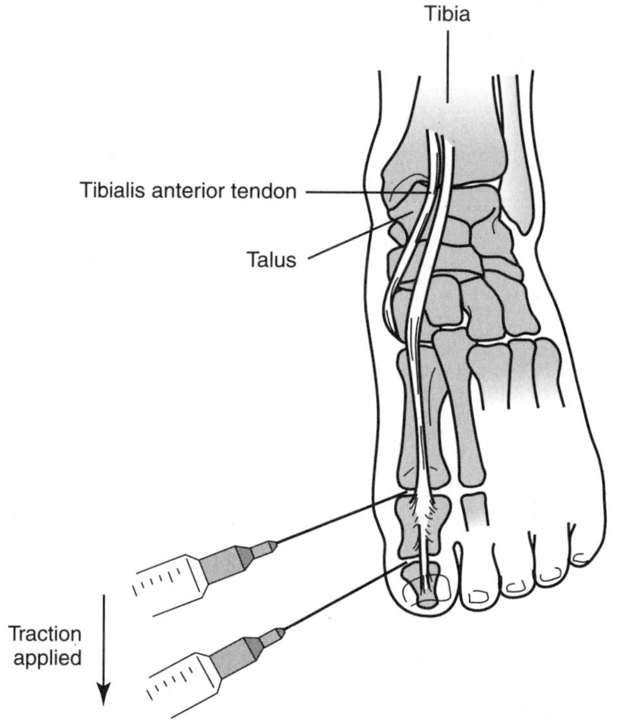

FIG. 11-25. Intraarticular finger/toe joint injection/aspiration.

SPECIAL PROCEDURES

Ring Removal

- Rings must be removed from any injured extremity in which significant swelling may be expected to occur. For example, a shoulder injury may cause hand swelling and, therefore, all rings must be removed before any immobilization.
- Occasionally, the amount of swelling in the digits exceeds the circumference of the ring, and despite the best efforts the ring will not come off.
- Similarly, the digit itself may be injured, thereby making it impossible to remove the ring directly.
- A ring cutter may be used to cut the ring in one or two places, and the pieces are removed.
- Another option is to perform the "string trick," in which a piece of string (or umbilical tape) is placed under the ring and then wrapped very tightly distally toward the tip of the finger, acting as a compressive finger tourniquet so that the ring can be pulled off over top of it (Fig. 11-26).

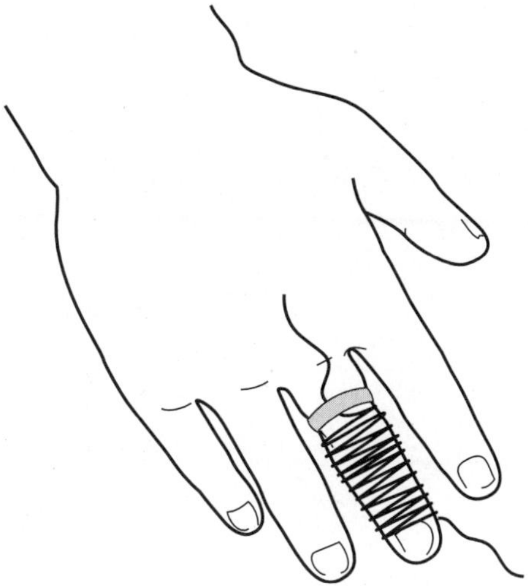

FIG. 11-26. String technique for removing rings.

Subungual Hematoma

- Occasionally, when a closed nailbed injury occurs, such as is seen with a crushing force (e.g., from being caught in a car door), a hematoma may develop between the nailbed and the nail plate (subungual hematoma).
- The pressure of this evolving hematoma often causes considerable pain, and there is an additional, smaller risk of infection (infected hematoma); therefore the subungual hematoma should be decompressed.
- A sterile preparation and tetanus prophylaxis are required. Antibiotics are reserved for associated open wounds.
- A simple and inexpensive method involves the use of a 20- or 22-gauge hypodermic needle.
- After sterile preparation of the nail, a drilling motion is applied to the nail overlying the hematoma. When the needle penetrates into the subungual space, the hematoma is decompressed.
- Another method involves the use of a handheld, disposable electrocautery device to burn a hole through the nail plate. This technique is quick and easy, does not require applying any pressure to an already painful nail, and is much less threatening than a needle to small children.
- In either case, anesthesia is generally not required because decompression results in immediate pain relief.
- A bandage dressing is all that is required because a small amount of continued bloody oozing usually occurs.
- Parents should be warned that nail discoloration will persist for several weeks, until the nail grows out, and that the nail plate may fall off completely. The nail

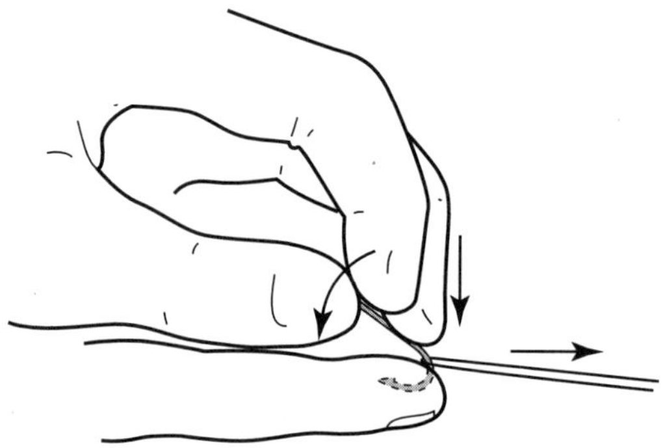

FIG. 11-27. Removal of fishhook using the string technique.

may or may not grow out normally; this depends on the type and amount of crush injury, and only to a lesser extent on whether or not the nail is trephinated.

Fishhook Removal

- Fishhooks that become embedded in the skin are a particular challenge because of the presence of their barbs.
- One manner in which hooks may be removed is by pushing the hook all the way through the skin and then cutting off the distal segment that contains the barb, thus allowing for an atraumatic removal.
- Another method is the "string technique," which uses the pull of a string at the bend of the hook to provide appropriate torque and removal without additional injury (Fig. 11-27).
- Wounds should be thoroughly cleansed and irrigated, and antibiotics should be considered because these objects are often dirty.

Hair Tourniquet Removal

- Hair tourniquets may occur on the fingers or toes of infants and are extremely difficult to remove because they often become deeply embedded.
- In general, hair-dissolving creams do not work.
- A better technique is to make a small but complete incision all the way down to and through the skin in the area in which the hair is embedded.
- The incision is best done along the midline in the dorsal aspect in order to avoid the neurovascular bundles along the medial and lateral aspects of the digits (Fig. 11-28).

Care of Amputated Segments

- Amputated parts should be wrapped in sterile gauze moistened with saline, placed into a bag, and the bag placed on ice.

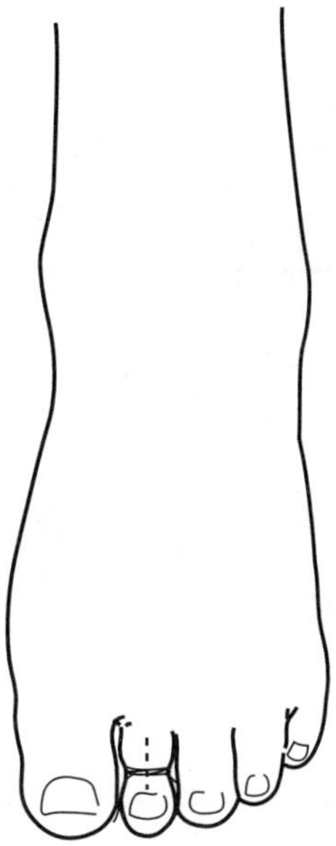

FIG. 11-28. Removal of hair tourniquet.

- The remaining stump should be dressed with sterile dressings that are moistened with saline.

SUGGESTED READINGS

Baker DG, Schumacher HR Jr: Acute monoarthritis, *N Engl J Med* 329:1013, 1993.

Barnett RC: Removal of fishhooks, *J Hosp Med* 70:56, 1980.

Cohen MS, Hastings H: Acute elbow dislocation: evaluation and management, *J Am Acad Ortho Surg* 6:15, 1998.

Curran C et al: Pediatric cervical-spine immobilization: achieving neutral position? *J Trauma* 39:729, 1995.

Hendey GW: Necessity of radiographs in the emergency department management of shoulder dislocations, *Ann Emerg Med* 36:108, 2000.

Huerta C, Griffith R, Joyce SM: Cervical spine stabilization in pediatric patients: evaluation of current techniques, *Ann Emerg Med* 16:1121, 1987.

Lipp EJ: Athletic physeal injury in children and adolescents, *Ortho Nurs* 17:17, 1998.

Macias CG, Wiebe R, Bothner J: History and radiographic findings associated with clinically suspected radial head subluxations, *Pediatr Emerg Care* 16:22, 2000.

Macias CG, Wiebe R, Bothner J: A comparison of supination/flexion to hyperpronation in the reduction of radial head subluxations, *Pediatrics* 102:e10, 1998.

Maffulli N, Baxter-Jones AD: Common skeletal injuries in young athletes, *Sports Med* 19:137, 1995.

Noonan KJ, Price CT: Forearm and distal radius fractures in children, *J Am Acad Ortho Surg* 6:146, 1998.

Nypaver M, Treloar D: Neutral cervical spine positioning in children, *Ann Emerg Med* 23:208, 1994.

Pang D, Wilberger JE Jr: Spinal cord injury without radiographic abnormalities in children, *J Neurosurg* 57:114, 1982.

Pfenninger JL: Injections of joints and soft tissue: part II. Guidelines for specific joints, *Am Fam Physician* 44:1690, 1991.

Rettig ME et al: Wrist fractures in the athlete. Distal radius and carpal fractures, *Clin Sports Med* 17:469, 1998.

Wall EJ: Practical primary pediatric orthopedics, *Nurs Clin North Am* 35:95, 2000.

Woodward TW, Best TW: The painful shoulder: part I. Clinical evaluation, *Am Fam Physician* 61:3079, 2000.

CHAPTER 12

Minor Ophthalmic Procedures

Robin R. Hemphill
Sally A. Santen

INTRODUCTION

- When patients present with complaints related to the eye, practitioners often focus on the abnormality, but it is important to perform a complete eye examination before making a final disposition.
- If possible, the examination should be performed at the beginning of the encounter. If pain or injury prevent this, it may be appropriate to wait until the patient has been provided with adequate analgesia.
- The eye examination for children is performed in essentially the same manner as for adults. Some modifications may be necessary, however, for the infant or young child.
- The best examination of the child is often observation while playing. Note if the child looks directly at objects, turns the head to view out of one eye, or covers eyes because of photophobia.
- Using the parents to assist in the examination is also often helpful. They may hold or distract the child during the examination, or they may assist by covering one of the eyes. This allows the child to trust the practitioner and the practitioner to complete an initial examination.

RELEVANT ANATOMY

Eye and Eyelids (Fig. 12-1)

- The eyelids are specialized folds of tissue that protect the eye from trauma and excessive light. The upper lid is more mobile than the lower, and they meet each other at the medial and lateral angles. The outermost layer of the eyelid is skin, composed of keritinized epidermis with little subcutaneous tissue. This is the thinnest skin of the body. Below this thin layer of skin is a striated muscle layer called the *orbicularis oculi.* The third layer of the eyelid is the *tarsus,* which is a dense fibrous tissue that gives the eyelid rigidity. The meibomian glands are located within the tarsus and produce an oily secretion onto the margin of the lid. The innermost layer of the eyelid is the *palpebral conjunctiva.*

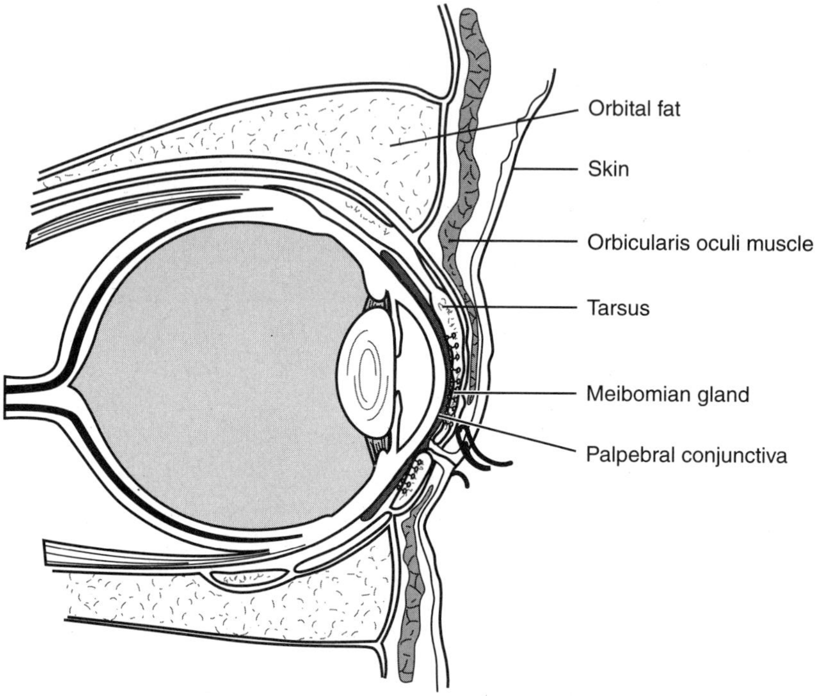

FIG. 12-1. Anatomy of the eye and eyelid.

- The eyelashes are present at the free edges of the eyelids. They are arranged in double and triple rows at the mucocutaneous junction. The sebaceous glands open directly into the eyelash follicles. Inflammation of the glands creates a hordeolum. The ciliary glands are modified sweat glands that open separately between each adjacent lash.
- The eye itself is embedded in orbital fat but is separated from this fat by the fascial sheath of the eyeball. The cornea is the clear, dome-shaped structure that extends across the anterior one fifth of the globe. The center of the cornea is about one half as thick as the peripheral portion. Within the cornea are sensory nerve endings but no blood vessels. This lack of vascularity and the regular arrangement of collagen fibrils renders the cornea transparent. The sclera is the "white" part of the eye. The collagen fibrils of the sclera are irregular and randomly arranged, which gives the sclera greater rigidity and makes it opaque rather than transparent. The sclera is pierced posteriorly by the optic nerve and is fused with the dural sheath of that nerve.
- The junction of the cornea with the sclera is called the *limbus*. This junction is also the transition zone between the corneal and conjunctival epithelium. The conjunctiva is a mucous membrane that covers the sclera and inner eyelids. Other structures lie nasally. The plica semilunaris is a conjunctival fold that is the

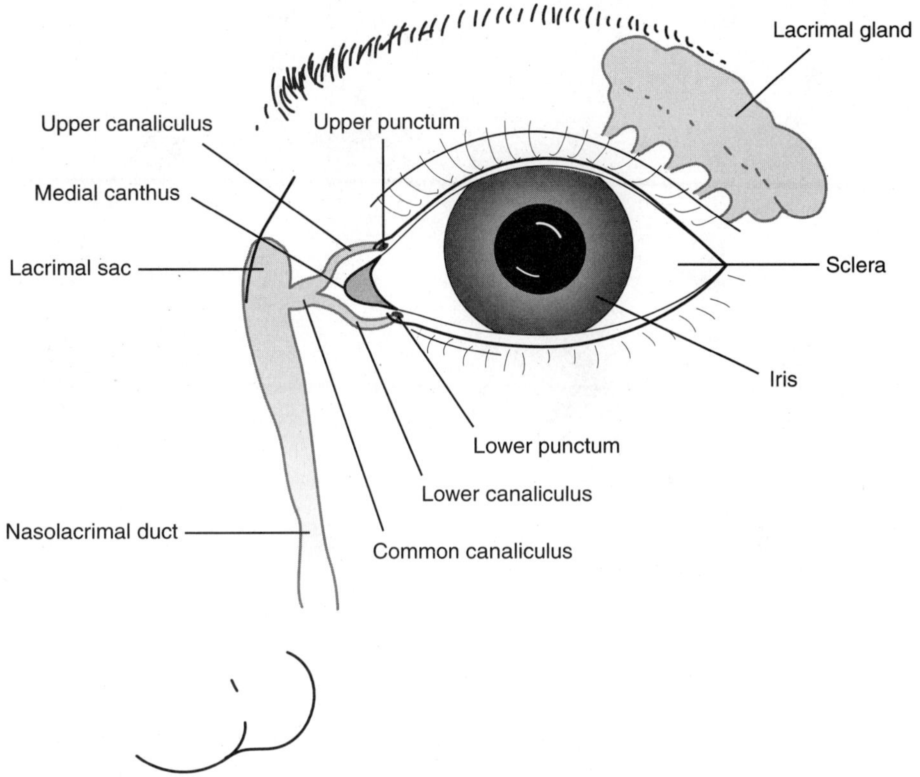

FIG. 12-2. Eye and lacrimal apparatus.

vestigial remnant of the nictitating membrane seen in lower animals. Just next to this structure is the caruncle, which is derived from a part of the lower eyelid and which contains hair and accessory lacrimal, sebaceous, and sweat glands.

The Lacrimal Apparatus (Fig. 12-2)

- The lacrimal gland is located at the anterior lateral portion of the orbit. The secretory ducts of the lacrimal gland empty into the superior conjunctival fornix. Tears pass down over the bulbar and palpebral conjunctiva. They then drain through the puncta of the eyelids that are located close to the medial canthus of the eye. Each of the punctum leads to a canaliculus that finally drains into the lacrimal sac.

Eye Chambers (Fig. 12-3)

- The anterior chamber is the area between the cornea and the anterior surface of the iris. The posterior chamber lies between the posterior surface of the iris and the anterior surface of the lens. Aqueous humor is secreted by the ciliary epithelium within the posterior chamber and passes into the anterior chamber at

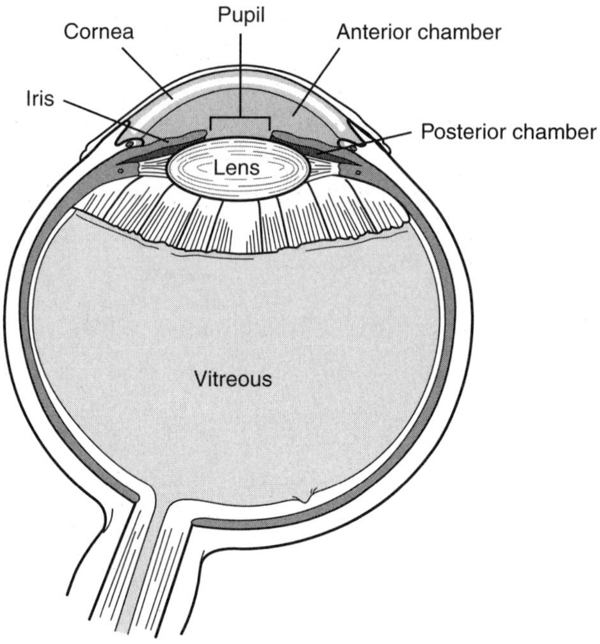

FIG. 12-3. Chambers of the eye.

the pupillary margin. Most of the aqueous humor is then reabsorbed at the anterior chamber angle. The iris controls the amount of light that enters the eye via action of dilator and sphincter muscles. The dilator muscles are innervated by the sympathetic system, and the sphincter muscles are innervated by the parasympathetic fibers of the third cranial nerve. The posterior segment of the eye is the vitreous cavity, retina, and optic disc.

Extraocular Muscles (Figs. 12-4 and 12-5)

- The muscles of the orbit are the levator palpebrae superioris, the four recti, and the two oblique muscles. The levator palpebrae superioris is a flat muscle that attaches to the superior tarsal plate and into the skin of the upper eyelid via two lamellae. This muscle receives innervation from the oculomotor nerve (CN3), but the smooth muscle fibers are innervated by sympathetic nerves from the superior cervical sympathetic ganglion. The levator muscle raises the upper eyelid.
- Four recti muscles act along with the two oblique muscles to give precise and coordinated control to eye movement. The four recti muscles share a common origin at the tendinous ring. As the muscles pass forward, the ring becomes wider and diverges from its neighbor. The tendon of each muscle pierces the fascial sheath of the eyeball and is inserted into the sclera. The superior, inferior, and medial recti are supplied by the oculomotor nerve (CN3), whereas the lateral rectus is supplied by the abducens nerve (CN6).

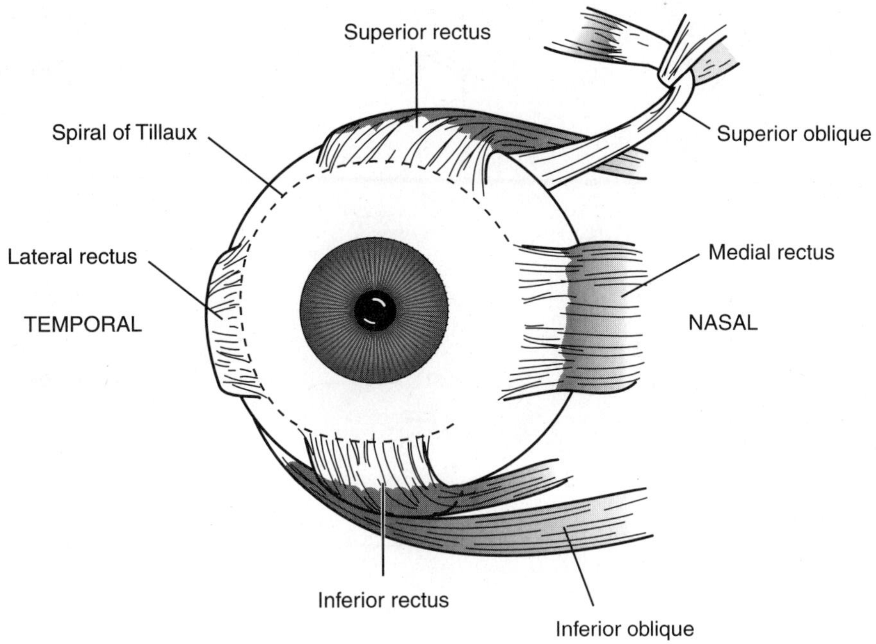

FIG. 12-4. Extraocular muscle attachments.

- The lateral rectus rotates the eyeball so that the cornea looks laterally, whereas the medial rectus rotates the eyeball so that the cornea looks medially. The superior and inferior recti are inserted on the medial side of the vertical axis of the eyeball. Therefore they not only raise and depress the cornea, but they also rotate in medially as well. For the superior rectus muscle to raise the cornea directly upward, the inferior oblique muscle must help. A similar principle holds true for direct downward motion of the cornea.
- The superior oblique muscle inserts into the sclera beneath the superior rectus muscle and is supplied by the trochlear nerve (CN4). The superior oblique muscle rotates the eyeball so that the cornea looks downward and laterally. The inferior oblique muscle is supplied by the oculomotor nerve and rotates the eyeball so that the cornea looks upward and laterally.

EXAMINATION

Visual Acuity

- Visual acuity is a simple, rapid test that should be performed on *all* patients presenting with eye or visual complaints. This single test can provide information about the status of the cornea, lens, and vitreous, which constitute the ocular media. Given the amount of information obtained by this single test, it should be considered the "vital sign" of the eye. Visual acuity is traditionally

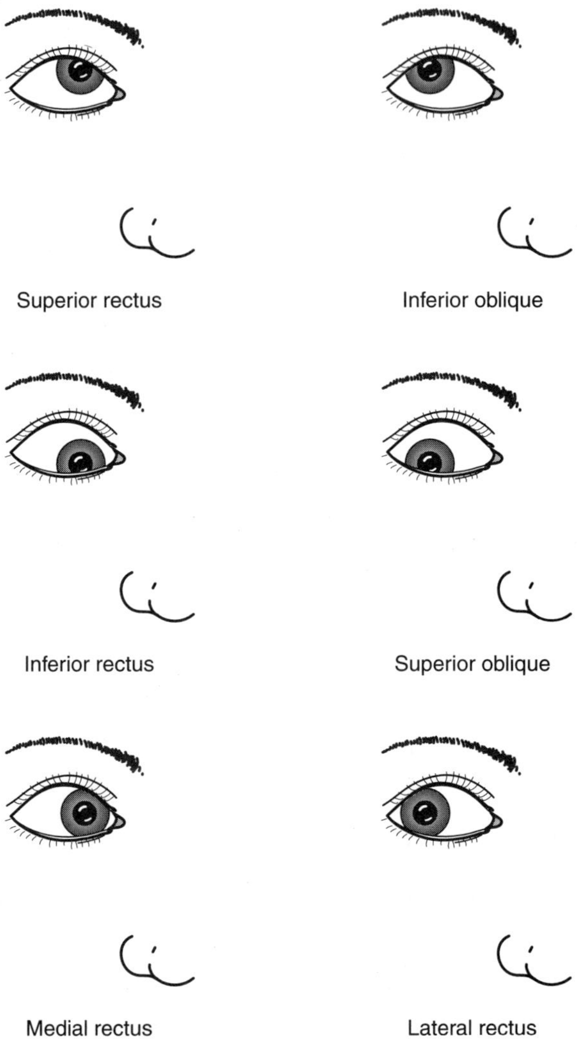

FIG. 12-5. Movements of the eye as controlled by each muscle.

measured at 20 feet and is expressed as a ratio of the patients' acuity as compared to that of a "normal" person. Acuity is commonly assessed with the Snellen chart, the illiterate E chart (i.e., patient indicates the direction of the letter E), or Allen cards of objects for young children who cannot yet read (Figs. 12-6 and 12-7). For injured or ill children, it may not be possible to have them stand, in which case a commercially available near card can be used. Although not as accurate as the Snellen chart, these cards allow a gross estimation of eyesight.

- "Twenty-twenty" (20/20) is considered normal vision, although 20/10 acuity is common; "twenty-forty" (20/40) means that the patient sees at 20 feet what the

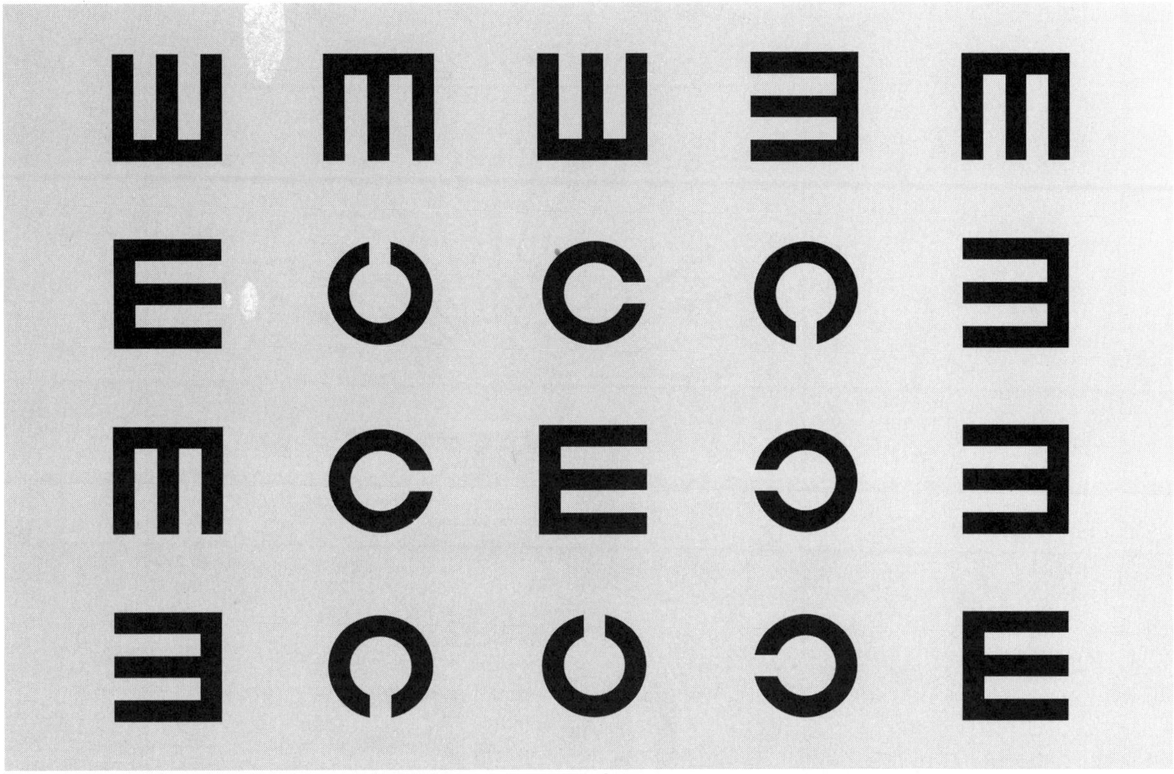

FIG. 12-6. Tumbling "E" and Landolt "C" illiterate eye chart.

"normal" person sees at 40 feet. If visual acuity is less than 20/200, move the patient closer to the chart and record the number of feet between the patient and the chart as the numerator at which he or she sees the largest letter, with the denominator remaining 200 (e.g., 5/200).

- This test should be done using the patient's glasses; however, use of pinhole testing usually corrects refractive error to at least 20/30 if the patient does not have his or her glasses available and no organic disease is present. Each eye should be tested separately, with the unaffected eye being tested first. This technique may help a child become familiar with the process before testing the affected eye.
- If the patient is unable to read the letters on the typical Snellen chart, even at close range, vision may be assessed in more gross terms. For example, documentation can be made of the patient's ability to count fingers at a certain distance. If vision is even worse than this, the chart should reflect whether the patient is able to see hand motion, light perception, or no light perception. When quantitative acuity is not possible, such as in a preverbal infant, attempts should be made to evaluate a preference for either eye and response of the infant to movements, lights, and so on.

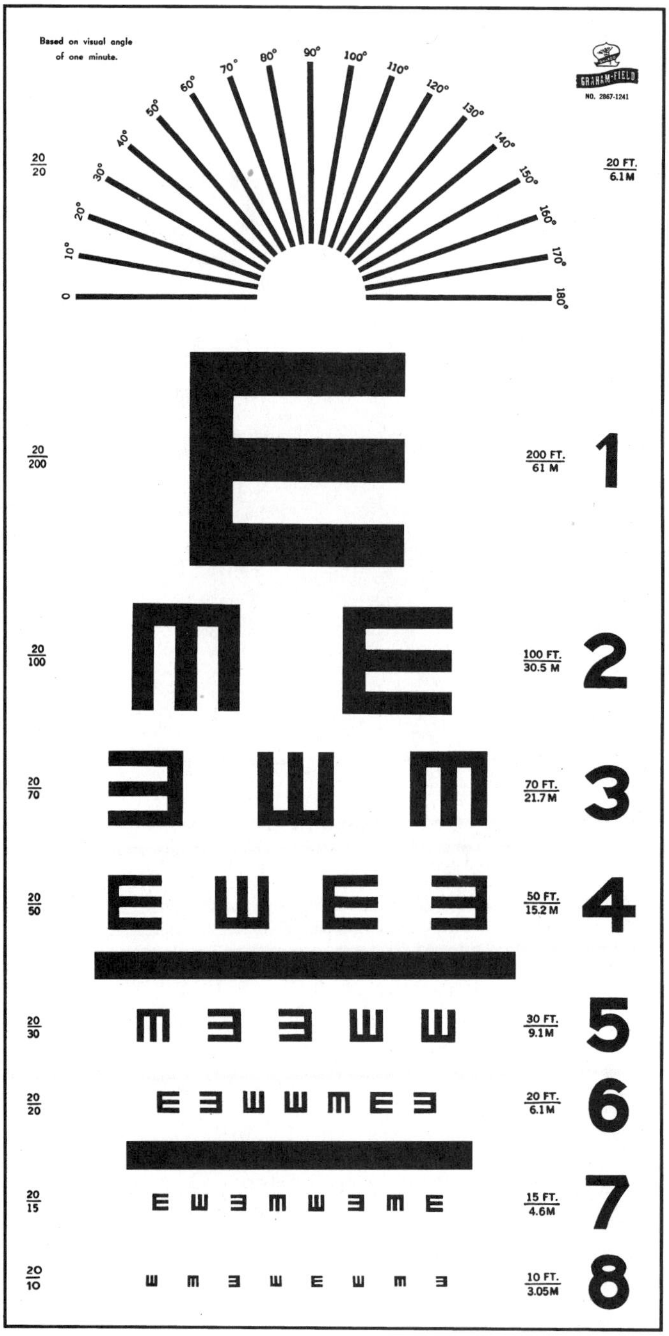

FIG. 12-7. Snellen visual acuity chart.

- Visual acuity is slow to develop and difficult to test in infants and young children. Visual acuity for neonates consists of eye contact and following the practitioner's face. Neonates see best at an arm's length (a fixed focal length). Testing is best performed by holding the neonate at arm's length and moving your face in front of the child for tracking. Repeat the examination with each eye covered. Vision can also be documented from birth through optokinetic nystagmus using alternating black and white bands.
- By 3 months of age, infants should focus on the practitioner's mouth and eyes and should be able to see colors. Visual acuity and field testing may be tested by covering one eye while moving a toy, light, or colored object in from the periphery. At 1 year of age, children have half the visual acuity of adults, and at 3 years of age, they usually have a visual acuity score (VAS) of 20/30. By 6 years of age, visual acuity should be normal.

Pupil Examination

- The pupil examination is another critical test, and the pupil shape, size, and reactions should be noted. This part of the examination is critical because it yields information about the anterior visual pathways and the afferent and efferent limbs of the pupillary reflex arc (Fig. 12-8).

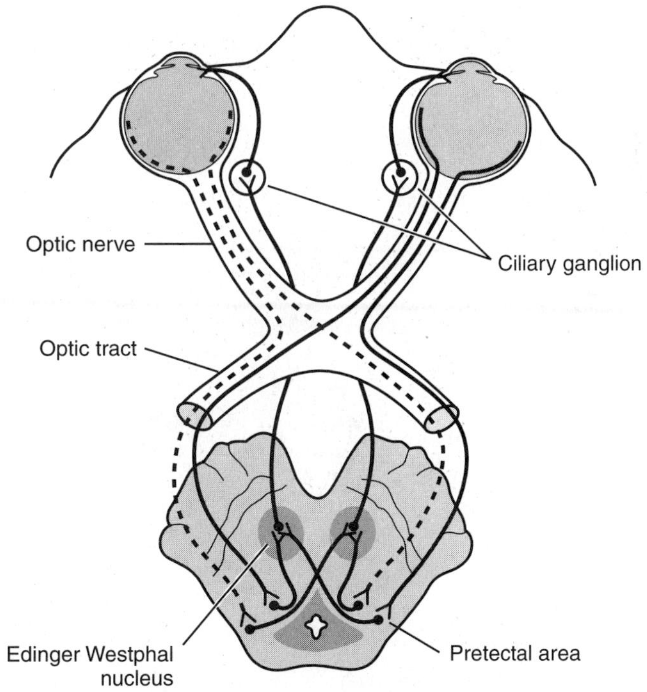

FIG. 12-8. Pupil response pathway.

- The patient's pupils should be round and change in size in response to direct and consensual light. In physiologic anisocoria, both pupils change in response to a change in the lighting conditions, but one is always smaller than the other. If one pupil does not change at all in response to different lighting conditions, this finding should be considered abnormal.
- The pupils should then be noted for both direct and indirect response to light. The swinging flashlight test provides information about a relative afferent pupillary defect or Marcus Gunn pupil. This test is performed by slowly swinging the light from one eye to the other, observing the direct response of each eye. A normal response is for the pupils to constrict at the same rate and extent. If one pupil constricts but the other does not, or if the other eye dilates slightly, then an afferent pathway defect is present in the eye that did not respond (Fig. 12-9). Finally, the pupils should be assessed for accommodative

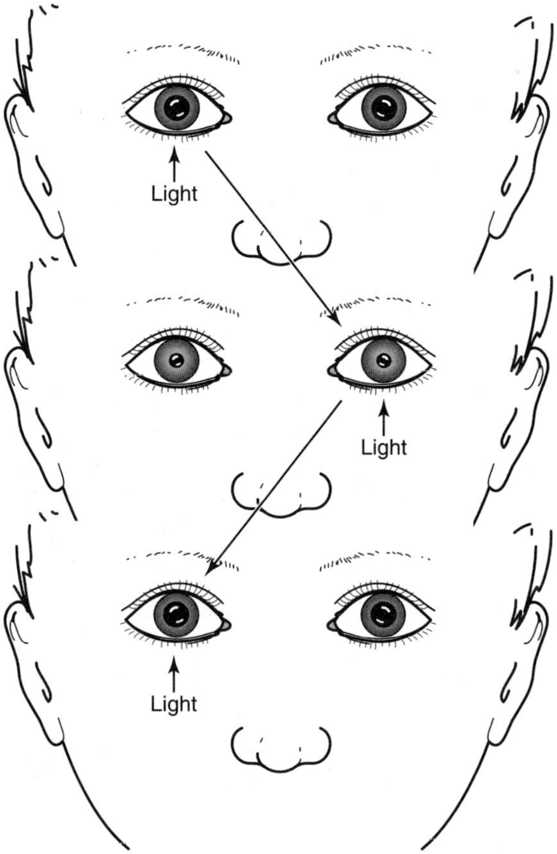

FIG. 12-9. Swinging flashlight test. Right optic nerve lesion causes right pupil to dilate as light is swung to right side.

response, keeping in mind that neonates do not have the ability to accommodate.

- In young patients, pupillary response and demonstration of a red reflex (from the choroid plexus) are also tested. Using the ophthalmoscope at the widest setting (or another light source), shine the light into the child's eyes from about 1 foot away. Equal red reflexes and corneal light reflexes should be observed. Abnormal red reflex indicates an obstruction such as opacified cornea, cataract, or retinoblastoma.

Ocular Motility and Alignment

- The patient should be able to move the eye through all six cardinal gaze positions. In children, this ability is tested by asking the child to look in different directions. In young children and infants, use a toy, the parent, or a light to stimulate the child to look in each direction. An infant can be held at arm's length and turned; the infant should move his or her eyes to stay fixed on the practitioner's face. Ocular motility is difficult to test in infants because eye movements may be disconjugate with esotropia or exotropia during the first 3 months. The eyes should remain parallel in all positions. If a patient cannot move the eyes through all positions, the muscle causing the dysfunction should be noted.

Visual Field Testing

- Confrontational field testing can be performed quickly in the emergency department and should be done on all patients with visual complaints (Fig. 12-10).

SPECIFIC PROCEDURES

Manual Lid Opening and Instillation of Medications

Indications

- This technique is useful in young children who are unable to comply with the need to keep their eyes open for the examination.
- Other indications are the need to place topical medications for pain control, to facilitate the eye examination, or to treat certain conditions.

Contraindications and indications for referral

- Open globe

Supplies and equipment

- Gauze pads (4 × 4) may facilitate the procedure when the child is crying or has moist skin.
- Cotton-tipped applicators, if this method is desired.

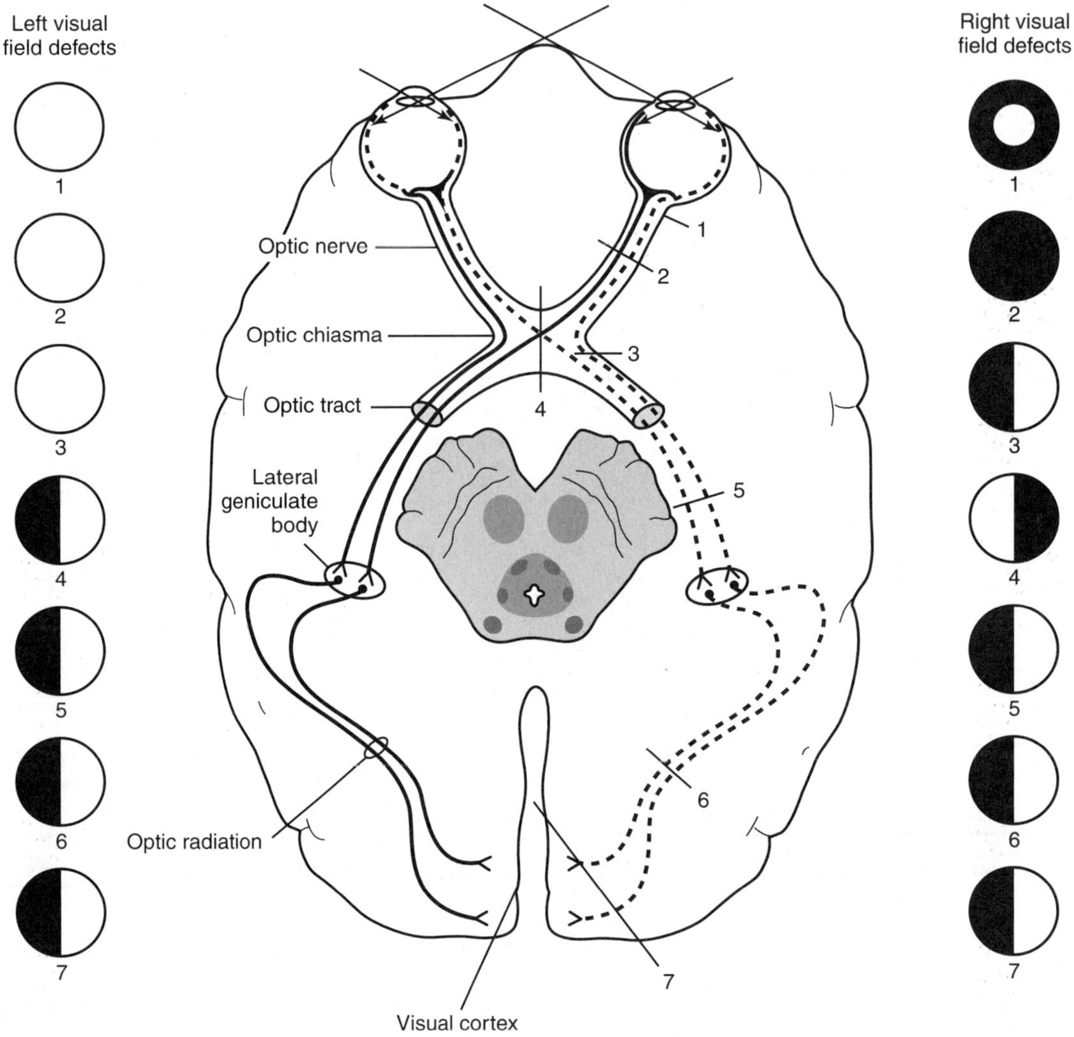

1. Right-sided circumferential blindness due to retrobulbar neuritis.
2. Total blindness of right eye due to division of right optic nerve.
3. Right nasal hemianopia due to partial lesion of right side of optic chiasma.
4. Bitemporal hemianopia due to complete lesion of optic chiasma.
5. Left temporal hemianopia and right nasal hemianopia due to lesion of right optic tract.
6. Left temporal and right nasal hemianopia due to lesion of right optic radiation.
7. Left temporal and right nasal hemianopia due to lesion of right visual cortex.

FIG. 12-10. Visual field defects.

Required nursing skills for procedure

- An assistant is helpful to hold either the child or the eyelids open as medication is applied.

Patient and family preparation and education

- The family should be informed about the need for examination and the placement of any medications. The parents should be made aware that the child may express discomfort.
- If the practitioner anticipates that the parents will need to apply medications to the child at home, it is helpful for them to observe and participate in this procedure.

Manual Lid Opening

1. Place infants in the lap of a seated parent or assistant, with the head directed toward the practitioner (Fig. 12-11) and gently restrained by the parent.
2. Using both thumbs, place pressure on the underlying skin while moving the thumbs in opposite directions. This technique should drag the lids apart, allowing examination (Fig. 12-12). The thumbs should not be placed on the eyelids; rather, they are placed on the tissues above the eyelids.
3. For extremely uncooperative children, place the child in a supine position while the head is held. A drop may then be placed in the medial canthus. When the child opens the eye to blink, the drop will flow into the eye.

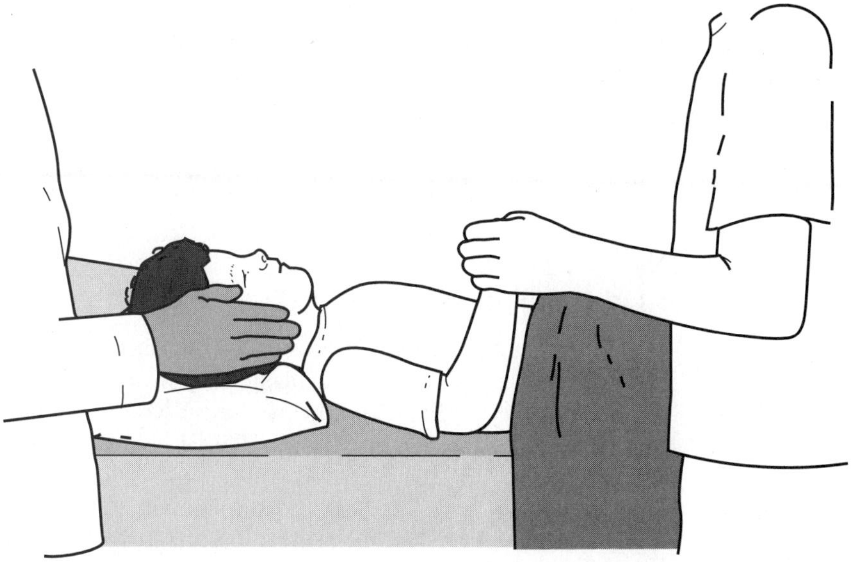

FIG. 12-11. Pediatric positioning for eye examination.

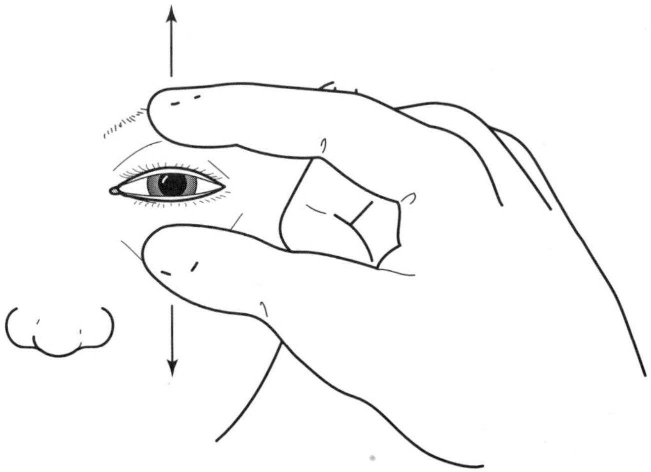

FIG. 12-12. Manual eye opening.

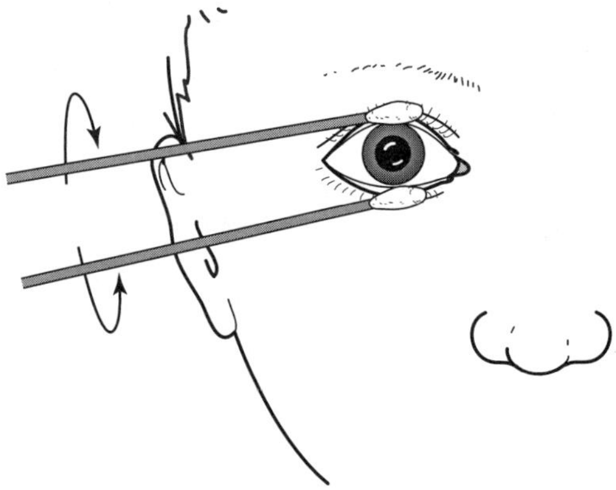

FIG. 12-13. Cotton-tipped applicators to open eyelids.

Lid Opening with Cotton-Tipped Swabs

1. Place the tip of one cotton swab applicator at the middle of the upper lid and another applicator in a similar position on the lower lid (Fig. 12-13). If long, wooden-tipped applicators are used, hold them with the fingers close to the tip to allow better control. The handles of the two applicators should be parallel to each other.
2. Rotate the applicators in the direction that begins to pull the eyelids open, while just enough force is used to engage the skin. The tips may be dampened with water to help with traction.

Aftercare Instructions

- If the patient requires medication application for a problem related to the eye, it is possible to teach the family how to perform the manual lid opening technique at home. It is helpful to watch the family attempt the procedure once after instruction.
- For extremely uncooperative children, parents may be instructed to place the eye drop in medial canthus as described previously. When the child opens the eye to blink, the drop will flow into the eye.

Lid Eversion

Indications

- Eversion of the lid is indicated when the practitioner needs to examine the palpebral conjunctiva of the upper lid and when more of the bulbar conjunctiva requires examination.
- Lid eversion allows better lavage after chemical injury and facilitates examination for foreign bodies adherent to the palpebral conjunctiva or physical findings specific to certain types of conjunctivitis.

Contraindications and indications for referral

- Open globe

Supplies and equipment

- Cotton-tipped applicator to facilitate the procedure.
- Handheld magnifier is useful, but not mandatory, to ensure that small foreign bodies are not missed.
- Topical anesthetic may facilitate the examination if the patient is very uncomfortable.
- Have equipment present to complete a foreign body removal if this is suspected (see following procedure).

Eversion of the Upper Eyelid (Fig. 12-14)

1. For cooperative patients, instruct them to look toward their feet.
2. Place the cotton-tipped applicator in the middle of the lid at the lid crease. This is the approximate position of the top of the tarsal plate. By applying pressure at this point, a fulcrum is created, which allows the lower portion of the lid to be rotated upward, thus folding the lid back on itself.
3. Place gentle pressure on the lid, and rotate the cotton-tipped applicator toward the lid margin, which will cause the lid margin and lashes to rotate away from the eye surface.
4. Grasp the eyelashes between your thumb and index finger.
5. Gently pull the eyelid out and upward (toward the forehead), while gently pushing the applicator downward. The palpebral conjunctiva will now be visible.

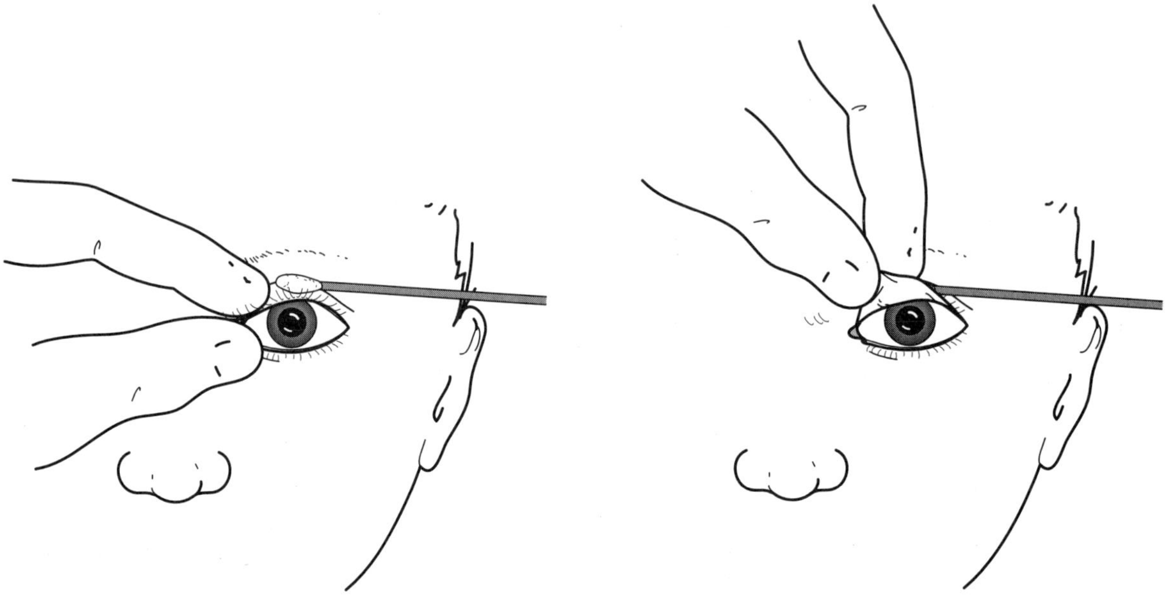

FIG. 12-14. Eyelid eversion.

6. Use the thumb of the hand that was holding the lashes to hold the lashes against the upper orbital rim to keep the eyelid in this position.
7. Remove the cotton-tipped applicator by gently pulling laterally away from the face.

Eversion of the Lower Eyelid

- The palpebral conjunctiva of the lower lid may be seen by placing the index finger near the margin of the lower lid and pushing downward and toward the back of the head.
- It is helpful to have the child look up during the examination.

Foreign Body Removal

Indications

- The presence of an extraocular foreign body mandates an attempt at removal.
- Although simple corneal abrasions may give patients a foreign body sensation, when the patient complains of this feeling, or if a young child presents with apparent eye irritation, a foreign body should be assumed.
- In uncomplicated cases, foreign body removal should be accomplished as soon as possible to prevent epithelialization over the foreign body or the formation of a rust ring if the foreign body is metallic.

Contraindications and indications for referral

- It is important not to create additional injury by aggressive examination or foreign body removal in an uncooperative child. Extremely uncooperative patients (young children) may require referral for removal with sedation.
- Complicated injuries involving multiple foreign bodies, an embedded foreign body, foreign bodies with coexistent infection, metal objects that have already been imbedded long enough to have formed a rust ring, or possible globe penetration require referral.
- If unsuccessful attempts have been made at foreign body removal, the patient should be referred.

Supplies and equipment

- Antibiotic ointment or solution
- Eye patches (2)
- Fluorescein strips
- Intravenous (IV) catheter (18- or 20-gauge)
- IV tubing
- Isotonic fluid for irrigation such as sterile normal saline
- Light source to facilitate examination
- Magnifier
- Needle (25- or 27-gauge)
- Sterile cotton-tipped applicators
- Syringe (1, 3, or 5 ml)
- Tape
- Topical anesthetic
- Wood's lamp
- Optional: slit lamp (nice to have but not present in most private offices), spud (blunt-tipped instrument), burr for removal of rust rings (if comfortable with this procedure)

Patient and family preparation and education

- For small children who are found to have a foreign body that appears easily removable (mobile or imbedded under an eyelid), inform the parents that the eye will be anesthetized, the child will be held by nursing assistants, and that an attempt will be made to remove the object. The eye will then be assessed for damage resulting from the foreign body.
- For those patients who are older and more cooperative, more detailed information about the procedure and what they can do to facilitate the process can be explained to both patients and parents.
- Let the patient know that the eye will be numbed during the examination.
- The patient and family should know that if attempts to remove the foreign body are unsuccessful, referral may be necessary. Even when removal is successful, subsequent findings of the examination may require follow-up or referral.

Preparation

- Obtain visual acuity before manipulating the eye.
- If available, obtain a history of the circumstance surrounding the injury. Objects that fall or blow into the eye are unlikely to result in severe injury to the globe. Metal striking metal or injuries that result from explosive forces may be associated with multiple foreign bodies or globe rupture. Length of symptoms is important to assess for the possibility of infection. Contact lens usage should be noted.
- Pupil size, shape, and reactivity are important because distortion or prolapse of the pupil indicate that a foreign body has penetrated the globe. Diffuse, chemotic hemorrhage of the conjunctiva may also indicate a globe laceration with penetration.
- If no foreign body is initially noted, the entire bulbar conjunctiva should be examined by having the cooperative patient look through the entire range of eye motion. Pain that continues after the application of anesthetic drips may indicate iritis, glaucoma, or another deeper injury.
- If no foreign body is seen at this point, evert the upper and lower lids to evaluate for the foreign body, which may be adherent to the underside of the eyelid.
- Foreign bodies may also be located in the upper fornix of the eye. A wetted cotton-tipped applicator may be swept up into the anesthetized fornix to remove entrapped material.
- If no foreign body is found, a fluorescein examination of the eye should be done.
- Tetanus immunization should be considered if a foreign body or corneal abrasion is found.

Removal of Eyelid Foreign Body

1. Anesthetize the eye.
2. Evert the upper eyelid as described previously.
3. Use a moistened cotton-tipped applicator to gently remove the foreign body from the everted eyelid.
4. Evert the lower lid as described previously and use a cotton-tipped applicator to remove any foreign body.
5. Complete a fluorescein examination of the eye to assess for conjunctival injury secondary to the foreign body.

Removal of Corneal Foreign Body

The examination and foreign body removal is best done with the aid of a slit lamp, if one is available. Large foreign bodies may be seen without a slit lamp and may be carefully removed as described.

1. Ancsthctize the eye.
2. Instruct patients to keep the head still, and for cooperative patients, have them fix their eyes on an object on the opposite side of the room.

3. Once a foreign body is located, the surrounding cornea should be inspected for edema, infiltration, abrasions, or rust ring using a magnifier.
4. If the foreign object is small and superficial, and the patient is a small infant or child who cannot cooperate with the procedure, the foreign body may be flushed from the eye using a syringe and saline or IV fluid, tubing, and an IV catheter. If this procedure is unsuccessful, and the child cannot cooperate, referral may have to be made for removal under sedation.
5. Embedded foreign bodies are best removed with a commercial spud, or with the use of a 25- or 27-gauge needle attached to a small syringe.
6. If a slit lamp is used, have patients press their forehead firmly against the slit lamp frame. If this is not available, position patients so that the conjunctiva is easy to reach, and have an assistant gently hold the patients' head.
7. Using the sterile needle attached to a syringe, approach the object from a direction tangential to the eyeball. Aim the needle bevel away from the eye (Fig. 12-15). Hold the syringe handle like a pencil.
8. Rest your hand on the patient's zygoma to help steady the hand. If the slit lamp is being used, rest the arm on the slit lamp table. The needle is brought into focus while close to the eye, then under direct examination, the foreign object is approached.
9. Use the needle tip to gently lift the object off the cornea. A spud may be substituted and is used in a similar manner.
10. If a rust ring (iron staining of the surrounding corneal epithelium) is present, it can sometimes be lifted off the eye using the needle technique. A burr is a device designed specifically for rust ring removal. It has a small, rotating head to "drill" out the rust ring. This should only be done for superficial rust rings. Deeply stained corneal rust rings should be referred. Alternatively, the iron of the rust ring may be left in place for 24 to 48 hours. During this time, the iron will kill the surrounding epithelial cells. At the end of this period, the rust ring is usually soft and can be lifted out in one solid plug. This technique can be attempted in the physician's office, or the patient can be referred to the ophthalmologist.
11. If, after several attempts, the foreign body or rust ring is still present, the patient should be referred.
12. After the foreign body is removed, the patient's vision should be tested again

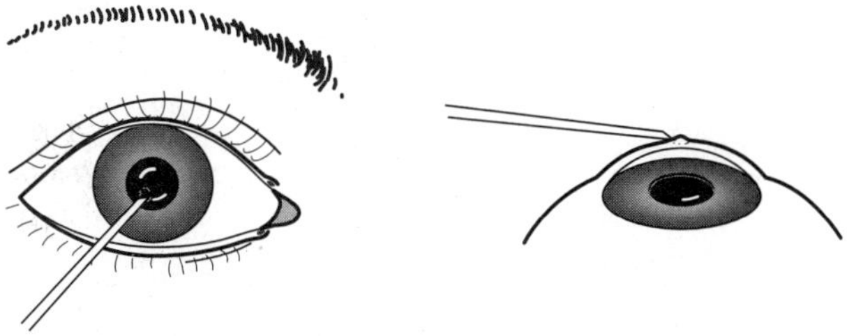

FIG. 12-15. Removal of foreign body.

and examined with fluorescein (see following procedure). It is likely that a corneal abrasion will be present.

Possible complications

- Not considering globe perforation in the patient with pertinent history
- Epithelial injury during removal
- Infection, usually introduced by patient rubbing the eye
- Scarring with vision defect if the foreign body is in the visual axis
- Perforation of the globe or cornea (rare)
- Unsuccessful or incomplete removal of the foreign body
- Incomplete healing because of retained rust ring

Modifications

- Use of the cotton-tipped applicator is controversial because, if used aggressively, it may increase corneal injury; however, if a foreign body is noted, and other materials are not available, it is reasonable to attempt removal of a small foreign body using cotton-tipped applicators.
- If used, the cotton-tipped applicator should be moistened and gently placed on the foreign body to try to lift the foreign body off the eye. Do not rub the swab across the cornea because this action will cause a corneal abrasion.

Irrigation

Indications

- Irrigation of the eye is a critical first step in treating chemical injuries to the eye. It is indicated immediately after exposure and is one of the few times that visual acuity testing should wait until after treatment.
- Significant injury to the eye requires irrigation to begin before the patient is brought to medical care. Parents and emergency medical technicians should be instructed to begin irrigating the eye before transporting the child.
- Irrigation is indicated for all chemical injuries to the eyes.
- Children who have sudden onset of burning, itching, or pain in the eye may have an unknown chemical exposure. Irrigation is indicated.
- Irrigation may also be used to remove small, nonimbedded foreign bodies in children's eyes.

Contraindications and indications for referral

- A perforating injury to the eye associated with chemical injury should still receive irrigation. It should be done gently in order not to put pressure on the globe.

Supplies and equipment

- Cotton-tipped swabs
- Fluorescein strips
- Gauze pads to help keep the eyes open
- Gloves

- IV tubing
- IV catheter (18- or 20-gauge)
- Papoose board may be necessary
- pH paper
- Sterile irrigating solution (normal saline solution, 500- to 1000-ml bag)
- Topical anesthetic
- Towels, emesis basin, and pail to collect fluid that drains from the eye
- Wood's lamp
- Optional: lids retractors, Morgan therapeutic lens, slit lamp

Required nursing skills for procedure

- An assistant may be necessary to help hold the child's head still even if the child is placed in a papoose board.

Patient and family preparation and education

- Inform parents and older children that rapid irrigation is necessary for chemical injury of the eye.
- Assure the patient that anesthetic is going to be placed in the eye to decrease the pain of the chemical as well as to ensure that the irrigation itself is painless.

Irrigation for foreign body removal

This procedure is most commonly used in young children who cannot cooperate with superficial foreign body removal using a needle, spud, or even a cotton-tipped applicator.

1. Have an assistant hold the child or place the child on a papoose board.
2. Turn the child's head slightly to allow fluid to drain toward the ear and away from the unaffected eye.
3. Place a drop of anesthetic in the eye.
4. Using a 500- or 1000-ml bag of sterile saline connected to IV tubing, and with an 18- or 20-gauge IV catheter, gently flush fluid across the eye from the nasal side laterally. This allows the foreign body to flow out of the eye or onto the lateral portion of the conjunctiva or lower eyelid. From this position, the foreign body can usually be safely swept from the eye using a moistened, sterile cotton-tipped applicator.

Irrigation after chemical exposure

1. Have an assistant hold the child or place the child on a papoose board.
2. Turn the child's head slightly to allow fluid to drain toward the ear of the affected eye and away from the unaffected eye.
3. Place towels and an emesis basin around the face and head to collect fluid flowing from the eye.
4. Older children can lie on the examination table with their head just beyond the edge of the table. This position allows irrigation fluid to drip into a pail placed below the head.
5. Place a drop of anesthetic in the eye.

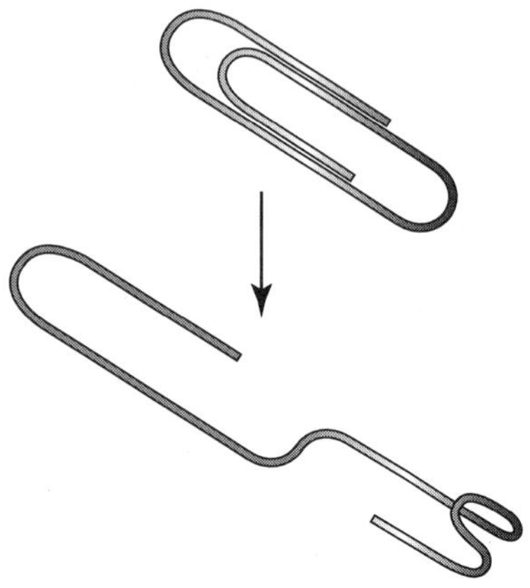

FIG. 12-16. Paper clip formed into eyelid retractor.

6. Using gloved hands to protect the practitioner from chemical injury, hold open the lids as described previously. Because the eyes will become wet and slippery, use gauze pads to get a grip on the slippery skin around the orbit. At times, blepharospasm is so severe that retraction using lid retractors or folded paper clips (Fig. 12-16) is necessary to keep the lids open. Special care should be used to prevent additional injury if paper clips are fashioned into lid retractors.
7. Perform irrigation using a 500- to 1000-ml bag of normal saline connected to IV tubing and an IV catheter (Fig. 12-17).
8. Hold the IV catheter just above the eyeball, allowing the fluid to flow across the eye from medial to lateral. Fluid should also be gently directed into the upper and lower fornices and over the canthi. This flow may be facilitated by everting the eyelids as described previously or by using retractors to hold the eyelids up while irrigation fluid is directed beneath the lids.
9. If one is available, insert a Morgan therapeutic lens into the eye. This device is a soft contact lens with an irrigation hole that extends from the center of the anterior section of the lens. The lens is connected to the bag of saline, thus allowing fluid to flush over and out of the eyeball.
10. Insert the lens by gently separating the eyelids and then placing the lens on the eyeball. The lens should be placed with water slowly dripping to create a water film and to prevent direct contact of the lens with the cornea. Some practitioners recommend that initial flushing be done with the IV catheter because of the possibility that the chemical may collect under the Morgan lens. Once traditional irrigation is done, remaining irrigation may be completed with the Morgan lens. If these lenses are used, the patient will probably require repeat instillation of anesthetic.
11. The duration of irrigation ultimately depends on the exposure. Most exposures require at least 2 liters of fluid over 20 to 30 minutes. Severe alkaline agents, hydrofluoric acid, and heavy metals may require much longer irrigation.

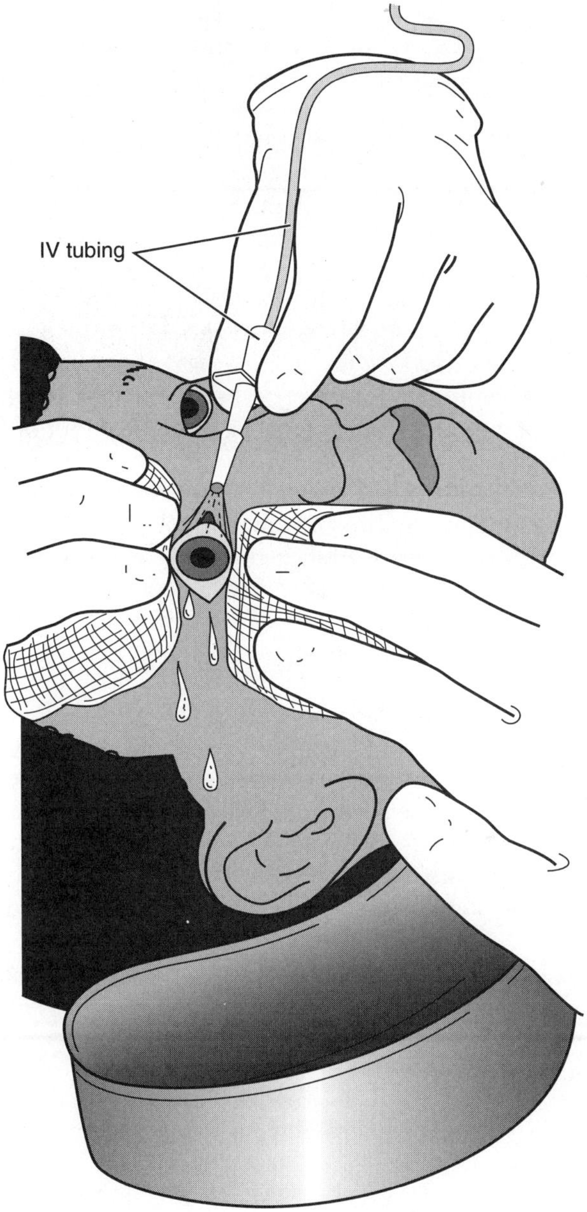

FIG. 12-17. Eye irrigation.

12. After this initial irrigation, evert the upper eyelid and use a moistened cotton-tipped applicator to sweep particulate matter from the upper and then lower fornices (if there is concern that the chemical exposure is particulate).
13. Two liters of irrigation will generally be adequate for minor chemical exposures. To ensure that this initial irrigation is sufficient, wait 10 minutes and then check the pH of the eye with pH paper. The normal pH of the eye is 7.4. The pH indicator on the urine multiindicator sticks can be used for this purpose if no pH paper is present. If the pH is at the extreme end of the indicator, remember that the pH may be higher or lower than the indicator can read. Ideally, the pH should be checked before and after irrigation as long as this does not delay irrigation.
14. Recheck the pH of the eye in 20 minutes if the initial pH was normal. The pH should also be checked in the superior fornix of the eye by double eversion of the eyelid.
15. If the pH begins to change, this indicates inadequate irrigation or retained material (usually within one of the fornices of the eye).
16. After irrigation is complete, check the eye for corneal abrasion or burn using fluorescein. Uptake can be looked for using the Wood's lamp or a slit lamp, if available.
17. Visual acuity should be checked before discharge.

Interpretation of results (if indicated)

- Irrigation is complete when the pH remains at 7.4 for 20 minutes and when no obvious corneal thickening or haziness is present.
- Fluorescein uptake indicates that a corneal abrasion or burn is present.

Possible complications

- Corneal abrasion may occur from attempts to keep the eye open in the uncooperative patient or from the irrigation itself.
- Deep corneal injury is most likely from the chemical agent and requires referral.

Modifications

- It is critical to start eye irrigation early after exposure. If sterile saline is not available, normal tap water flushed across the eyes is appropriate to not delay irrigation.

Hard Contact Lens Removal

If possible, check visual acuity before contact removal. The lens can generally be identified by shining a light on the eye from the side. Several methods are recommended to attempt removal of hard contact lenses. If patients are cooperative, the following series of steps may be taken:

1. Have patients lean slightly forward with their face over a clean cloth.
2. Wear gloves that have been rinsed so no powder is left on them.

3. Place your thumbs on the upper and lower eyelids and pull apart and then bring down the eyelids, trapping the lens between the eyelids.
4. Have patients look toward the nose and then downward. This movement works the lower eyelid under the contact lens, and the motion of the eye works the contact out of the eye.

If patients cannot cooperate or must remain flat, a different technique may be used:

1. Use a drop of anesthetic to minimize discomfort.
2. Place one thumb on the upper eyelid and the other on the lower eyelid near the margin of each lid.
3. With the lens centered over the cornea, gently force the eyelids open until the lid margins are beyond the edges of the lens.
4. Press both eyelids gently down on the eyeball and move the lids downward until they are just touching the upper edges of the contact lens.
5. At this point, place greater pressure on the lower eyelid so that the lid margin works under the contact lens edge.
6. Press the two lids together, and the contact should slip out of the eye and can be grasped.

Other methods of removal:

- The hard contact lens can also be removed using a cotton-tipped applicator. After a drop of anesthetic is placed in the eye, the lens is moved laterally onto the sclera (to prevent accidental corneal abrasion). The tip of the applicator is then gently worked under the side of the contact lens, and the lens is gently removed from the eye.
- The lens can also be removed using a suction cup device, if available. The suction device is moistened and applied directly to the contact lens. This device easily removes the contact with little pressure to the eyelid.
- Once the lens is removed from the eye, it should be stored in a sterile saline solution. If patients have their lens case with them, this may be used. Otherwise, the lens may be placed in a sterile container (urine cup).

Soft Contact Lens Removal

1. Place a drop of anesthetic in the eye for comfort.
2. Identify the lens by shining a light on the eye from the side.
3. Wear gloves that have been rinsed to remove powder.
4. Pull down the lower eyelid using the middle finger. Place the tip of the index finger on the lower edge of the contact lens. Slide the lens down onto the sclera and pinch it between the index finger and thumb of the opposite hand.

The Lost Contact Lens

- Check visual acuity. Decreased acuity below normal suggests that the contact is not properly located on the cornea.
- Anesthetize the eye.

- Soft and hard contact lenses are generally visible on the surface of the eye with a good light source located over the cornea.
- If the contact is not visible, evert the lids as described earlier. If the lens is seen, it may be gently swept out of the eye using a wetted cotton-tipped applicator.
- Even if the lens is not seen, the upper fornix may be gently swept to try to dislodge the lens.
- If the contact is still not visible and the patient still believes that the contact is in the eye, fluorescein may be placed in the eye. This will discolor the soft lens, so the patient must be warned that the contact will be ruined.
- The fluorescein will pool around the outside of the lens, usually making it possible to visualize the contact.
- If the lens is still not found, the patient should be told that it cannot be found and most likely is not present in the eye.
- Fluorescein staining and an examination with a Wood's lamp or slit lamp should be done to evaluate the eye for injury.

Possible complications

- Corneal abrasion may result from contact removal. It can be treated as discussed in a following section.
- Soft contact lenses may be ruined by fluorescein staining.

Eye Cultures

Indications

- Grossly purulent discharge
- Evidence of corneal ulcer

Contraindications and indications for referral

- Corneal ulceration requires urgent referral to an ophthalmologist.

Supplies and equipment

- Bacterial culture media (blood agar, chocolate agar, and Thayer-Martin media)
- Steel spatula or blade
- Sterile applicators (dacron-tipped or calcium alginate-tipped)
- Sterile saline solution
- Topical anesthetic

Specimen collection for conjunctivitis

1. Moisten a Dacron-tipped or calcium alginate–tipped swab with sterile saline before use.
2. Evert the unanesthetized lower lid (see previous discussion on lid eversion) and wipe the swab along the conjunctival surface of the lower lid, avoiding large collections of discharge.
3. Plate the specimen onto a blood or chocolate agar plate and onto Thayer-Martin media if gonococcal conjunctivitis is being considered as the cause of conjunctivitis.
4. Place smear on slide for Gram stain.

5. If a chlamydial test is desired, sample the conjunctival surface of the lower lid as described previously.

Specimen collection for corneal ulcer

This procedure is best performed by an ophthalmologist.

1. Organize culture media and slides.
2. Anesthetize the cornea.
3. Scrape the base of the ulcer with a sterile blade.
4. Inoculate the media and smear onto slides.
5. Send slides to a laboratory for Gram, Giemsa, and fungal stains.

Interpretation of results

- Depending on the results of the Gram stain or culture, treatment may be directed toward a specific organism.
- The Giemsa stain is used to provide information concerning the inflammatory cell type and the presence of cytoplasmic inclusion bodies (chlamydia).
- Gram stain may show Gram-negative intracellular diplococci if gonococcal conjunctivitis is present.
- If corneal ulcer is suspected and Gram stain cannot be immediately obtained, discuss the patient's condition with an ophthalmologist. Treatment may begin with ciprofloxacin drops every hour until the patient can be seen.
- More common organisms are *Staphylococcus aureus, S. epidermidis, Streptococcus pneumoniae,* and *Haemophilus influenza* and may be suspected by the Gram stain.

Possible complications

- Corneal injury may occur during the procedure, particularly the scraping of the base of the corneal ulcer.
- Introduction of infection may occur during the procedure.

Fluorescein Staining

Indications

- Foreign body sensation, photophobia, and pain in the eye
- Red eye or evidence of infection
- Eye trauma
- Known foreign body to the eye
- Eye irritation in a contact lens wearer
- Chemical exposure to the eye that appears mild after irrigation is complete
- Painful eyes after exposure to ultraviolet light
- To help find a lost contact lens
- Neonates or small infants with persistent crying or obvious irritation to an eye

Supplies and equipment

- Cobalt-blue light source (Wood's lamp) or slit lamp (nice to have)
- Isotonic ophthalmic solution for irrigation (normal saline is adequate)

- Light source
- Sterile cotton-tipped applicators
- Sterile fluorescein sodium strips or equivalent
- Topical anesthetic

Patient and family preparation and education

- The family and older children should have the procedure explained to them and should be told that some mild burning may be felt when the fluorescein is first placed in the eye.
- Children should be told that the eye will be yellow for several minutes after the procedure, but this will resolve. Any of the fluorescein that leaks onto the skin may cause staining and be present for a few days.
- Parents should be told that follow-up referral may be necessary depending on the findings of the examination.

Procedure

1. Remove the patient's contacts, if necessary.
2. Position the cooperative child seated or lying in front of the practitioner. Young children may be held in the lap of a parent or an assistant, with the head facing the practitioner. This position will help immobilize the child, and the lids can then be opened as described previously.
3. Place a drop of anesthetic in the eye (if needed to control pain and facilitate the examination).
4. Carefully inspect the eye with a light source, looking at the sclera, iris, the anterior chamber, and the reactivity of both eyes.
5. Have the child lean the head back and look at the ceiling if sitting, or gaze upward if lying down.
6. Wet the orange end of the fluorescein strip with sterile saline, water, or a drop of anesthetic solution.
7. Place the tip of the wetted fluorescein strip gently onto the lower conjunctival sac for a few seconds or against the palpebral conjunctiva of the lower lid. Have patients blink their eyes after the strip is removed.
8. Examine the cornea with the cobalt-blue light source and magnification (Wood's lamp or slit lamp). Those areas of the cornea that are injured will be highlighted by the fluorescein. The entire cornea should be examined.
9. If a defect is found, document the defect with a drawing in the patient's records for comparison to later examinations.

Interpretation of results

- Patients with uptake of fluorescein indicate injury to the cornea. In general, all corneal injuries are best visualized with a slit lamp, if one is available.
- If multiple vertical injuries are found, a foreign body adherent to the upper eyelid should be suspected and the lid everted.
- Dendritic (treelike branching) pattern of uptake indicates a herpes infection and needs immediate referral to an ophthalmologist.
- Corneal ulcers need immediate referral to an ophthalmologist. This should be

suspected if the area of corneal staining has an infiltrate or opacification around the lesion.

- If there appears to be a flowing stream of fluorescein (Seidel's sign), this indicates a leak of aqueous fluid caused by a corneal perforation and open globe. This requires immediate referral to an ophthalmologist.

Modifications

- Examination is best done with a slit lamp; however, if one is not present, it is possible to use a Wood's lamp or any pen light with a blue filter to determine whether the patient has a corneal defect.

Tonometry

Indications

- To investigate eye pain or headache with suspicion of increased ocular pressures.
- Evidence of primary or secondary infantile (congenital) glaucoma; these infants may present with tearing, sensitivity to light, and eyelid squeezing. Corneal enlargement and clouding may be noticeable, but the aforementioned symptoms do not always occur together.
- To measure eye pressures in those patients with history of glaucoma who need follow-up examinations or who have new symptoms.
- After blunt ocular injury, baseline ocular pressure may need to be determined because intraocular pressure may increase after injury. This can be done only if penetrating eye injury has been ruled out.

Contraindications and indications for referral

- Tonometry is relatively contraindicated when eye infection is present unless a device is used that has individual covers (Tono-Pen or noncontact tonometer). The contact portion of any device that does not have a specific cover should be cleaned with alcohol and hydrogen peroxide. Preferably, the device should be sterilized between uses.
- The presence of a corneal defect is a relative contraindication to tonometry.
- Children who cannot hold the eye still cannot have tonometry done and should be referred.
- Tonometry should not be done when globe perforation is suspected.

Supplies and equipment

- Anesthetic drops
- Schiotz tonometer kit (the kit comes with the measurement device, three weights, and a conversion chart), Tono-Pen XL, or Goldman application tonometry on all slit lamps

Patient and family preparation and education

- Because the Schiotz tonometer is somewhat frightening to look at, assure the family and patients that the eye will be anesthetized and the procedure will not be painful.

Procedure

1. Check the visual acuity and complete the relevant eye examination.
2. Assemble the tonometer with the 5.5-gram weight in place and test for accuracy on the test block. If the tonometer does not calibrate to zero on the test block, it should be sent for repair.
3. Place patients in a supine or semirecumbent position.
4. Place a drop of anesthetic in each eye.
5. Instruct patients to keep their eyes wide open and stare at one spot on the ceiling. Encourage patients to relax and hold the eyes very still.
6. Gently hold (or have an assistant help) the upper and lower eyelids apart. The eye should be checked on the side that the practitioner is standing on. To check the other eye, the practitioner should move to the other side (Fig. 12-18).
7. When holding the lids open, be careful not to place additional pressure on the globe because this will increase the ocular pressure.
8. While the eyelids are held open, hold the tonometer by the handles with the thumb and index or middle finger. Lower the tonometer over the cornea until it is gently resting on the cornea. The tonometer should be held perpendicular to the cornea.
9. If the pressure is below 5 units, this indicates a high intraocular pressure.

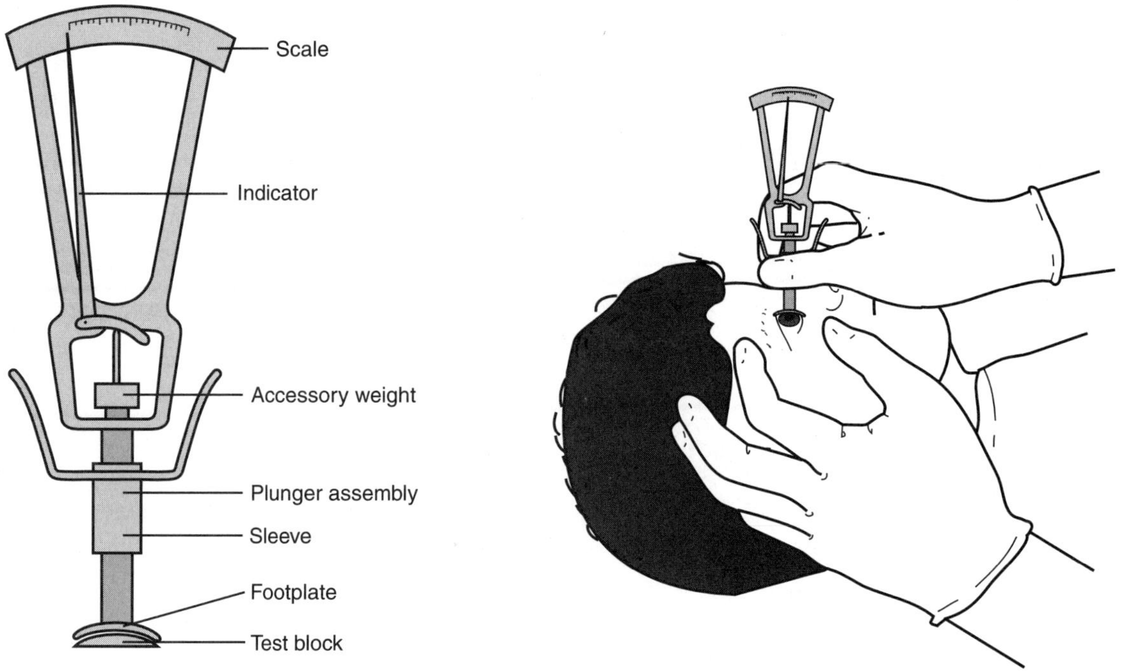

FIG. 12-18. Tonometer and examination with tonometer.

To get a better idea of the exact degree of pressure elevation, remove the tonometer and place the 7.5-unit or 10-unit weight on the tonometer and repeat the procedure.

10. To convert the unit reading to a mm Hg reading of intraocular pressure, use the conversion chart that comes with the Schiotz tonometer (Table 12-1).

TABLE 12-1
Intraocular pressure (mm Hg) by Schiotz tonometry

Tonometer scale reading	Plunger Weight (g)			
	5.5	7.5	10.0	15.0
0.0	41.4	59.1	81.7	127.5
0.5	37.8	54.2	75.1	117.9
1.0	34.5	49.8	69.3	109.3
1.5	31.6	45.8	64.0	101.4
2.0	29.0	42.1	59.1	94.3
2.5	26.6	38.8	54.7	88.0
3.0	24.4	35.8	50.6	81.8
3.5	22.4	33.0	46.9	76.2
4.0	20.6	30.4	43.4	71.0
4.5	18.9	28.0	40.2	66.2
5.0	17.3	25.8	37.2	61.8
5.5	15.9	23.8	34.4	57.6
6.0	14.6	21.9	31.8	53.6
6.5	13.4	20.1	29.4	49.9
7.0	12.2	18.5	27.2	46.5
7.5	11.2	17.0	25.1	43.2
8.0	10.2	15.6	23.1	40.2
8.5	9.4	14.3	21.3	38.1
9.0	8.5	13.1	19.6	34.6
9.5	7.8	12.0	18.0	32.0
10.0	7.1	10.9	16.5	29.6
10.5	6.5	10.0	15.1	27.4
11.0	5.9	9.1	13.8	25.3
11.5	5.3	8.3	12.6	23.3
12.0	4.9	7.5	11.5	21.4
12.5	4.4	6.8	10.5	19.7
13.0	4.0	6.2	9.5	18.1
13.5		5.6	8.6	16.5
14.0		5.0	7.8	15.1
14.5		4.5	7.1	13.7
15.0		4.1	6.4	12.6
15.5			5.8	11.4
16.0			5.2	10.4
16.5			4.7	9.4
17.0			4.2	8.5
17.5				7.7
18.0				6.9
18.5				6.2
19.0				5.6
19.5				4.9
20.0				4.5

Interpretation of results

- Pressures above 21 mm Hg are elevated, and the patient requires referral to an ophthalmologist.
- Patients with pressures greater than 30 mm Hg require urgent evaluation by an ophthalmologist.
- Patients with symptoms or signs of acute pressure elevation and elevated intraocular pressures require emergent referral to an ophthalmologist.

Possible complications

- Corneal abrasions may be caused by this procedure.
- Infections may be transmitted by a poorly sterilized Schiotz tonometer.

Modifications

- If no equipment is available, the pressures of the two eyes can be compared by palpating the eyeballs through the eyelids.
- It should be possible to distinguish the asymmetry of a very firm eye present on one side compared to the other.

Patching/Eye Shield Placement

Indications for an eye patch

- Patching may provide comfort and facilitate healing of a corneal injury by preventing the eyelid from moving over injured areas.
- A patch may protect a dilated eye from bright light.

Indications for eye shield placement

- An eye shield is placed when globe perforation is suspected.

Contraindications and indications for referral

- If a penetrating injury to the eye is present, placing a patch on the eye may increase the injury.
- Patching is contraindicated when a corneal injury is the result of an infection or the presence a dirty foreign body.
- Patches should not be placed on patients diagnosed with glaucoma.
- Patches should generally not be placed on patients who have corneal abrasions caused by contact lens wear.
- Use of the patch has not conclusively been proven to improve the healing of a corneal abrasion. Therefore if a child is likely to be distressed or constantly pull at the patch once it is in place, it may be preferable to proceed without the patch and use drops instead.
- No specific contraindications exist for use of an eye shield unless use of a patch is better for the injury.

Supplies and equipment

- Antibiotic ointment
- Dilator eyedrops (cyclopentolate 1% or homoatropine 5%)

- Fox eye shield or other fenestrated metal guard that places no pressure on the eye
- Gauze eye patches (2)
- Tape (1-inch paper tape is best to minimize allergic reaction)
- Tincture of benzoin

Eye patch procedure (Fig. 12-19)

1. Before patching a corneal abrasion, place a drop of dilating agent in the eye. This will help decrease ciliary spasm that may be present with some corneal abrasions.
2. After this, place an antibiotic ointment in the eye before patching.
3. Have the patient close both eyes. Infants will need to have the lid manually closed, and then pressure should be maintained on the lid for the entire procedure. The patch needs to be applied tightly enough to keep the eyelid closed.
4. Fold the first patch in half. Place the patch with the folded edge just below the superior orbital rim, to fit securely against the eyelid. If a gauze pad is used, it may be trimmed to be an oval shape and then double-folded to fit in the orbit.
5. The second eye patch is placed horizontally across the eyelid and first patch.
6. Tape strips should be placed across the face from the middle of the forehead to the cheek. The skin of the cheek should be pulled upward or toward the nose so that when it is released it pulls the tape tight.
7. Tincture of benzoin may help hold the tape in place, but it should not be placed near the eye.

Eye shield procedure

1. Place an eye guard over the injured eye without anything underneath. Care should be taken to prevent pressure to the eye.
2. Align the edges of the guard against the bone of the surrounding orbit.
3. Apply tape from the forehead to the cheek, ensuring that the metal guard is not putting pressure on the eye.

Modifications

- Gauze pads (4×4) may be folded over on themselves and used as eye patches in place of gauze eye patches. They will fit better if cut to an oval shape.
- A Styrofoam cup may be substituted for an eye shield if a patient has a penetrating eye injury.

Slit Lamp Examination

Indications

- The slit lamp is used to examine the anterior segment of the eye. It should be used to examine the eye for all but the simplest of injuries or complaints. The fact that many private offices may not have this device is the limiting factor in completing a thorough eye examination.

- The slit lamp is useful to diagnose corneal ulcers, foreign body, iritis, and microscopic hyphema.
- For practitioners who are comfortable using the slit lamp, it helps with foreign body removal.

Contraindications and indications for referral

- Patients with other injuries that preclude the upright position cannot have this examination.

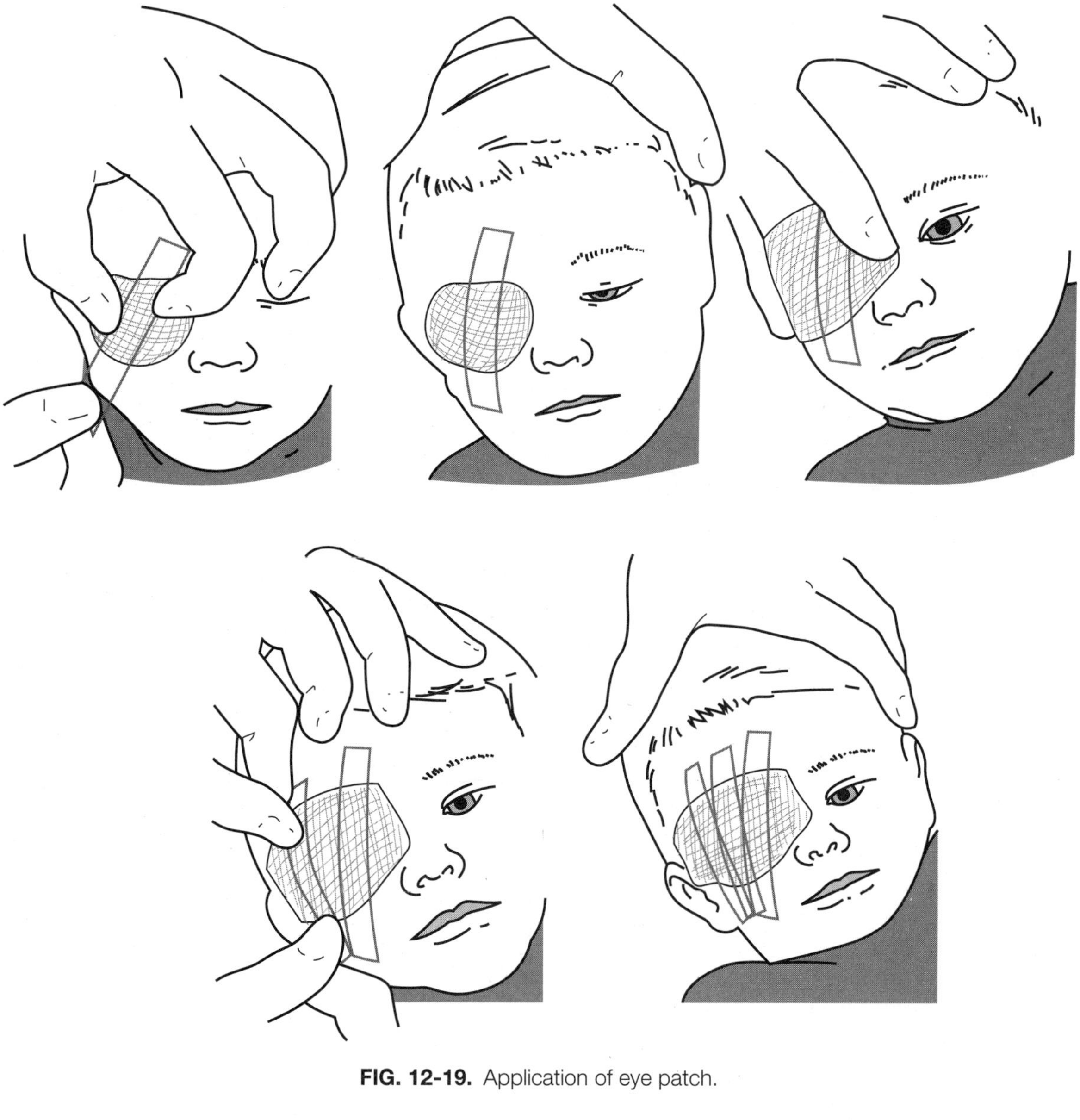

FIG. 12-19. Application of eye patch.

Supplies and equipment

- Cotton-tipped applicators
- Fluorescein strips
- Slit lamp (each model has different knob locations, so familiarize yourself with the slit lamp before placing the child in position)
- Topical anesthetic

Required nursing skills

- Infants can be examined using the slit lamp if an assistant holds the child with the head in slight extension. The infant's head is placed against the head strap of the slit lamp. Another assistant will need to hold the head still. Although this position will not allow a detailed examination, it will allow reasonable evaluation of the cornea and a fluorescein examination.
- Young children may respond better if they are held on their parent's laps. Tell children that they are looking into a special television or telescope and engage them in conversation to decrease anxiety. Having the parent behind the practitioner to focus the child is helpful to reduce motion.

Procedure

1. If the patient is having discomfort in the eye, place a drop of anesthetic in the eye to facilitate the examination.
2. Place the patient's chin in the chin rest and the forehead against the forehead bar. Adjust the height of the chin rest so that the canthus of the eye are at the same level as the indicator line on the side bar of the slit lamp.
3. When the child is in position, turn on the slit lamp. Use the least amount of light possible to limit discomfort. Filter switches on the lamp change the intensity of the light. A knob on the slit lamp changes the height of the light beam, and another knob adjusts the width of the beam. A beam of 2 to 3 mm width and full vertical height is useful to complete the examination. Another knob is present to adjust the degree of magnification. The lowest magnification is generally the easiest to examine the eye.
4. Place the light source at approximately a 45-degree angle to facilitate examination of the cornea and anterior chamber. For example, to examine the patient's right eye, the light source should be swung toward the practitioner's left side at approximately a 45-degree angle with the light beam at full height and minimal width.
5. Focus the beam of light on the patient's cornea by moving the base of the slit lamp back and forth along its tract using the controlling stick. This stick can be rotated to move the slit lamp light source up or down as needed to facilitate complete examination of the cornea and conjunctiva.
6. Scan across the eye first at the level of the cornea and sclera. Then by pushing forward slightly at the base, scan across the eye at the level of the iris. This examination should show conjunctival injury, inflammation, or foreign body. Abnormality of the eyelid and lashes can also be noted.
7. The slit lamp is useful for evaluating cells in the anterior chamber. This is one of the more difficult uses of the slit lamp to master, however. Decrease the height of the white light beam to 3 to 4 mm and make it as narrow as possible.

Increase the magnification for this part of the examination. The angle of the light beam should be approximately 45 degrees.

8. Focus the beam of light on the center of the cornea. Then push the base of the slit lamp gently forward to focus on the anterior surface of the lens. Move the slit lamp very slightly back so that it is in the center of the anterior chamber. The light beam should remain over the pupil so a black background acts as contrast against floating white or red blood cells.
9. Look specifically at the beam of light as it traverses the anterior chamber. Normally, there are no cells in the anterior chamber, so if small flecks are seen floating in this area (like dust in a projector beam), then either white or red cells are present. If the light beam appears to light up the aqueous like a light in a fog cloud, this indicates that protein is present in the anterior chamber. This is called flare. Evaluation for red blood cells needs to be done over the entire anterior chamber because blood may clot anywhere in this chamber.
10. If identification of the cells as either red or white blood cells is difficult, the green light that is available on all slit lamps may be used. Using this light, red blood cells become invisible, and any remaining cells are white blood cells or pigment cells that have been broken free from trauma.
11. The slit lamp is equipped with a cobalt-blue beam to evaluate for corneal abrasion. As described previously, stain the eye with a fluorescein strip and examine it using a cobalt beam for uptake of fluorescein, indicating a corneal injury. Using the slit lamp for this procedure allows the examination to be done under a magnifying lens that also allows for depth perception.

Interpretation of results

- Fluorescein uptake in the cornea indicates corneal injury.
- White blood cells in the anterior chamber indicate iritis, and referral is needed.
- Protein in the anterior chamber suggests iritis, and the patient requires referral to an ophthalmologist.
- Red blood cells in the anterior chamber indicate hyphema, and immediate referral is appropriate.

GENERAL CONTRAINDICATIONS TO EXAMINATION AND INDICATIONS FOR REFERRAL

- If a child is suspected of having a globe rupture based on the injury or mechanism, referral should be made rather than risking further damage by trying to examine the eye.
- Perforation should be suspected in patients exposed to metal hammering or heavy machinery. If severe pain is present with this history, referral is appropriate.
- Other findings suggestive of globe penetration include hyphema, irregularity of the pupil, lens opacification, or an abnormal anterior chamber examination.
- Any examination or procedure is difficult in small and uncooperative children.

If attempts have been made to complete an examination or perform a procedure with no success, and there is a significant possibility that a foreign body, injury, or infection is present, a child should be referred for sedation and complete examination.

- Exposure to all but the mildest acids should be referred to an ophthalmologist after immediate irrigation.

USEFUL MEDICATIONS

Tetracaine 0.5% to 1.0% (topical anesthetic agent) lasts approximately 15 to 20 minutes
Proparacaine 0.5% (topical anesthetic agent) lasts approximately 10 to 15 minutes
Phenylephrine 2.5% (dilating agent) lasts approximately 3 hours
Cyclopentolate 1% (dilating agent) lasts approximately 24 hours
Homoatropine 5% (dilating agent) lasts approximately 24 hours
Gentamycin ointment or drops, many brands (antibacterial)
Erythromycin ointment 0.5% (antibacterial)
Ciprofloxacin 0.3% drops (antibacterial)
Sulfacetamide sodium 10% drops and ointment (antibacterial)

GENERAL AFTERCARE INSTRUCTIONS

- Many procedures on the eye have minimal postprocedure instruction. Rather, the findings of the examination may require specific instruction.
- Typically, after manipulation of the eye (e.g., foreign body removal, contact lens removal, irrigation for foreign body or chemical exposure), injury may be present on the cornea. As the anesthetic used for the procedure wears off, the injury may be painful and cause photophobia and tearing.
- If a small abrasion is present, patching is not necessary, and the eye generally heals within 24 to 36 hours.
- If a corneal abrasion is present after chemical injury, patching should not be done in case additional chemical is left on the eye.
- A topical antibiotic (e.g., sulfacetamide drops or ointment, polytrim drops, polysporin ointment) may be used but has not been proven to improve healing or outcome.
- Patching is more useful in larger abrasions or for patient comfort. If a patch is placed, it should not be left in place for longer than 24 to 36 hours without a recheck.
- If a corneal ulcer is found, the patient requires immediate referral.
- If bacterial conjunctivitis is present, antibiotic ointment or drops may be started directed at the suspected organisms, and the eye should *not* be patched.
- Oral pain medications may be appropriate for painful eye injuries or infection.
- Follow-up for repeat examination should be arranged for most eye injuries.

- The parents should be instructed to bring the child back for increasing pain, discharge from the eye, swelling of the eye, or new visual complaints.
- Adolescents who may be driving need to be informed that they cannot drive or attempt other tasks requiring depth perception while one of the eyes is impaired or while a patch is in place.

SUGGESTED READINGS

Catalano RA, Nelson LB, editors: *Pediatric ophthalmology,* Norwalk, Conn, 1994, Appleton and Lange.

Catalano RA, editor: *Ocular emergencies,* Philadelphia, 1992, WB Saunders.

Goldbloom RB, editor: *Pediatric clinical skills,* New York, 1997, Churchill Livingstone.

Kay-Wilson LG: Localization of corneal foreign bodies, *Br J Ophthalmol* 76:741, 1992.

Leat SL, Shute RH, Westall CA, editors: *Assessing children's vision,* Oxford, 1999, Butterworth.

MacCumber MW, editor: *Management of ocular injuries and emergencies,* Philadelphia, 1998, Lippincott-Raven.

Rhee DJ, Pyfer MF, editors: *The Wills eye manual,* Philadelphia, 1999, Lippincott Williams and Wilkins.

Samples JR, Hedges JR: Ophthalmologic, otolaryngologic, and dental procedures. In Roberts JR, Hedges JR, editors: *Clinical procedures in emergency medicine,* Philadelphia, 1998, WB Saunders.

Santen SA, Scott JL: Ophthalmologic procedures, *Emerg Med Clin North Am* 13:681, 1995.

Trobe JD, editor: *The physician's guide to eye care,* San Francisco, 1993, American Academy of Ophthalmology.

CHAPTER 13

Minor Ear, Nose, and Throat Procedures

Terry A. Adirim

This chapter delineates how to perform minor procedures involving the ears, nose, and throat (ENT) in the outpatient setting.

EAR FOREIGN BODY AND CERUMEN IMPACTION REMOVAL

Background and Introduction

The external auditory canal is a convenient and appealing place for children to place foreign objects; it is also the site of considerable accumulation of cerumen. Therefore removal of foreign bodies and impacted cerumen is a fairly common procedure in pediatrics, and it may often be performed in the office or emergency department setting.

Relevant Anatomy

The ear is divided into the external ear, the middle ear, and the inner ear. The external ear is composed of the pinna (or auricle) and the external auditory canal. The external auditory canal has its narrowest point at the isthmus, which is the bony portion of the canal. The external canal ends at the tympanic membrane, where the middle ear begins. The middle ear consists of the tympanic membrane, the tympanic cavity, three ossicles, two muscles, several tendons, and the eustachian tube. The eustachian tube connects the middle ear to the nasopharynx (Fig. 13-1).

The external auditory canal is very sensitive, and the skin is very thin. Therefore the canal bleeds easily with manipulation. Because local anesthesia is difficult and obscures the practitioner's view, it is not practical; therefore the patient's cooperation is essential. In most young children this is impossible, so prevention of movement, such as with a papoose or conscious sedation, is important in performing foreign body removal.

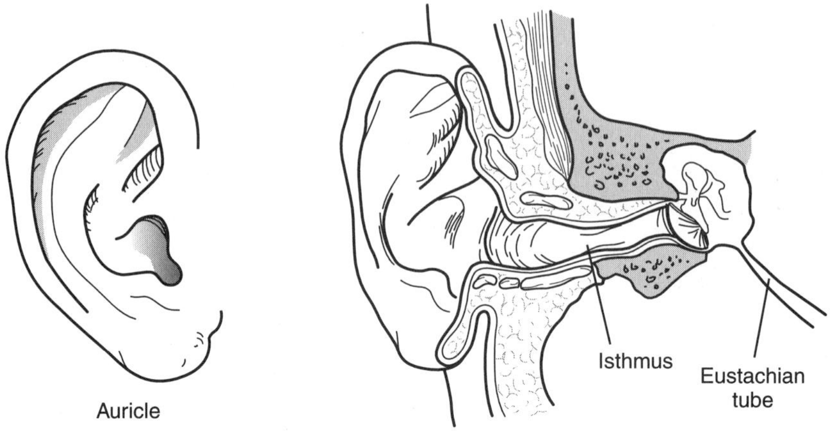

FIG. 13-1. Anatomy of the ear.

Indications

Any foreign body (FB) in the external auditory canal needs to be removed. The decision to be made is whether the removal procedure should be performed in the office, the emergency department setting, or the operating room (referral to an ENT surgeon). An attempt can be made in the office if (1) the FB is easily visible, (2) the FB is in the outer portion of the external canal, and (3) the practitioner has appropriate instruments.

Contraindications and Reasons for Referral to a Specialist

Do not attempt an in-office removal if the FB is lying against the tympanic membrane, the patient has a bleeding diathesis, or the practitioner is unable to adequately restrain or sedate the patient. Any of these conditions warrant referral either to a fully equipped pediatric emergency department or to an otolaryngologist. Although FBs in the ear canal must ultimately be removed, removal is rarely an emergency, making it inadvisable to attempt removal under any but the most ideal circumstances.

Supplies and Equipment

- Alligator or Hartmann forceps
- Assistant
- Good light source
- Otoscope or headlamp with separate specula
- Papoose board and/or sheet
- Sedation medications when indicated
- Suction and catheters
- Wire loops or blunt hooks of varying sizes

Procedure

1. Explain the procedure to the child and parents.
2. Physically restrain or adequately sedate the child. If placing the child in a papoose, wrap the child in a sheet first.
3. Have an assistant hold the child's head in place to prevent movement that can cause injury to the external canal during instrumentation.
4. In order to see the FB in the canal, pull the pinna posterior and lateral, which straightens the canal.
5. Choose an instrument depending on the nature of the FB. For a smooth, round object, such as a bead that is difficult to grasp with an alligator forceps, use a blunt hook between the object and the canal wall.
6. Attempt to get the hook behind the object and withdraw the hook with the object in front of that (Fig. 13-2, *A*). If the instrument cannot get behind the object or this attempt fails, try a suction catheter with a smooth tip (Fig. 13-2, *B*).
7. Apply low suction to draw the object out of the canal. Alligator forceps are best for those objects that can be grasped (Fig. 13-2, *C*).
8. If the object is a live insect, use mineral oil or lidocaine to kill it. When the insect has stopped moving, removal can be attempted by either irrigation with saline or with forceps. If fragments of the insect are embedded in the wall of the canal, forceps are necessary to remove the parts.

Irrigation with warm saline is a less invasive technique for removing FBs from the ear; however, do not use this technique with vegetable matter, such as seeds or beans, because they absorb the saline and swell, complicating their removal. To use the irrigation technique, the following equipment is needed: a 20-ml syringe and a 16- to 18-gauge intravenous (IV) catheter without the needle (or a butterfly needle tubing with needle removed). Complete the following procedure steps:

1. Attach the IV catheter or the tubing to the syringe.
2. Using warm saline or tap water, insert the catheter approximately 1 cm into the canal.
3. Infuse the solution steadily.

Cerumen that obscures the view of the tympanic membrane can be removed in three ways: (1) A metal or plastic cerumen spoon/curette can be used to scoop out the cerumen from the canal; (2) for hard and impacted cerumen, the canal can be flushed with warm saline, using a syringe to effect removal; and (3) a cerumenolytic (e.g., Cerumenex, Debrox, Waxsol, Exterol, Cerumol, Burosol, mineral oil, or hydrogen peroxide) can be instilled in the ear to dissolve the cerumen. Then, using a cerumen spoon, the cerumen is easier to remove.

Possible Complications

Complications of ear FB removal include perforated tympanic membrane, laceration or abrasion to the ear canal, and postprocedure inflammation. Warn the parents that the canal may bleed. For a perforated tympanic membrane and/or

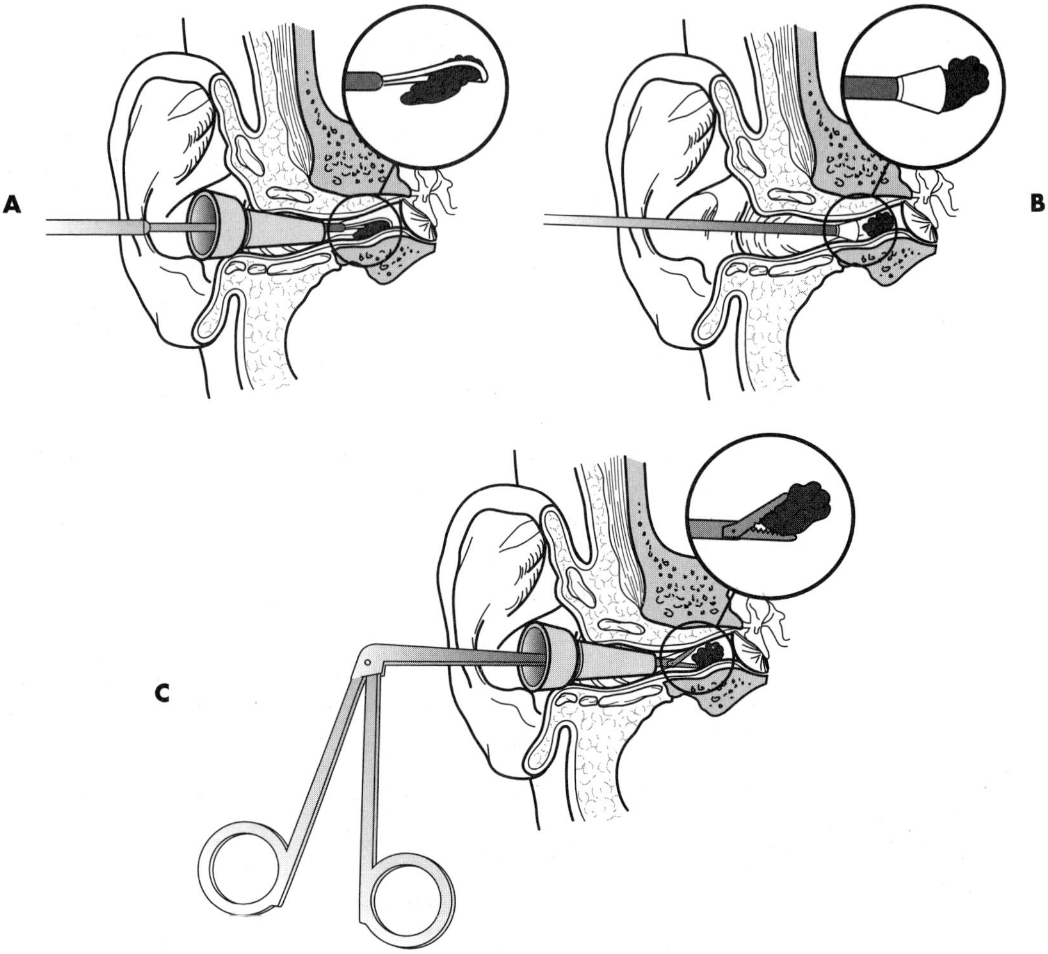

FIG. 13-2. Foreign body removal procedure.

inflammation, prescribe an antibiotic/steroid suspension. For a residual FB or an FB that cannot be removed, refer the patient to an emergency department or ENT surgeon.

Aftercare Instructions

No special instructions are required after easy removal of an FB. If the canal has become abraded, is bleeding, or is inflamed, then antibiotic/steroid suspension should be used every 6 hours for 5 days. If the ossicles may have been disrupted, either by the procedure or by the FB itself, prompt referral is indicated.

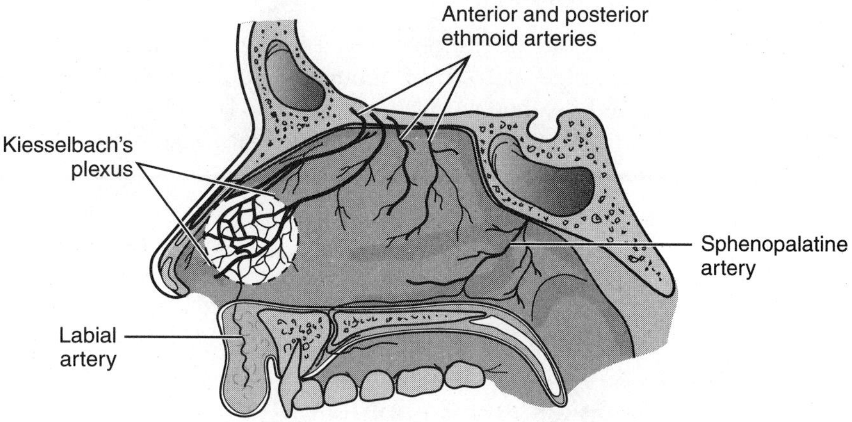

FIG. 13-3. Anatomy of the nose.

EPISTAXIS AND NASAL PACKING

Background and Introduction

Epistaxis is a common complaint in pediatric practice that is most commonly seen in toddlers and school-aged children. The bleeding usually resolves before medical intervention; however, persistent bleeding requires intervention.

Relevant Anatomy

Most of the distal and lateral portions of the external nose consist of nasal cartilages. Inside the nose, the nasal septum is composed of cartilaginous and bony areas. The septum is formed by (1) the perpendicular plate of the ethmoid bone, (2) the vomer, and (3) the cartilage of the nasal septum. The anterior ethmoid artery supplies the posterior lateral wall of the nose, which includes the superior turbinate, and the superior aspect of the nasal septum. The terminal branch of the internal maxillary artery supplies the posterior septum and the posterior inferior and middle turbinates. The lower midseptum is supplied by the descending palatine artery.

The Kiesselbach plexus, which supplies the anterior septum, is the coalescence of several arteries from the internal and external carotid systems. The anterior septum is richly vascularized and is covered by a thin mucosal layer (Fig. 13-3); therefore this is the site of most nosebleeds in children. The mucosal layer in children is even thinner than in adults and is, therefore, more likely to bleed. In addition, children are apt to pick their noses. Other factors influence the incidence of nosebleeds, including viral infections, allergic rhinitis, and the dry air in winter, which irritate the nasal mucosa and can promote bleeding.

Indications

Before consideration of nasal packing, a trial of anterior nasal pressure should be attempted. If 10 to 15 minutes of squeezing the nares together does not stop the bleeding, then nasal packing should be performed. Bleeding from the anterior site indicates the need for an anterior nasal pack. Blood in the hypopharynx without an anterior nasal source indicates the need for a posterior nasal pack.

Contraindications and Reasons for Referral to a Specialist

In a patient with a known bleeding disorder, intranasal lesion, or with unstable vital signs, an ENT surgeon should be consulted.

Supplies and Equipment

- Alligator forceps
- Bayonet forceps
- Cotton pledgets
- Foley catheters (10 to 16 French)
- Gauze (2 × 2)
- Hemostat
- Hoffman clamp
- Light source
- Nasal speculum
- Nasal tampon (Rhinorocket)
- Oxycellulose (Surgicel)
- Plastic cuff
- Silver nitrate sticks
- Syringe (30 ml)
- Topical antibiotic ointment
- Topical vasoconstrictors (e.g., Lidocaine [2-4%], Epinephrine [1:1000], Oxymetazoline [Afrin], Phenylephrine [Neosynephrine])
- Vaseline gauze

Procedure

Anterior nasal packing

1. Position the child in an upright sitting position. A very young child may need to be supine and physically restrained.
2. Apply topical vasoconstrictor and anesthetic to the nasal mucosa.
3. If possible, locate the site of bleeding and cauterize it with silver nitrate sticks.
4. Apply antibiotic ointment onto gauze or use Vaseline gauze.
5. Insert a nasal speculum into one nostril and open to expose the septum.
6. Using bayonet forceps, clasp the gauze and insert it into the nostril, leaving a tail of gauze of approximately 1 to 2 cm.
7. Pack down gauze as well as possible to create tamponade.

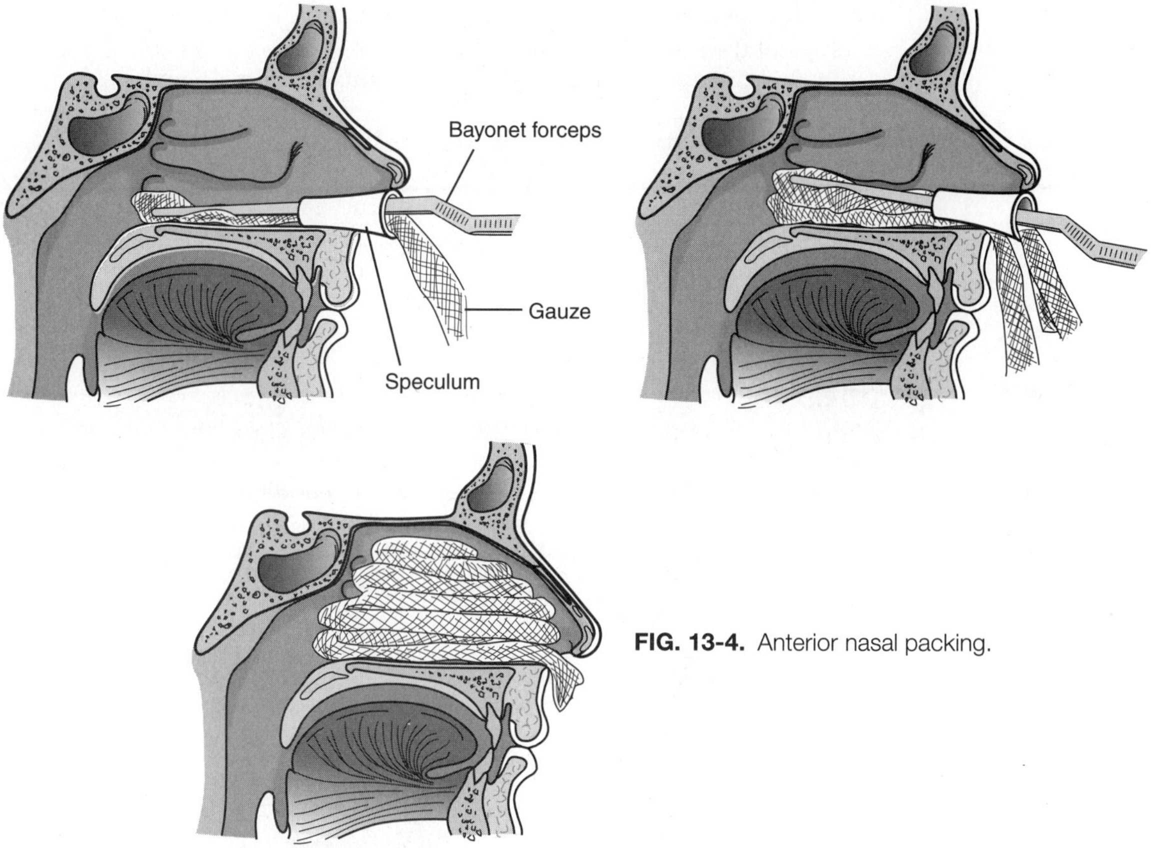

FIG. 13-4. Anterior nasal packing.

8. Continue this procedure with as many layers as necessary until the nasal cavity is filled (Fig. 13-4).
9. Place a piece of tape over the gauze to stabilize the packing.
10. An alternative to gauze is Surgicel, which can be used as packing and inserted as described previously. Surgicel dissolves within 24 hours.

Posterior nasal packing

Posterior nasal packing is a more complicated procedure; therefore it is important that the patient be adequately sedated and that analgesia is used because this procedure is painful and uncomfortable. The Foley catheter technique involves the insertion of a 10- to 16-French catheter.

1. Before inserting the Foley catheter, check that the balloon is intact by inflating it.
2. Apply antibiotic ointment or another form of lubrication to the catheter to facilitate insertion.
3. Anesthetize the nasal mucosa.
4. Insert the catheter into the nostril until the balloon can be seen in the posterior pharynx.

5. Inflate the balloon with 10- to 15-ml of water, and then pull on the catheter gently until the balloon is snug.
6. Secure the catheter in place with tape, a Hoffman clamp, an umbilical clamp, or a hemostat.
7. Place an anterior pack around the catheter (Fig. 13-5).

Patients with posterior packing should be referred to an ENT surgeon and should be monitored in the hospital setting. All patients with posterior nasal packing in place should be started on antibiotics to cover *Staphylococcus aureus,* to prevent the rare but potentially serious complication of toxic shock syndrome.

Complications

Anterior packs can potentially cause ischemia to the nasal septum and, therefore, possible necrosis of the nasal mucosa. Infection is another possibility, so topical and, in some cases systemic, antibiotics are recommended. Nasal packing should

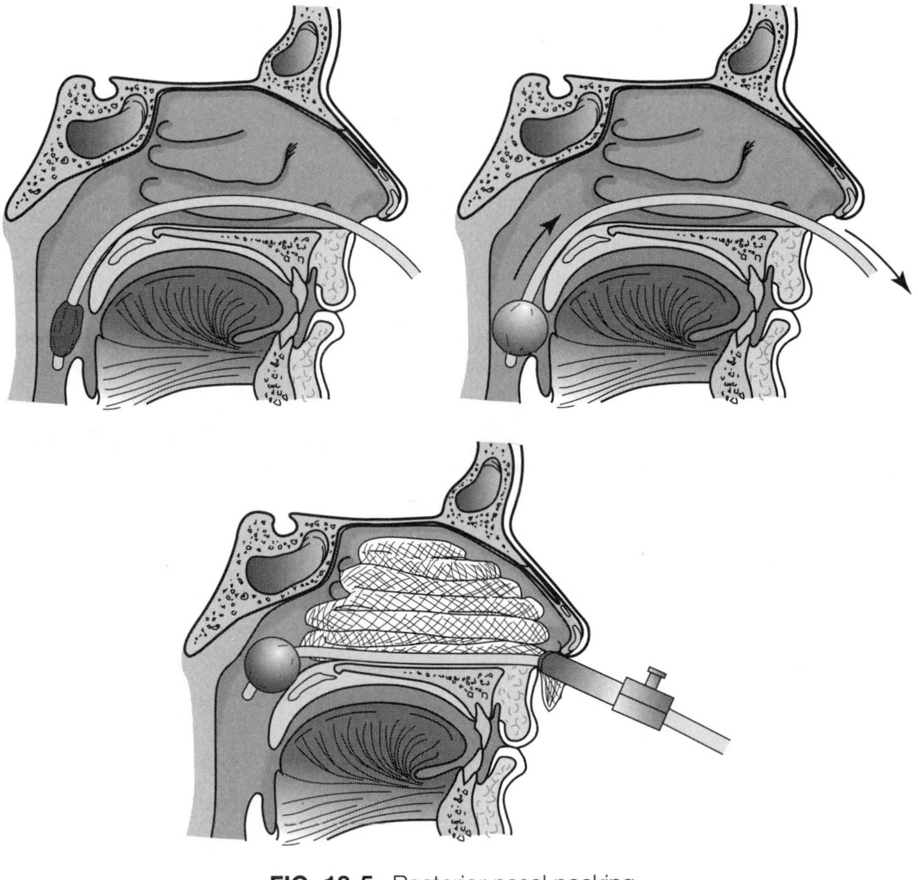

FIG. 13-5. Posterior nasal packing.

be removed within 3 days. Posterior packs pose risks if they become dislodged. They can obstruct the airway, so these patients need to be closely monitored, especially if they received sedation.

Aftercare Instructions

Patients with nasal packings in place should be instructed not to remove the packing themselves, but rather should see their physician for follow-up removal. Persistent bleeding, foul odor, or a sense that the packing has shifted its position require immediate return for evaluation.

NASAL FOREIGN BODY REMOVAL

Background and Introduction

Nasal FBs are common in the pediatric population. Sometimes the act is not witnessed, and the child presents with purulent nasal discharge, foul breath, or chronic sinusitis. The most common objects placed in the nose by children include tissue, foam, beads, seeds, beans, and parts from toys.

Relevant Anatomy

See previous section on nasal packing.

Indications

All FBs in the nose should be removed. If a child presents with unilateral persistent nasal discharge, then inspection and examination of the nose with suspicion of an FB is indicated.

Contraindications and Reasons for Referral to a Specialist

Although all nasal FBs must be removed, in some instances this procedure cannot be safely accomplished in an office environment. These circumstances are usually an uncooperative child or a very high placement of the FB that makes it difficult to remove. In either instance, referral to a pediatric emergency department or an otolaryngologist is indicated, both for adequate sedation and the availability of better equipment. Children with bleeding disorders should generally also be managed in a more technically advanced environment.

Supplies and Equipment

- Adequate lighting (overhead light, lamp, or operating microscope)
- Alligator forceps
- Assistant

- Lidocaine 2% to 4%
- Nasal speculum
- Neosynephrine
- Papoose and a sheet
- Right-angled instrument, such as cerumen spoon or loop
- Suction

Procedure

1. Examine the child's nose to determine the nature and location of the FB.
2. Explain to the family the procedure for removal. Warn the parents of the likelihood of some mucosal bleeding.
3. For a young child who is unlikely to cooperate, decide whether either physical restraint or sedation may be necessary.
4. Ask the assistant to hold the child's head steady.
5. Insert the nasal speculum and directly visualize the object.
6. Apply a topical anesthetic (lidocaine) and a vasoconstrictor (neosynephrine).
7. If the object is smooth, insert the right-angle instrument so that the tip is behind the object, and draw the object out.
8. If the object is soft or graspable, grab it with the forceps and remove it from the nose.
9. Reexamine the nasal cavity after removal to ensure that the entire object was removed and that no trauma has been inflicted on the nasal mucosa.

Complications

The most common complication of nasal FB removal is trauma to the nasal mucosa with a possible bleed. If the object has been in the nasal cavity for a long time, the risk of epistaxis is greater because of the formation of granulation tissue around the FB. If a bleed occurs, pinch the nares together for 10 minutes. Care should be taken not to push an instrument too deeply within the nasal cavity because the cribriform plate that lies medial to the middle turbinate could be punctured. If the FB cannot be removed, referral to the local emergency department or to an ENT surgeon is indicated.

Aftercare Instructions

Routine care can be provided after removal of a nasal FB. Use of a humidifier in the child's bedroom may help soothe irritated or inflamed mucosa.

TONGUE LACERATIONS

Background and Introduction

Tongue lacerations are common in children and usually arise as a result of a fall or a sudden blow to the head, while the child's tongue is between the teeth.

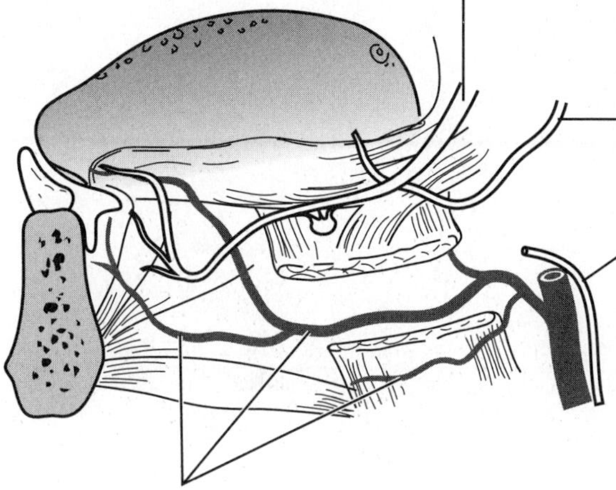

FIG. 13-6. Anatomy of the tongue.

Relevant Anatomy

The tongue's primary blood supply is from the lingual arteries. Innervation of the tongue is through the lingual nerve. The anterior part of the tongue is innervated by the lingual nerve, and the posterior portion is innervated by the glossopharyngeal nerve and the superior laryngeal nerve (Fig. 13-6).

Indications

The tongue heals quickly because of its high vascularity; therefore not all tongue lacerations need to be sutured. A deep or gaping wound should be considered for repair, however, especially if food can get caught inside. If a laceration does not naturally fall into good opposition, or if the tongue is lacerated deeply for more than 50% of its width, suturing is indicated. Similarly, if a through-and-through laceration is present or the laceration penetrates the full thickness of the tongue in any area, suturing should be performed.

Contraindications and Reasons for Referral to a Specialist

There are few absolute contraindications to suturing a tongue laceration. A near-amputation for which there is a risk of completing the amputation in an uncooperative patient merits referral to a pediatric emergency department, where both sedation and otolaryngologists are readily available. Any situation in which adequate patient cooperation is in question also merits referral.

Supplies and Equipment

- Forceps
- Gauze

- Good light source
- Lidocaine without epinephrine
- Needle holders
- Papoose board and sheet
- Sedation medications, if indicated
- Suture material (4-0 vicryl, gut, chromic or rapide)
- Suture material for a "stay stitch" (3-0 silk)
- Syringe, 3-ml with a 25- to 26-gauge needle

Procedure

1. After determining that the patient needs suturing, assess the need for sedation. In general, the younger the child, the more likely sedation medications are needed to complete the procedure.
2. Papoose a child that is unlikely to be fully cooperative.
3. With a 3-ml syringe and a 25- to 26-gauge needle, infiltrate the tip of the tongue with lidocaine.
4. Place a "stay stitch" (3-0 silk) through the tip of the tongue to keep the tongue out of the mouth.
5. Infiltrate the laceration with 2 to 3 ml of lidocaine to anesthetize the wound.
6. Suture deep lacerations that do not approximate well in the muscle layer to close the dead space. For this layer, use 4-0 vicryl and bury the knots. The outside sutures should be interrupted, using 4-0 chromic, gut, or rapide. These sutures dissolve over time.
7. Prophylactic antibiotics are not indicated because of the excellent blood supply of the tongue.

Complications

If the knots are not buried, they can become untied and the wound can open.

Aftercare Instructions

After repair of a tongue laceration, the child should be given a soft, bland diet for several days. Daily rinses with half-strength hydrogen peroxide 3% solution may help cleanse the mouth. The family should be told to watch for excessive swelling, discharge, or pain, all of which signal the possibility of infection.

REDUCTION OF TEMPOROMANDIBULAR JOINT DISLOCATION

Background and Introduction

Although temporomandibular joint (TMJ) dislocations are not common in young children, they do occur occasionally in school-aged children and adolescents. The earlier the reduction is performed, the better the likelihood of success. Some

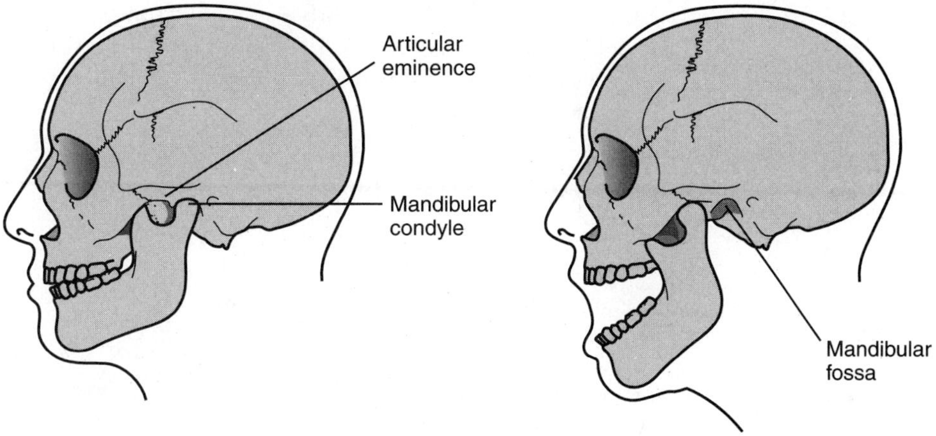

FIG. 13-7. Mandibular anatomy and dislocation.

people are predisposed to TMJ dislocation because they have a shallow mandibular fossa or underdeveloped condyle or ligamentous laxity. Most cases occur spontaneously when the jaw is opened wide when yawning, eating, or during prolonged dental work.

Relevant Anatomy

The TMJ is composed of the head of the mandibular condyle within the mandibular fossa of the temporal bone. The structure of the joint allows for multiple motions, such as hinge movement and side-to-side movement, because the articular surfaces are lined with a synovial membrane and separated by a meniscus composed of connective tissue. The joint is supported by two ligaments on the medial surface (the sphenomandibular and stylomandibular ligaments) and one on the lateral surface (the temporomandibular ligament). Dislocation of the TMJ often occurs in the anterior direction, causing the mandibular condyle to become locked in front of the articular eminence (Fig. 13-7). Posterior dislocations are usually seen as a result of trauma and are associated with trauma to the auditory system.

Indications

Simple dislocations of the TMJ that have occurred within a few hours of presentation may generally be reduced manually by closed reduction. The sooner reduction is attempted, the more likely it is to succeed.

Contraindications and Reasons for Referral to a Specialist

Before reduction is attempted, radiographs should be obtained both to confirm the dislocation and to diagnose any associated fracture. TMJ dislocations with fractures of the mandibular condyles often require open reduction and internal fixation by an oral surgeon. A variety of radiologic views can be obtained, but the panorex view is considered the best. Closed reduction should not be attempted in the presence of a bony fracture.

Supplies and Equipment

- Gauze
- Gloves
- Lidocaine 1% to 2% without epinephrine
- McGill forceps
- Needle, 25-gauge
- Suction
- Syringe, 3-ml

Procedure

1. Consider conscious sedation. Many patients are anxious, and sedation aids in completing the procedure successfully. You may also consider using local analgesia into the TMJ region—either into the joint space (intraarticular) or into the masseter muscle itself, which may aid in relaxing the muscles in spasm.
2. Seat the patient in a chair facing you.
3. Swathe both of your thumbs with gauze.
4. Place gloved thumbs on the retromolar pad on either side of the mandible and grasp the inferior surface of the mandible with the fingers on each side.
5. Apply pressure with a downward motion to free the condyle from its entrapped position anterior to the articular eminence.
6. Ease the mandible posteriorly to return to its normal anatomical position (Fig. 13-8).

Another method involves the practitioner's approach from behind the patient, as follows:

1. Seat the patient upright in a chair.
2. Press downward with your thumbs over the posterior lower molars.
3. Use your fingers to pull upward along the inferior aspect of the patient's anterior mandible.

If the joint relocation fails, consultation with an oral surgeon is indicated. All patients with TMJ dislocations should be referred to an oral maxillofacial surgeon for follow-up care.

Complications

Inability to reduce the dislocation is the most common complication and mandates immediate referral. Because the force with which the muscles surrounding the joint can spring back into place is considerable, fracture of the mandible or the

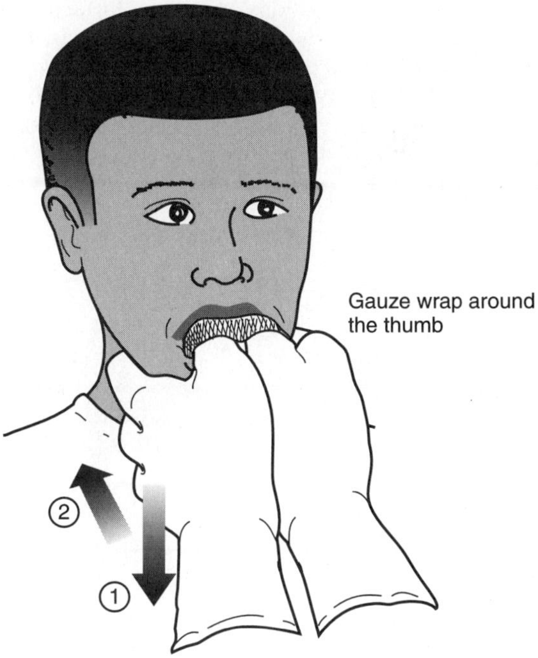

FIG. 13-8. Reduction of mandibular dislocation.

patient's teeth can occur. Also, if practitioners are not careful, their fingers can be crushed during the procedure. Aspiration of the gauze around the practitioners' thumbs can also occur.

Aftercare Instructions

After successful reduction of a TMJ dislocation, patients should follow a soft diet for 1 to 2 days, avoid widely opening the jaw, and use a nonsteroidal antiinflammatory agent such as ibuprofen. All patients should be seen within 1 week by an oral maxillofacial surgeon.

SUGGESTED READINGS

Clemente CD: *Anatomy: a regional atlas of the human body,* Baltimore, 1981, Urban and Schwartzenberg.

Henretig FM, King C, editors: *Textbook of pediatric emergency procedures,* Baltimore, 1997, Williams & Wilkins.

Manning SC, Culbertson MC Jr: Epistaxis. In Bluestone CD, Stool SE, Kenna MA, editors: *Pediatric otolaryngology,* Philadelphia, 1996, WB Saunders.

Newton E: Dislocations, mandible. In Keany J et al., editors: www.e-medicine.com.

Park AH, Stankiewicz J: Pediatric epistaxis. In Souza C, Stankiewicz JA, Pellitteri PK, editors: *Textbook of pediatric otorhinolaryngology—head and neck surgery,* San Diego, 1998, Singular Publishing Group.

Sculerati N: Foreign bodies of the nose. In Bluestone CD, Stool SE, Kenna MA, editors: *Pediatric otolaryngology,* Philadelphia, 1996, WB Saunders.

CHAPTER 14

Dental Procedures

Robert J. Berkowitz
Robert Shapiro

INTRODUCTION

This section focuses on technical dental procedures that can be performed by primary care pediatricians, including storage and reimplantation of avulsed permanent incisors and repair of certain oral soft tissue injuries. Technical procedures utilized in the management of fractured and displaced teeth, facial fractures, toothache, facial infection, and extensive orofacial soft tissue injury require the expertise of a subspecialist. All children with such injuries should be referred to a pediatric subspecialist or pediatric emergency department, where specialist care can be obtained.

STORAGE AND REIMPLANTATION OF AVULSED PERMANENT INCISOR TEETH

Indications/Contraindications

The likelihood that an avulsed permanent incisor can be normally reattached to alveolar bone is related to the viability of the periodontal ligament. The longer the extraoral dry storage, the greater the likelihood that the periodontal ligament is nonviable. Therefore immediate reimplantation of avulsed permanent incisors is indicated, unless the patient presents with either or both of the following contraindications: (1) Children who are medically compromised and/or developmentally disabled must be given special consideration; and (2) the alveolar socket must be structurally intact to provide proper support for the avulsed tooth.

Procedure

1. Place the avulsed permanent incisor into saline immediately. If saline is not available, an alternative storage medium is cow's milk.

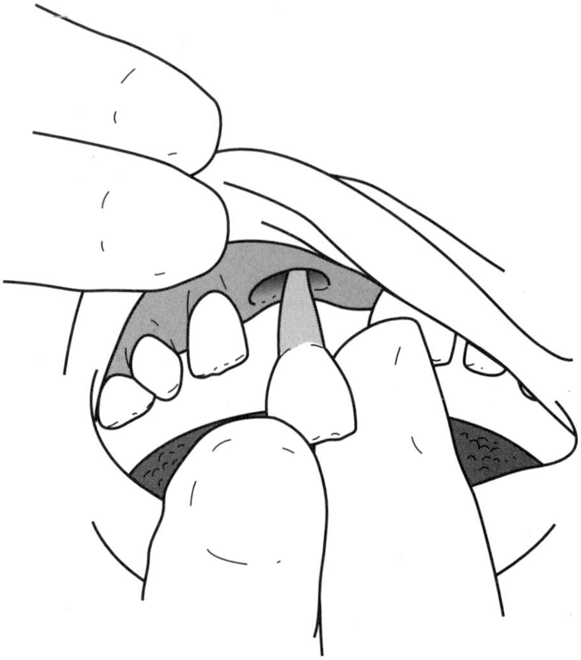

FIG. 14-1. An attempt should be made to gently replant the tooth as soon as possible, preferably within 30 minutes.

2. If the root of the tooth has visible debris on it, irrigate it with a stream of saline. Irrigation can also be accomplished with running tap water (close the drain).
3. Hold the tooth by the crown; do not touch the root.
4. Gently reinsert the tooth into the socket (Fig. 14-1). If resistance is met, do not force the tooth. Resistance to gentle reinsertion usually means that alveolar bone has been displaced and/or a blood clot is present.
5. Solicit involvement of a dental specialist to reduce displaced alveolar bone and/or to remove a blood clot before reinsertion.
6. After the tooth is reinserted, the emergent phase of treatment is completed.
7. Immobilize the tooth with an acrylic splint to facilitate reattachment. Splint fabrication necessitates the expertise of a dental specialist.
8. Avulsed teeth with incomplete root formation may revascularize their severed neurovascular bundle, eliminating the need for endodontic (root canal) therapy, but this procedure is mandatory if root development is complete.

REPAIR OF ORAL SOFT TISSUE INJURIES

Indications/Contraindications

Extensive orofacial soft tissue trauma requires the clinical expertise of an oral-maxillofacial surgeon or plastic surgeon. Simple oral soft tissue injuries can usually be managed by a primary care pediatrician. Accordingly, guidelines for treatment of nonextensive oral puncture wounds and lacerations are presented in the following sections.

Treatment

Puncture wounds

Most oral puncture wounds in children occur in toddlers and preschoolers and involve the hard or soft palate. History usually reveals that children fell or were bumped while holding an object in their mouths. Puncture wounds of the hard palate are usually small (less than 5 mm in diameter) and involve only the mucosa. No treatment is necessary because these wounds heal by secondary intention. Puncture wounds of the soft palate may be through-and-through or just penetrating. Small penetrating wounds usually heal by secondary intention; however, large penetrating wounds and through-and-through wounds require surgical repair. Surgical repair requires good visualization, access, no mobility, and a stable airway; therefore a general anesthetic is required. Accordingly, these types of injuries need to be managed by a surgical specialist.

Another common site for puncture wounds is the lower lip. The mechanism of injury is chin trauma; the lower incisor teeth penetrate the oral labial mucosa, and the upper incisor teeth penetrate the extraoral skin covering the obicularis oris. If a through-and-through injury occurs, surgical repair is indicated. If repair involves the vermillion border, a surgical specialist must perform the procedure to enhance the likelihood of a favorable cosmetic outcome. If the wound involves labial mucosa and skin, closure can be done by a primary care pediatrician. The wound should be repaired from the inside out after copious irrigation and inspection to remove foreign bodies. Adequate local anesthesia can be achieved by injecting into the vestibule (the area where alveolar mucosa becomes labial mucosa) with 2% lidocaine containing 1/100,000 epinephrine (Fig. 14-2).

Injection of anesthesia into the wound is not indicated because it will distort the tissue, thereby interfering with surgical repair. If sedation is needed, oral midazolam (0.5 mg/kg) is usually effective. Closure of the labial mucosa is performed first. A resorbable suture material should be used (e.g., 4-0 chromic). Penetration of the suture into the underlying muscle facilitates repair of the torn obicularis oris and labial mucosa (Fig. 14-3). The skin wound is then treated; its anatomy dictates the method of repair. Large wounds with separated margins need to be sutured (6-0 nylon); skin sutures should be removed 3 to 4 days after placement. The closed wound should be coated with an antibiotic ointment. Small wounds with little tissue separation can usually be repaired with a steri-strip or surgical glue.

Lacerations

Lacerations of the tongue can cause significant hemorrhage. Early (within a few hours after the injury) primary closure is usually indicated for most tongue lacerations. Strong resorbable sutures (e.g., 4-0 chromic) should be used. Tissue bites should be deep to obliterate any dead space. Before closure, local anesthesia should be injected into the depth of the wound; the wound should then be

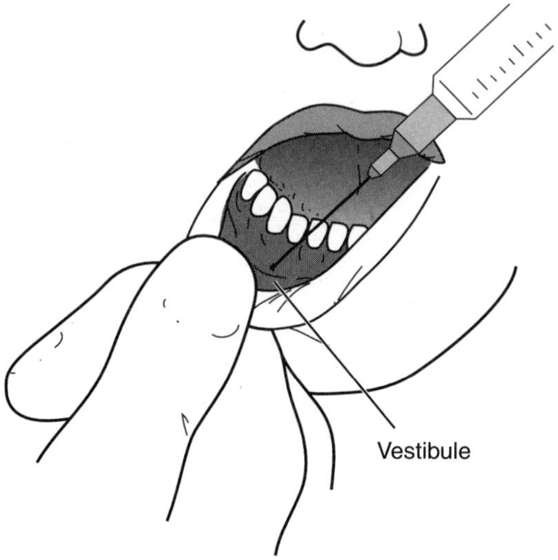

FIG. 14-2. Injection into the vestibule for treatment of oral lacerations.

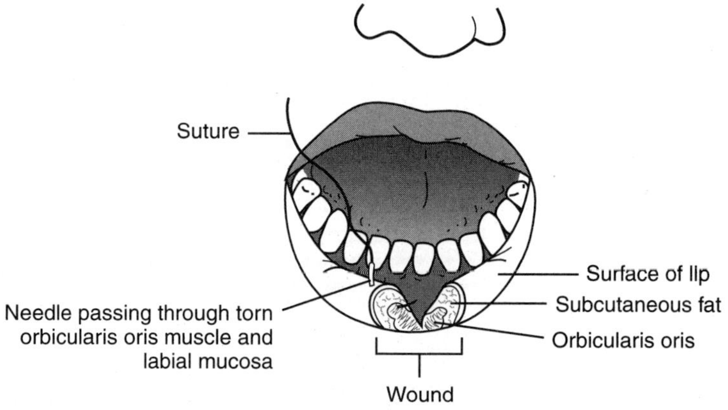

FIG. 14-3. Suture of oral puncture lacerations to repair torn obicularis oris and labial mucosa.

copiously irrigated and inspected for foreign bodies. Suture knots should be buried because they are an annoyance, particularly for young children. This technique is accomplished by suturing from the "inside out and the outside in," resulting in a tie that places the knot in the wound.

Cheek lacerations, unless superficial, are best managed by a subspecialist because they may involve the facial nerve and/or parotid duct. Likewise, lacerations of the floor of the mouth should be managed by a subspecialist because such wounds may involve Warthon's duct.

ADDITIONAL COMMENTS

Orofacial soft tissue injuries usually do not require systemic antibiotic prophylaxis unless the wound is grossly contaminated or more than 6 hours old. Pain control is usually adequate using acetaminophen or ibuprofen.

SUGGESTED READINGS

Andreasen JO et al: *Traumatic dental injuries—a manual,* Copenhagen, 1999, Munksgaard.

Kaban L: *Pediatric oral and maxillofacial surgery,* Philadelphia, 1990, WB Saunders.

CHAPTER 15

Dermatology Procedures

Alison Ensor Dunn
Bernard A. Cohen

SKIN BIOPSY

Background and Introduction

A skin biopsy is usually performed to establish or confirm a clinical diagnosis. When a neoplasm is suspected, histological findings help direct further surgical intervention and/or long-term follow-up care. In patients with inflammatory dermatoses, histological diagnosis allow for more precise medical management and counseling regarding prognosis.

Relevant Anatomy

Consideration should be given to the site of the biopsy. Bullae and ulcerations should be biopsied at the border in order to include some intact skin, whereas definitive findings are most likely to be found in the middle of plaques, nodules, and tumors.

Indications

Skin biopsy may be performed for several reasons, most commonly for diagnostic purposes. Biopsy of lesions that are a part of a systemic illness may provide the diagnosis in a definitive fashion or may at least indicate a diagnostic category. Occasionally, fungal or bacterial culture of lesions provide critical diagnostic information. Certain lesions are excised in their entirety, especially when they are cosmetically important or when malignancy is suspected.

Contraindications and Reasons for Referral to a Specialist

There are few reasons not to obtain a biopsy when indicated. When lesions are present on the face as well as other sites, nonfacial sites are preferred. Biopsies from nonhealing ulcers should be avoided unless absolutely necessary. Although it was initially thought that biopsies of melanomas could increase the risk of metastasis, recent evidence shows that this is untrue. Consequently, immediate biopsy to establish the diagnosis is warranted even when complete excision is not possible initially. Large excisional biopsies, or those in cosmetically sensitive areas, are best managed directly by a dermatologist or plastic surgeon. Biopsy can be performed by three techniques: punch, shave, or excision.

Punch Biopsy

A punch biopsy is the simplest and most commonly used biopsy method to obtain tissue for histology, immunofluorescence, culture, or electron microscopy. If the lesion is smaller than 6 mm and complete excision is desired, the clinician should use a punch that is 0.5 to 1 mm larger than the lesion. If the biopsy is being taken for diagnostic reasons, a 3- to 4-mm-diameter punch is adequate regardless of the lesion size.

Supplies and equipment

- Aluminum chloride solution
- Cotton-tipped applicator
- Fine-toothed forceps
- Iris scissors
- Lidocaine 1%
- Reusable sterile punch or a sterile, disposable punch (2 to 8 mm diameter)
- Sterile drape and preparation
- Sterile gloves
- Suture material (if primary closure desired)

The use of absorbable suture (polyglactin, polyglycolic acid, or mild chromic gut) 6-0 is preferable in younger patients. In older patients, 4-0 or 5-0 monofilament nylon suture can be used, with suture removal planned at 7 to 10 days depending on the biopsy site.

Procedure

1. Don sterile gloves.
2. Clean the skin with antiseptic.
3. Inject 1% lidocaine HCl intradermally. Lidocaine HCl 1% with epinephrine 1:100,000 (10 μg epinephrine/1 ml lidocaine) may be used to decrease bleeding and prolong analgesia. The concurrent use of epinephrine should be avoided on the fingers, toes, and the tip of the nose and penis.
4. Minimize the pain of the needlestick by applying topical anesthesia, such as eutectic mixture of local anesthetics (EMLA) cream, 2 hours before the procedure. In addition, 8.4% sodium bicarbonate (1 meq/1 ml) may be added in a 1:10 (1 part sodium bicarbonate to 9 parts lidocaine HCl) ratio to the lidocaine to decrease its sting.
5. Hold the punch between the thumb and forefinger, perpendicular to the lesion's surface. With slight downward pressure, rotate the punch approxi-

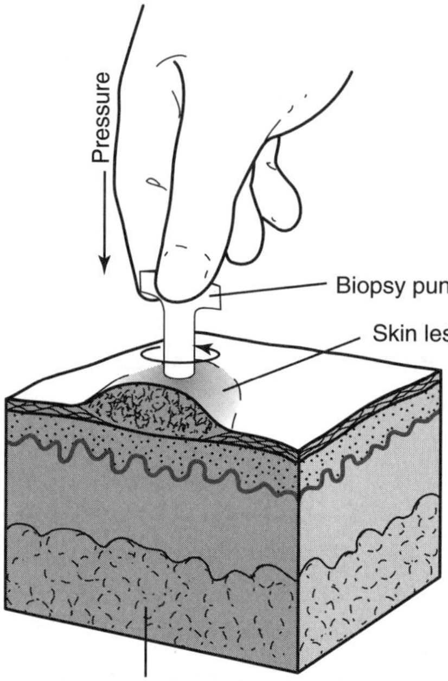

FIG. 15-1. Punch biopsy.

mately one complete turn until it "pops" through the dermis into the subcutaneous fat (Fig. 15-1).

6. When the punch is removed, the specimen will often protrude through the hole. If it does not come out of the wound, carefully lift it out with a pair of fine-toothed forceps. Alternatively, the needle used for the lidocaine injection can be used to pierce the specimen and lift it out.
7. Divide any remaining attachments between the biopsy and the wound with iris scissors.
8. Apply pressure for 1 to 2 minutes to control bleeding, which is usually light.
9. Apply aluminum chloride topically to the wound (use very carefully around the eyes) with a cotton-tipped applicator to provide hemostasis.
10. To speed wound healing, or for the best cosmetic results, close the wound with a suture or staples. Before obtaining the biopsy, stretch the skin slightly, 90 degrees away from the anticipated line of closure. While the skin is stretched, perform the biopsy. This maneuver results in an oval wound, rather than a round one, which facilitates surgical closure (Fig. 15-2). The wound can also be undermined with blunt-tipped scissors to create an elongated opening.

What the patient and family should know

Clean the wound twice daily with 3% hydrogen peroxide or soap and water. Then apply antibacterial ointment and a bandage. The crust usually falls off

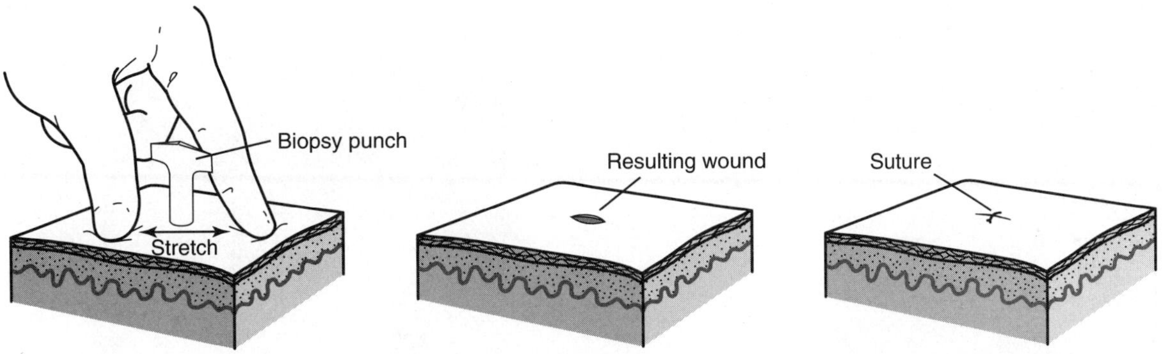

FIG. 15-2. Stretch for suturing.

in 8 to 10 days. No restriction of activity is needed. When stitches are placed, they will need to be removed in 6 to 10 days, depending on the location of the biopsy.

Shave Biopsy

A shave biopsy can be used to remove benign lesions, such as molluscum contagiosum, verruca vulgaris, intradermal nevocellular nevi, skin tags, and seborrheic keratoses.

Supplies and equipment

- Aluminum chloride solution
- Bard-Parker blade #15 attached to a scalpel handle (a razor blade may be used instead)
- Fine-toothed forceps
- Lidocaine 1%
- Sterile preparation and drape

Procedure

1. Prepare the skin with antiseptic and anesthetize with intradermal lidocaine 1%.
2. With the blade and scalpel, use a sawing, back-and-forth motion to remove the lesion flush with the surrounding skin (Fig. 15-3).
3. When the lesion is nearly completely severed, hold the free edge of the specimen with a pair of fine-toothed forceps and apply hemostasis with topical aluminum chloride solution. Alternatively, light electrocautery can be used to stop bleeding at the base of the lesion.

What the patient and family should know

Clean the wound twice daily with 3% hydrogen peroxide or soap and water. Then apply antibacterial ointment and a bandage. The crust usually falls off in 8 to 10 days. No restriction of activity is needed. When stitches are placed,

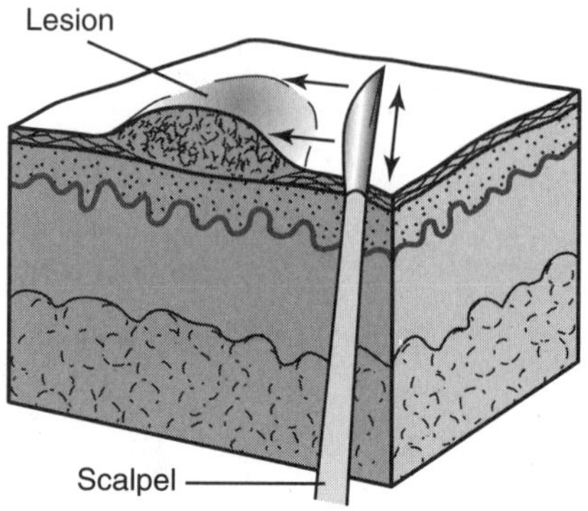

FIG. 15-3. Shave biopsy.

they will need to be removed in 6 to 10 days, depending on the location of the biopsy.

Scissor Biopsy

A scissor biopsy can be used to remove small, pedunculated lesions, such as an intradermal nevi and skin tags. This can often be done without intradermal anesthesia or with topical anesthesia, such as EMLA cream. Hold the pedunculated lesion with a pair of fine-toothed forceps and snip the lesion flush with the surrounding skin with a pair of iris scissors. The wound heals in 7 to 10 days.

Excisional Biopsy

An excisional biopsy is used to completely remove lesions that are too large or deep to remove with either the punch-biopsy or shave-biopsy techniques. This procedure is generally best performed in consultation with a dermatologist or a surgeon.

CRYOSURGERY

Background and Introduction, Anatomy, and Indications

Cryosurgery uses cryogenic agents such as liquid nitrogen to create both intracellular and extracellular ice crystals that cause injury to the cell membrane or that result in cell death. It has been successfully used to treat verruca vulgaris, acne vulgaris, adenoma sebaceum, keloids, pyogenic granulomas, epidermal nevi, and dermatofibromas.

Contraindications

Pretreatment biopsy is recommended for all atypical lesions. Treatment is painful and should be avoided in young or uncooperative children for benign, self-limiting lesions such as molluscum or warts.

Supplies and Equipment

- Cotton-tipped applicator
- Liquid nitrogen

Procedure

1. Dip cotton-tipped applicator in liquid nitrogen. For better results, additional raw cotton (from a cotton ball) may be wrapped around the applicator tip to increase the amount of liquid nitrogen on the tip of the swab.
2. Apply the applicator to the lesion long enough to turn the lesion white. Avoid freezing surrounding tissue, especially near digital vessels and nerves at the sides of fingers.
3. For recurrent warts, a "double freeze-thaw" technique may be employed. In this technique, a frozen area 0.5 to 1 mm larger than the lesion is created (usually takes 10 to 25 seconds); the area is then allowed to thaw, and a second freeze is performed. The double-freeze method is more painful and may require anesthesia (e.g., EMLA, lidocaine).

What the Patient and Family Should Know

Postoperative pain, atrophic scarring, and wart recurrence are the most common side effects. Permanent nail dystrophy, temporary hypopigmentation, and cutaneous nerve injury may also occur.

DIAGNOSTIC TECHNIQUES

Background and Introduction

Without performing a biopsy, certain diagnostic procedures may be performed to shed light on the cause of many skin conditions. Several of these procedures are easily performed in the primary care setting, including potassium hydroxide preparations for fungal diagnosis, skin scrapings for scabies, Tzanck preparations for diagnosis of herpes viral infections, and Wood's lamp examination of the skin, as well as various forms of skin testing.

Relevant Anatomy

With the exception of intradermal Mantoux testing for tuberculosis, these procedures all involve access to only the most superficial skin layers, are readily accomplished with minimum discomfort to the patient, and require only very basic equipment.

Indications

These diagnostic procedures are generally performed in order to establish a rapid diagnosis before initiation of prolonged treatment. Culture of the organisms involved is time-consuming and usually unnecessary if proper diagnostic studies are used.

Contraindications

There are no absolute contraindications to these simple procedures. Caution should be used in obtaining scrapings of skin in patients with coagulopathies.

Potassium Hydroxide Preparation

Potassium hydroxide (KOH) preparation is a quick, simple technique that can be useful for diagnosing fungal infections of the skin, hair, or nails (e.g., tinea corporis, tinea capitis, tinea versicolor), or molluscum contagiosum. KOH dissolves keratin found in skin cells, allowing the typical microscopic features of fungal organisms to become apparent.

Supplies and equipment

- Glass slide with cover slip
- Matches
- Microscope
- Potassium hydroxide solution 20%
- Scalpel blade #15

Procedure

1. Obtain scales, hair, or nail fragments with a curved blade and place them on a glass slide. This can be done by gently scraping the loose scale at the margin of a skin lesion; gently scraping the surface of a superficially infected fingernail; extracting subungual material; or extracting the small, pearly globule from the center of a lesion of molluscum. The short, residual hair stubs of tinea capitis also may be shaved off and examined.
2. When scraping the skin, angle the scalpel blade so that the sharp edge is directed away from the direction in which the skin is being scraped, and hold the slide just under the lesion to allow for most efficient collection of material (Fig. 15-4).
3. Place one to two drops of KOH on the specimen on the slide.
4. Heat the slide gently with a match or allow it to quick dry on the microscope stage with the light turned on. Do not allow the KOH to come to a boil. If the sample is not heated, the keratin will still dissolve in 15 to 20 minutes.
5. Place a cover slip on top of the specimen.
6. Absorb extra KOH with a paper towel blotted at the edge of the cover slip. A pencil eraser may be used to flatten thick specimens by applying pressure to the cover slip.
7. Allow the slide to sit for 10 to 15 minutes after heating while the epithelial cells dissolve.
8. Scan the slide under low (10x to 20x) power for hyphae or yeast. Then examine suspicious areas under higher power.

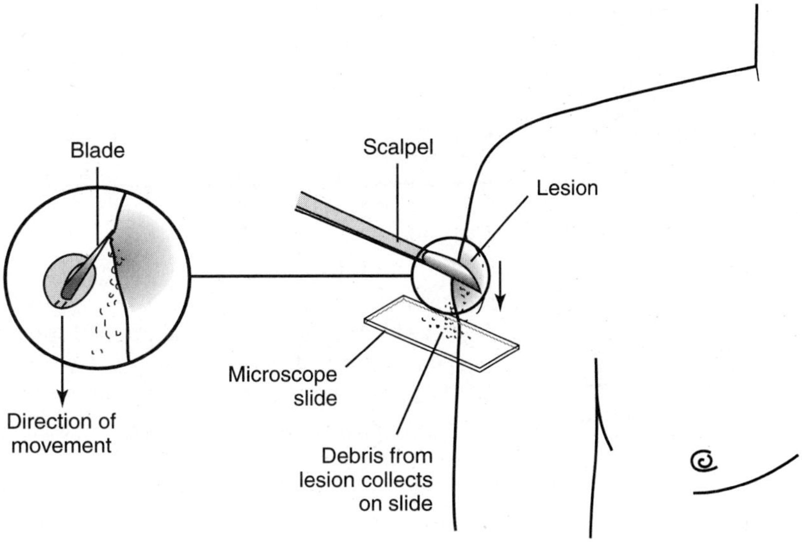

FIG. 15-4. Scraping for potassium hydroxide (KOH) preparation.

Interpretation of results

True hyphae of fungal infections are long, green, branching rods of a uniform width that cross epithelial cell borders. They may contain septae. Yeast infections may also show budding yeast and pseudohyphae. A molluscum body is a homogeneous oval disc consisting of an aggregate of multiple keratinocytes (squamous stem cells). In fungal infections of the scalp, small, round spores are packed within or surrounding the hair shaft, and hyphae are rarely seen.

What the patient and family should know

Children under 2 years of age may need to be restrained. For older children, it may be helpful to demonstrate the scraping technique on your own hand so they know it is not painful.

Scabies Preparation

A scabies preparation can be helpful for diagnosing scabies infection. This infection is characterized clinically by burrows on the wrists, intertriginous areas, interdigital spaces, scrotum, penis, palms, and soles. In infants, lesions may occur on the head and neck. Because of the highly pruritic nature of this infestation, the characteristic rash may be altered secondary to excoriation, scarring, and topical or oral medications, thus making the scabies preparation a useful tool.

Supplies and equipment

- Glass slide with cover slip
- Microscope

- Mineral oil
- Scalpel blade #15

Procedure

1. Try to identify a fresh burrow. Classically, these are 3- to 10-mm elongated papules with a vesicle or pustule at one end. A small, dark spot may be seen in the vesicle, which represents the mite and can be lifted out of the burrow with the scalpel tip or a needle.
2. Apply a drop of mineral oil to the burrow with a cotton-tipped applicator. This will help the scrapings to adhere to the scalpel.
3. With multiple, short, quick stokes, scrape along the burrow with the scalpel blade while holding the skin taut between the index finger and thumb. A small amount of bleeding may occur.
4. Place the scrapings on the slide and apply a second drop of mineral oil.
5. Cover the specimen with a cover slip.

Interpretation of results

The scabies mite is an eight-legged arachnid that can be seen with low power. Focus through thick areas of skin scrapings. Eggs may be seen in or nearby the female mite and are smooth ovals. The eggs are about half the size of the adult mite. Mite feces, which appear as red-brown pellets in clusters, are also diagnostic.

Tzanck Smear

The Tzanck smear is used to look for the multinucleated giant cells diagnostic of herpes simplex or varicella zoster virus infections. This test can be helpful in differentiating these viral infections from other causes of vesiculobullous diseases in newborns (e.g., transient neonatal pustular melanosis, acropustulosis of infancy, and erythema toxicum) and older infants and children (e.g., bullous erythema multiforme, toxic epidermal necrolysis, or staphylococcal scalded skin syndrome).

Supplies and equipment

- Giemsa or Wright stain
- Glass slide with cover slip
- Microscope
- Scalpel blade #15
- Sterile gauze
- Optional: 95% alcohol

Procedure

1. Unroof the blister or eschar with a scalpel blade or a pair of scissors.
2. Blot the fluid from the blister with sterile gauze.
3. Gently scrape the base of the blister or the erosion with the blade.
4. Spread the material thinly on a glass slide.
5. Air dry and, if possible, fix it with 95% alcohol for 2 minutes.

6. Stain with Giemsa or Wright stain. Toluidine blue or crystal violet may also be used.
7. Scan the slide and isolate an area of epithelial cells. Then examine for giant cells under high power.

Interpretation of results

Multinucleated giant cells or balloon cells (discrete rounded-up keratinocytes) are diagnostic of virus infection. Unfortunately, a positive finding does not distinguish between herpes simplex and varicella zoster infection. Further studies, including double-fluorescent antibody, polymerase chain reaction, and electron microscopy, can be performed when warranted. Eosinophils are seen in eosinophilic pustular folliculitis, erythema toxicum, or incontinentia pigmenti. Polymorphonuclear leukocytes are seen in neonatal pustular melanosis, acropustulosis of infancy, or pustular psoriasis.

Wood's Lamp

Wood's lamp examination can be useful in screening for possible fungal infections with certain microsporum species. Unfortunately, *Trichophyton tonsurans* is now the most common cause of tinea capitis, and it does not fluoresce. *Microsporum canis* is the only fungal cause of tinea capitis in the United States that fluoresces. In addition, the Wood's lamp can facilitate visualization of hypopigmented or depigmented lesions, such as the ash leaf macules of tuberous sclerosis, the linear and swirling hypopigmentation of hypomelanosis of Ito, the truncal hypopigmented macules and plaques of tinea versicolor (which will fluoresce a green-yellow color), and the hypopigmentation and depigmentation of vitiligo. Wood's lamp examination is particularly useful in individuals with light complexions.

SKIN TESTING

Patch Testing

Patch testing can be useful in determining the causative allergen in allergic contact dermatitis, which is the result of a T-lymphocyte cell-mediated, type IV immune response. This response consists of two phases: the induction phase and the elicitation phase. The induction phase consists of the first contact with the allergen and is completed when the subject is sensitized to it and able to produce an elicitation phase, in which the allergic dermatitis is produced on reexposure to the antigen. The induction phase typically takes 5 to 25 days to occur, whereas the elicitation reaction occurs in 24 to 48 hours.

To obtain a positive patch test, an individual must have completed the induction phase and be able to produce an elicitation phase. In this test, the suspected agent is applied to the skin, which is then reexamined 48 hours later to look for a reaction. If the allergen is unknown, a battery of common allergens, standardized by the North American Contact Dermatitis Group, can be used initially.

Contraindications

Recent studies suggest that, if performed properly, this study can be reliable even in children under 2 years of age.

Supplies and equipment

- Hypoallergenic tape
- Suspected allergen or, if unknown, a standard patch test kit (North American Contact Dermatitis Group)

Procedure

1. Apply the suspected allergen or patch test onto the skin, usually the back. Special aluminum chambers are generally used for consistent application of a standard quantity of the antigen.
2. Occlude the area with the hypoallergenic tape.
3. Leave the patches in place and kept dry for 48 hours.
4. Remove the patches and read the results a few hours later and again at 72 hours.

Interpretation of results

A patch test should be interpreted with caution because both false-positive and false-negative results occur commonly. A definitively positive patch test consists of erythema, edema, and small vesicles set closely together, which extend beyond the patch's border. Severe pustular or bullous reactions are rare and usually are the result of an irritant reaction. Interpretation of the patch testing is as follows:

0	negative reaction
?	doubtful reaction: faint erythema
+	weak positive reaction: erythema, infiltration, and possibly papules
++	strong (vesicular) positive reaction: erythema, infiltration, papules, and vesicles
+++	extreme positive reaction: bullous reaction

Mantoux Test-PPD (Purified Protein Derivative)

The Mantoux Test-PPD (purified protein derivative) is a delayed hypersensitivity, type IV reaction, which can be used to screen for a past or present tuberculosis infection. It becomes positive 12 to 36 hours after exposure and is caused by activation of sensitized lymphocytes after antigen contact. In performing the procedure, it is critical that the PPD be injected intradermally, not subcutaneously, in order to attain the standardized result. Proper intradermal injection is confirmed by the observation of a blanched raised bleb, rather than a rounded weal, at the site of the injection. Tuberculin skin testing can be done concurrently with the administration of the measles, mumps, and rubella vaccine (MMR); however, if the two are not done concurrently, the PPD must be given at greater than a 4- to

6-week interval after the administration of the MMR to be valid because MMR can induce anergy during the several weeks after its administration.

Contraindications

Previous Bacillus Calmette-Guerin (BCG) vaccination is not a contraindication to Mantoux skin testing. BCG is a live vaccine prepared from attenuated *Mycobacterium bovis*. It is currently used in more than one hundred countries in an attempt to prevent disseminated disease; however, BCG does not prevent *Mycobacterium tuberculosis* infection.

Supplies and equipment

- Alcohol swab
- Pen for marking positive area
- Purified protein derivative (PPD), 5 tuberculin units (TU), usually 0.1 ml
- Small-gauge needle (25 to 27) with 1-ml syringe

Procedure

1. Cleanse the flexor surface of the forearm with alcohol.
2. With the bevel up, introduce the needle into the skin's superficial layers, and inject 0.1 ml of PPD intradermally. A white bleb approximately 10 mm in diameter should be seen (Fig. 15-5). This bleb will disappear soon. No bandage is needed.
3. Mark the test site with a pen.

Interpretation of results

Examine the injection site at 48 to 72 hours. Measure the area of induration, *not erythema*. A negative Mantoux test never excludes tuberculosis infection. Approximately 10% of immunocompetent children with culture-documented disease do not react to the standard Mantoux test. Young age, malnutrition,

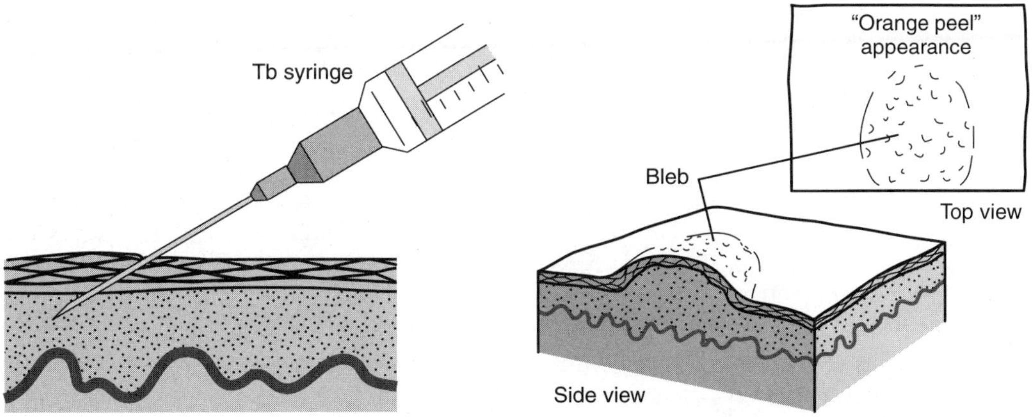

FIG. 15-5. Intradermal purified protein derivative (PPD).

BOX 15-1 DEFINITIONS OF POSITIVE MANTOUX SKIN TEST RESULTS IN CHILDREN

Induration Greater than or Equal to 5 mm

Children in close contact with known or suspected infectious cases of tuberculosis:

Households with active or previously active cases if treatment cannot be verified as adequate before exposure, treatment was initiated after the child's contact, or reactivation is suspected

Children suspected to have tuberculosis:

Chest radiograph consistent with active or previously active tuberculosis

Clinical evidence of tuberculosis

Children receiving immunosuppressive therapy or with immunosuppressive conditions, including HIV infection*

Induration Greater than or Equal to 10 mm

Children at increased risk of disseminated disease:

Age less than 4 years

Other medical risk factors, including Hodgkin's disease, lymphoma, diabetes mellitus, chronic renal failure, or malnutrition

Children with increased environmental exposure to tuberculosis:

Those who were born, or whose parents were born, in high prevalence regions of the world

Frequently exposed to adults who are HIV-infected, homeless, users of illicit drugs, residents of nursing homes, incarcerated or institutionalized persons, and migrant farm workers

Travel and exposure to high prevalence regions of the world

Induration Greater than or Equal to 15 mm

Children 4 years of age or older without any risk factors

*Including immunosuppressive dose of corticosteroids.

immunosupression, other viral infections (e.g., measles, varicella, influenza), and severe disseminated tuberculosis can also result in decreased skin reactivity. Children with human immunodeficiency virus (HIV) may be anergic; therefore in the case of suspected or known immunosuppression or severe disease, placement of an anergy panel (see following section) is recommended. The classification of a test response as positive depends on clinical and epidemiological factors (Box 15-1).

After BCG administration, it is difficult to distinguish between a true positive result and that which results from the vaccination. Some BCG-vaccinated individuals may not demonstrate any skin test reactivity. Because no reliable criteria have been established for distinguishing a positive test from BCG vaccination from those of tuberculosis infection, the same guidelines are generally applied to both groups. Typically, if Mantoux skin test reactivity occurs after BCG vaccination, it is unlikely to be greater than 10 mm. It is also unlikely to persist for longer than a few years postvaccination in the absence of exposure to and infection with *M. tuberculosis* or repeated skin testing. The degree of Mantoux reaction after BCG depends on the child's age at vaccination, the quality and strain of BCG used, the number of doses received, nutritional and immunological status, time interval elapsed since BCG vaccination, and frequency of Mantoux testing. If the BCG is given a few months after birth, a larger reaction will be seen than when an infant is immunized soon after birth. A positive Mantoux (larger than 10 mm) in a child 5 years of age or older is unlikely to have resulted from a BCG received in infancy alone, and other sources of infection should be explored.

Patients with nontuberculosis mycobacterium (NTM) infections can also have a false-positive Mantoux result because the PPD preparation derived from *M. tuberculosis* has several antigens in common with NTM species. These false-positive results occur in otherwise well children with no known tuberculosis exposure and usually, but not always, result in a skin reaction with less than 10 mm of induration. These false-positive results may be more common than true positives in a population with a high NTM prevalence and low tuberculosis prevalence. A positive Mantoux result of less than 10 mm of induration, the presence of cervical adenitis or other symptoms consistent with NTM infection, normal chest radiograph, negative PPDs in family members, and the absence of an index case make NTM infection probable.

Anergy Panel

Use of an anergy panel is based on the assumption that patients have been exposed previously to certain common antigens and that, if patients are immunocompetent, they should mount a reaction to them. Candida, mumps, and trichophyton are some of the common antigens used. They are applied and read in the same fashion as the PPD (an area of erythema larger than 1.5 cm is considered positive and normal).

SUGGESTED READINGS

Cohen BA: *Pediatric dermatology,* London, 1999, Wolfe.

Peter G: *1997 red book: report of the Committee on Infectious Disease,* ed 24, Elk Grove Village, Ill, 1997, American Academy of Pediatrics.

Schachner LA, Hansen RC: *Pediatric dermatology,* ed 2, New York, 1995, Churchill Livingstone.

CHAPTER 16

Cardiopulmonary Procedures

Allen Walker

GENERAL INTRODUCTION

This comprehensive chapter covers the most common or most important procedures involving the cardiac and pulmonary systems. Some information overlaps with the Emergency Procedures chapters. This chapter mainly addresses procedures that are considered elective or semielective but that are often performed to prevent the rapid deterioration in status that might lead to the need for an emergency procedure.

ELECTROCARDIOGRAPHY

Background and Introduction

Electrocardiography, the recording of electrical activity from the heart during the cardiac cycle, is a common method of assessing the size of various components of the heart, determining the presence of abnormal rhythms or conduction abnormalities, and obtaining clues about the health of the myocardium or pericardium. The science underlying the actual process of converting cardiac electrical signals into a recorded pattern of activity that can be interpreted is beyond the scope of this book.

Newer methods of assessment of cardiac function, especially the echocardiogram, have resulted in somewhat less emphasis on the electrocardiogram (ECG) recently, but intelligent, organized interpretation of the ECG can yield significant diagnostic insights, and an ECG is generally more easily obtained.

Relevant Anatomy

The heart occupies the anterior portion of the chest and undergoes a significant change in anatomy as a child ages. During the early years of life, the right ventricle is dominant, and the ECG reflects this, demonstrating "right axis deviation." The right heart border may lie to the right of the right edge of the sternum, leading to a different lead placement for ECGs in young children.

The ECG is obtained by placing electrical leads on the chest wall and then recording electrical activity arising from the surface of the heart. Extreme obesity may make accurate placement of leads difficult and may reduce the amplitude of the tracings obtained.

Indications

An ECG is indicated when concern arises about a cardiac abnormality and assessment of specific aspects of cardiac function is expected to be useful in determining the nature and effects of the abnormality. Broadly considered, ECG tracings should be obtained for the following reasons:

- To determine the heart rate (tachycardia, bradycardia)
- To determine abnormalities of rhythm (atrial ectopy, ventricular ectopy)
- To assess the presence or absence of ischemia of cardiac muscle
- To assess the possibility of electrolyte imbalance (hyperkalemia, hypercalcemia, hypocalcemia)
- To assess relative size of cardiac chambers (congenital heart disease, ventricular hypertrophy)
- To assess the possibility of toxin-induced changes (tricyclic antidepressant overdose, cocaine ingestion)

Contraindications and Reasons for Referral to a Specialist

There are essentially no contraindications to performing an ECG. Referral to a specialist is indicated when the underlying condition being evaluated requires care that is beyond the expertise of the general pediatrician or when local interpretation of the ECG tracing is in question.

Required/Recommended Nursing Skills and Procedures

The most important nursing skill in obtaining ECGs is consistency. Anyone obtaining ECG tracings must have specific training in the procedures, particularly lead placement. Specific locations must be used for each electrode, and failure to place leads appropriately can lead to ECGs that are uninterpretable or, perhaps worse, misleading. It is also important that children lie still while ECG tracings are obtained; nursing expertise in reassuring and comforting infants and children leads to better results. For these reasons, experienced pediatric nurses are critical to obtaining reliable ECG results.

Supplies and Equipment

The only equipment needed is an ECG recorder, which is available in several configurations, ranging from the relatively old, but reliable, strip recorder, which records one lead at a time, to modern machines that record all leads simultaneously, print out the results, and provide a suggested interpretation of the ECG quickly. Supplies required include the following:

- Alcohol swabs, for cleaning the area to which the electrodes are applied
- Electrodes, which often include a conducting substance already applied
- Electrode wires, normally a part of the ECG machine
- Paper for recording the ECG

Procedure

Children should be lying down in the supine position because the electrode positioning and the resulting pattern on the ECG has been standardized in this position. Other positions may lead to results that cannot be interpreted. Children must be calm and quiet; in this instance, nursing and child life personnel can be invaluable in distracting children during the brief time needed to obtain a tracing.

Proper electrode placement is critical to successfully recording an ECG. The limb leads (i.e., RA [right arm], LA [left arm], RL [right leg], and LL [left leg]) are generally recorded by the electrodes at the wrists and ankles. Placement of the leads closer to the torso (e.g., upper arm for the arm leads, and thigh for the leg leads), however, may decrease artifactual recordings without changing the interpretability of the tracing.

Fig. 16-1 illustrates the recommended sites of electrode application for the chest leads and the names for those leads. Accurate placement of the chest leads is critical to successfully recording and interpreting the ECG. Normally, in adults and older children, electrodes are placed in six different positions on the chest wall, with only one electrode to the right of the sternum (V1). In infants and young children, however, placement of at least two, and sometimes three, electrodes to

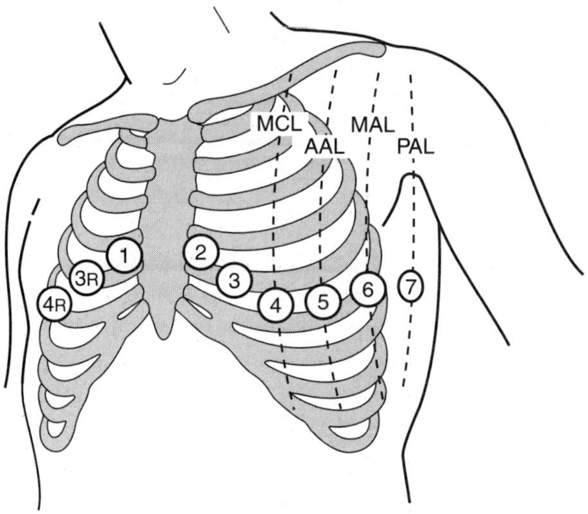

FIG. 16-1. ECG lead placement.

the right of the sternum is recommended (V1, V3R, V4R). ECG machines may have only six electrode wires, and the recommended leads for infants and young children are V1, V2, V3R, V4, V5, and V6.

Once the leads are in place, the tracing is obtained in different ways depending on the specific ECG machine in use. Modern ECG machines are small computers that record a patient's name, medical record number, age, height, weight, location, as well as automatically obtaining, recording, and displaying the tracing. Older machines may record only one lead at a time and may require manual entry of markers identifying the origin of each part of the tracing.

On any machine, two variables must be identified and recorded correctly. ECG machines can record tracings at different speed; the routine speed is 25 mm of paper per second. Any change in paper speed will lead to major difficulties in interpretation if a speed other than 25 mm/sec is used and not appropriately noted. The amount of deflection in the vertical direction is a direct measure of voltage; ECG machines can record at several different sensitivities to allow easier display of the full range of deflection. Standard deflection is 1 mV (millivolt) per 10 mm. Any changes in the sensitivity of recording must be clearly identified and marked on the tracing. Significant errors in interpretation may be made if assumptions about the sensitivity setting at the time of recording are incorrect.

Interpretation of Results

Interpretation of ECGs has filled entire books, and specifics will not be repeated here. Accurate interpretation of ECGs depends on a systematic approach to the information contained on the ECG tracing, and one approach is outlined here. The following steps should be undertaken in interpreting an ECG:

1. Assess the rhythm (sinus rhythm, abnormal rhythms).
2. Assess the rate.
3. Determine the QRS axis.
4. Measure the important intervals (PR, QRS, and QT).
5. Determine the P-wave amplitude and duration.
6. Determine the QRS amplitude; look for abnormal Q-waves; compute R/S ratios.
7. Examine the ST segment and the T-wave.

Interpretation of the ECG by a general pediatrician often reveals significant abnormalities, which often leads to direct referral to a pediatric cardiologist. In general, ECGs should be reviewed by a specialist who is experienced in interpreting pediatric ECGs soon after the patient is evaluated and the ECG is obtained; the haste with which this review must be sought varies with the patient's clinical condition.

What the Family and Patient Should Know

Perhaps most significant, patients and parents should be told that the process of obtaining an ECG is painless. Young children should be reassured that the wires and leads do not produce electricity and that no pain will be experienced with the procedure. Patients and parents should also be told that the most successful ECG tracing is obtained when children lie as still as possible during the procedure.

Parents should also understand that interpretation of the ECG by the primary care pediatrician is not a definitive reading and that the interpretation may change in subtle ways once the tracing is reviewed by a pediatric cardiologist. They can be reassured that major abnormalities will be identified and that, if they or the pediatrician have any unresolved questions, arrangements can be made to transmit the tracing electronically to a specialist for immediate interpretation.

Possible Complications

No complications are expected during or after the process of obtaining an ECG tracing.

Aftercare Instructions

Instructions for aftercare depend on the underlying abnormality or presenting problem. No specific aftercare instructions are necessary relative to having obtained an ECG tracing.

Modifications for Situations of Limited Resources

The only possible modification for situations of limited resources is that the machine used to obtain the ECG tracing may be older and less automated than current units. The processes of lead placement and interpretation, however, remain the same.

DYSRHYTHMIA AND CARDIOVERSION, NONPHARMACOLOGIC

Background and Introduction

Discussion of the electrical approach to resolution of various dysrhythmias is given in the Emergency Procedures section of this book. The following section focuses on nonpharmacologic maneuvers that may be performed to attempt to convert supraventricular tachycardia into a stable rhythm.

Supraventricular tachycardia (SVT) is a tachyarrhythmia that may develop throughout childhood but is most common in infants. Most children who develop SVT have accessory pathways between the atria and the ventricles that allow for transmission of electrical energy along the conducting pathways much more rapidly than normal. SVT is the most common tachyarrhythmia in children. It may lead to congestive heart failure rapidly (within hours), or it may be tolerated relatively well over a period of days.

The diagnosis of SVT is generally straightforward. The hallmarks are a heart rate greater than 240 beats per minute (bpm) and usually less than 300, along with a narrow QRS complex on the monitor or ECG display. The two significant conditions that must be differentiated from SVT are sinus tachycardia (ST) and ventricular tachycardia (VT). ST is a physiologic response to changes in the vascular system; it is often caused by a combination of dehydration and fever, but it may also result from the effects of toxins, trauma, infection, or cardiac conditions causing a decrease in cardiac output (e.g., cardiogenic shock caused by congenital heart disease or myocarditis). ST rarely results in a pulse rate above 220 bpm, whereas children in SVT typically have a heart rate greater than 240 bpm. ST is generally preceded by signs and symptoms caused by the underlying disorder (e.g., gastroenteritis with dehydration and fever), whereas SVT typically has an abrupt onset.

Distinguishing VT from SVT depends on observing the waveform on the monitor or ECG tracing. SVT is a narrow-complex tachycardia, with a QRS interval that is normal and preceded by a P-wave, although the P-wave may not be visible because of the rapid heart rate. VT is a wide-complex tachycardia, with an abnormally wide QRS interval and an absence of preceding P-waves. Differentiating VT from SVT is usually straightforward, whereas differentiating ST from SVT may occasionally be difficult and may rely on response to therapy as a diagnostic tool.

Once SVT is diagnosed, a crucial distinction is whether patients with SVT are stable or unstable. In this instance, stability refers to the patients, not to the propensity of the rhythm to degenerate into a lethal rhythm. Unstable patients with SVT have the following signs and symptoms of congestive heart failure:

- Tachypnea, retractions, nasal flaring
- Rales on auscultation
- Hepatomegaly
- Prolonged capillary refill time (more than 2 seconds)
- Mental status changes suggesting decreased perfusion of the brain

Relevant Anatomy

Patients may have an accessory pathway between the atria and ventricles, allowing for rapid transmission of electrical impulses.

Indications

Children with SVT who are unstable must receive immediate synchronized cardioversion. Nonpharmacologic maneuvers are inappropriate in managing these patients, and neither are pharmacologic agents suitable unless the episode is recurrent, children are already in the hospital, a physician and a nurse are ready to assist, and a prefilled syringe of adenosine, which can be given rapidly through a functional intravenous (IV) catheter, is available at the bedside.

Nonpharmacologic maneuvers may be used in patients with SVT who are stable. The intent of all of the maneuvers is to increase vagal tone, slowing the heart rate through the parasympathetic pathways. The vagal maneuvers discussed here often have temporary effects and are variably effective. Although they may be worth trying as a temporizing measure, practitioners must be ready to move to pharmacologic therapy rapidly.

Contraindications

The major contraindication to these maneuvers is the presence of signs of congestive heart failure; such children need to be provided with synchronized cardioversion immediately.

Required/Recommended Nursing Skills and Procedures

The major nursing skill required is monitoring the patient. Recognizing the tachycardia, quickly attaching a monitor to the patient, recognizing the signs and symptoms of congestive heart failure, and careful monitoring of the patient during and after the attempts at nonpharmacologic rhythm conversion are all critical nursing skills required when these maneuvers are attempted. Specific skill at recognizing narrow-complex and wide-complex tachycardia is helpful in the initial presentation.

Supplies and Equipment

Even though stable at the initial decision point, patients with SVT can deteriorate relatively rapidly. They require full cardiorespiratory monitoring from the moment their dysrhythmia is recognized. If patients are stable and a monitor is not immediately available, the preferred procedure (e.g., in the office) is to call "911." In most instances, that maneuver should not only summon an appropriate transport vehicle (compared to the family car) but should also provide a monitor and personnel trained in its use.

Because a more complex rhythm can result from vagal maneuvers, supplies and equipment that allow for full resuscitation and for pharmacologic treatment of any complications should be immediately available. Patients should have a functioning IV line in place. Appropriate airway equipment, especially a bag-valve-mask, oxygen, and suction equipment, must be present and functioning. Resuscitation medications most likely to be needed are epinephrine (1:10,000), lidocaine, and atropine.

Equipment capable of delivering electrical energy for cardioversion or defibrillation must be available in the event that the vagal maneuvers produce unstable SVT or a ventricular tachyarrhythmia (either VT or ventricular fibrillation). In general, ambulances are equipped with units that can fulfill both the monitoring and the cardioversion/defibrillation functions. With a stable patient, however, the safest option may be to simply transport the patient to the nearest available facility that can render definitive care safely and efficiently.

Equipment for the vagal maneuvers themselves is fairly simple and readily available. It includes the following items:

- gloves and lubricant
- ice

- plastic bag or large basin
- tongue depressor
- water

Procedure

Several vagal maneuvers can be employed in attempts to convert SVT to a stable rhythm. All of these maneuvers require that patients be monitored and under the direct, bedside care of pediatricians and nurses who can provide resuscitation if necessary.

The most widely used vagal stimulus is applying a plastic bag of ice to the patient's face. Recall that the intent is to provoke the "diving reflex." A large bag of ice applied to the entire face is required, not simply applying a small bag of ice to the forehead. For the ice to work, frank immersion of the child's face into a basin of iced water or saline is often necessary; this technique is more effective than applying a bag of ice to the face but more difficult to carry out, especially if the child is uncooperative. Pressure on the eye is not recommended because of the possibility of injury to the eye itself.

A gentle rectal examination may provide some vagal stimulus, as might a gag produced by a tongue blade, but neither maneuver is very effective. If the child is old enough, a Valsalva maneuver may terminate the tachycardia.

Carotid massage may also be tried. Massage of the carotid artery at the level of the upper border of the thyroid cartilage and at the anterior edge of the sternocleidomastoid muscle may be tried for no longer than 5 to 10 seconds. The massage should be gentle and should not occlude the pulse. Simultaneous bilateral carotid massage should not be employed because of the potential for interfering with blood flow to the brain. Carotid massage should also not be performed in a patient in whom digitalis toxicity is a possibility.

Interpretation of Results

With the child on a cardiac monitor, results of the vagal maneuvers will be immediately apparent. Conversion from SVT to sinus rhythm may be abrupt, and careful attention to the monitor is crucial.

What the Family and Patient Should Know

The family, and patients if they are old enough to understand, must be told that the maneuvers that are about to be applied are generally safe but may be ineffective in converting the rhythm. Each of the procedures is unpleasant, and parents should be prepared for the patients' discomfort, which is unavoidable.

Most important, family and patients should know that whether the maneuvers are successful or not, patients will need to be evaluated by a pediatric cardiologist immediately. The possibility of an aberrant, accessory atrioventricular pathway, and the possibilities for treatment to avoid a recurrence, make a full evaluation by an experienced pediatric cardiologist mandatory.

Possible Complications

The major potential complication of these maneuvers is the conversion of a stable, perfusing rhythm into an unstable, nonperfusing rhythm, particularly asystole or a ventricular tachyarrhythmia. Such an outcome is possible, although rare, with any of the maneuvers.

Other complications include those that stem from the procedures themselves. Vomiting while provoking a gag reflex, with subsequent aspiration, is unlikely but possible. Apnea resulting from applying a bag of ice to the face is similarly rare but possible. Carotid massage can theoretically cause interference with blood flow to the brain, with subsequent brain injury, although this outcome is vanishingly rare.

Aftercare Instructions

The only aftercare instruction directly related to these maneuvers is the absolute necessity for evaluation by a pediatric cardiologist, whether the episode of SVT is the initial episode or is a recurrence. If the episode is the initial one, full evaluation by the current sophisticated techniques often reveals a treatable cause of the SVT and prevents recurrences. If the episode is a recurrence of the SVT, its occurrence may indicate the need for reevaluation and the institution of, or change in, medication.

It may be helpful to obtain a full ECG immediately after sinus rhythm is achieved. Evidence of an accessory atrioventricular pathway in the form of a delta wave may be more evident just after conversion than at other times.

Modifications for Situations of Limited Resources

At certain times and circumstances, these maneuvers are the best that can be done for children in distress. In that case, it may be beneficial to teach children and their families how to perform some of the less invasive maneuvers themselves. If no pediatric cardiologist is available, and no chance of further evaluation is forthcoming, then these maneuvers may represent the standard of care for children in some locations at some times.

DYSRHYTHMIA AND CARDIOVERSION, PHARMACOLOGIC

Background and Relevant Anatomy

See discussion in the preceding section on nonpharmacologic dysrhythmia and cardioversion.

Indications

Any child with SVT who is unstable must receive immediate synchronized cardioversion. Nonpharmacologic maneuvers are inappropriate in managing these patients, and neither are pharmacologic agents suitable unless the episode is recurrent, children are already in the hospital, a physician and a nurse are ready to assist, and a prefilled syringe of adenosine, which can be given rapidly through a functional IV catheter, is available at the bedside.

The primary indication for using adenosine to treat stable SVT is a desire to end the tachycardia quickly. Failure of vagal maneuvers to convert SVT to sinus rhythm is not a necessary prerequisite for using adenosine, which is considered first-line therapy for SVT in infants and children.

Contraindications and Reasons for Referral to a Specialist

There are few contraindications to using adenosine to treat SVT. A relative contraindication is a history of asthma in patients because adenosine may provoke bronchoconstriction.

Children who receive adenosine to treat SVT must be immediately referred to a pediatric cardiologist, whether the adenosine is effective or not. Diagnostic and treatment options have become more available and safer over the past decade. Many children with SVT can be evaluated and treated electrophysiologically, by ablating their aberrant pathway and preventing recurrence of the SVT.

If adenosine fails to convert the SVT to a normal rhythm, consultation from a specialist should be sought. Several medications can be used after adenosine, including digoxin and beta-blockers. Esophageal overdrive pacing may be required. These medications and procedures require the consultation, if not the active management, of a specialist in such problems.

One contraindication must be pointed out: Although the therapeutic armamentarium for adults with SVT includes verapamil, this drug should not be used in infants or young children because it can cause cardiac arrest, from which infants cannot be resuscitated.

Required/Recommended Nursing Skills and Procedures

The major nursing skill required is that of monitoring the patient. Recognizing the tachycardia, quickly attaching a monitor to the patient, recognizing the signs and symptoms of congestive heart failure, and careful monitoring of the patient during and after the attempts at pharmacologic rhythm conversion are all critical nursing skills required when conversion is attempted. Specific skill at recognizing narrow-complex and wide-complex tachycardia is helpful in the initial presentation.

Because adenosine often causes a period of asystole after injection, the team caring for these patients must be capable of resuscitating children in asystole. Adenosine must be given as a rapid bolus. Although it is routinely given in a peripheral vein with success, the IV line should be a secure, relatively large catheter that can tolerate a very rapid IV bolus pushed with pressure.

Supplies and Equipment

Even though stable at the initial decision point, patients with SVT can deteriorate relatively rapidly and require full cardiorespiratory monitoring from the moment their dysrhythmia is recognized. If patients are stable and a monitor is not immediately available, the preferred procedure (e.g., in the office) is to call "911." In most instances, that maneuver should not only summon an appropriate transport vehicle (compared to the family car) but should also provide a monitor and personnel trained in its use.

Because a more dangerous rhythm can result from using adenosine, supplies and equipment that allow for full resuscitation and for pharmacologic treatment of any complications must be immediately available. Patients should have a functioning IV line in place. Appropriate airway equipment, especially a bag-valve-mask set, oxygen, and suction equipment, must be present and functioning. Resuscitation medications most likely to be needed are epinephrine (1:10,000), lidocaine, and atropine.

Equipment capable of delivering electrical energy for cardioversion or defibrillation must be available in the event that the adenosine produces unstable SVT or a ventricular tachyarrhythmia (either VT or ventricular fibrillation). In general, ambulances are equipped with units that can fulfill both the monitoring and the cardioversion/defibrillation functions. With a stable patient, however, the safest option may be to simply transport the patient to the nearest available facility that can render definitive care safely and efficiently.

The actual equipment for delivering adenosine is simple, readily available, and includes the following:

- Active drug
- Saline for preparing IV boluses
- Syringes and needles for accessing the port on the IV tubing

The initial dose of adenosine is 0.1 mg/kg, to a maximum of 12 mg as a single dose or a total cumulative dose for an infant or young child. If the first dose is not effective, a second dose of 0.2 mg/kg can be given, as long as the total dose given is not more than 12 mg.

Procedure

Adenosine must be given as a true bolus dose and must be infused rapidly in order to be effective. The recommended technique is as follows:

1. Insert both the syringe containing the active drug and a syringe containing a 3- to 5-ml dose of normal saline into one port in the IV line, as close to the bloodstream as possible.
2. Occlude the IV tubing proximal to the site of the injection port to prevent the reflux of adenosine retrograde through the tubing.
3. Administer the dose of adenosine by rapidly depressing the plunger of the syringe containing the active drug and, once that syringe is empty, immediately depressing the plunger of the syringe containing normal saline, pushing the adenosine into the bloodstream as rapidly as possible.
4. As soon as the adenosine is given, focus on the child and the monitor. Older

children may complain of chest pain, shortness of breath, facial flushing, nausea, lightheadedness, or dyspnea shortly after the infusion. The monitor generally shows a period of asystole lasting from 5 to 15 seconds and then may show sinus rhythm.

5. If the rhythm is sinus, continue to monitor the patient. Adenosine is cleared from the bloodstream in one pass through the system, which takes a matter of seconds. Improvement after adenosine may be brief, and children must be watched carefully.

Interpretation of Results

The monitor provides the information needed and can graphically illustrate to patients and the family the success, or lack of success, in converting the SVT to sinus rhythm. A brief initial period of sinus bradycardia may occur, which is generally followed by mild ST, which is easily differentiated from SVT.

What the Family and the Patient Should Know

Patients and family should be informed that adenosine does have some unpleasant, brief side effects. They should also understand that adenosine may not convert the tachycardia and that other treatments may be necessary. If the family is present during the adenosine infusion, they should be warned about the appearance of asystole on the monitor and the likelihood of monitor alarms going off; such alarms can be worrisome to patients and family members if they occur unexpectedly. They should also be warned about the very small chance that an arrhythmia may occur, which requires more active treatment, including cardioversion or defibrillation. The steps that might be taken if such an event occurs should be briefly reviewed before the procedure.

Possible Complications

The most significant complication is bronchoconstriction, which occurs rarely after using adenosine. The other side effects listed previously may be viewed as complications but simply represent the action of the drug.

Aftercare Instructions

The only aftercare instruction that is directly related to using adenosine is the absolute necessity for evaluation by a pediatric cardiologist, whether the episode of SVT is the initial episode or a recurrence. If the episode is the initial one, full evaluation by the current sophisticated techniques often reveals a treatable cause of the SVT and prevents recurrences. If the episode is a recurrence of the SVT, its occurrence may indicate the need for reevaluation and the institution of, or change in, medication.

It may be helpful to obtain a full ECG immediately after sinus rhythm is achieved. Evidence of an accessory atrioventricular pathway in the form of a delta wave may be more evident just after conversion than at other times.

Modifications for Situations of Limited Resources

Presumably, in a developing country or in remote areas, the opportunities to monitor children undergoing treatment with adenosine may not be ideal. Monitoring with a stethoscope or with a finger on the pulse provide much of the same information as monitors; however, palpating an infant's pulse, especially one with a short, full neck, can be difficult for practitioners who do not attempt this task regularly. In a situation of limited resources, trusting one's powers of observation (i.e., inspection, palpation, percussion, auscultation) is crucial; practicing each skill during routine visits can help make one more certain of one's abilities during a crisis. Practicing feeling pulses in infants refines a skill that many practitioners take for granted.

Referral to a pediatric cardiologist may be more difficult in situations where resources are limited. The goal of diagnosis and definitive treatment for the individual child should not change, but the means of getting to the goal may be different and much more difficult.

PULSE OXIMETRY

Background and Introduction

Noninvasive measurement of one aspect of oxygenation by pulse oximetry has accounted for changes in the way many children are diagnosed and monitored. The ease with which a measurement of oxygen hemoglobin saturation can be made has led to the widespread employment and acceptance of the percentage oxygen saturation by pulse oximetry. Although this widespread acceptance has contributed to the care of children, misinterpretation or overinterpretation of the numbers that are obtained so easily can occasionally be misleading and lead to either undertreatment or overtreatment.

Pulse oximeters are designed to measure the difference in absorption of light at two specific wavelengths by oxyhemoglobin and deoxyhemoglobin. Deoxyhemoglobin absorbs more light than oxyhemoglobin at wavelengths in the 600 to 750 nm range, whereas oxyhemoglobin absorbs more light than deoxyhemoglobin at wavelengths in the 850 to 1000 nm range. The probe measures the difference in absorption of light generated by two light-emitting diodes (LEDs) at specific wavelengths and then converts that difference in absorption to a percentage oxygen saturation number using algorithms built into the machinery. The number is subsequently displayed as percentage hemoglobin saturation.

Relevant Anatomy

Patients must have a pulse in order for the pulse oximeter to function effectively. Although this requirement seems self-evident, pulse oximeters do not function accurately when patients have weak or nonexistent pulses. Pulse oximeters rely on changes induced by a pulse to accurately measure changes in hemoglobin saturation caused by arterial flow rather than local tissue conditions, venous flow, and the like. Areas with pulsatile flow adequate for pulse oximetry include the fingers, toes, earlobes, hands, feet, and penis.

Indications

Indications for pulse oximetry include monitoring children in whom it is important to assess adequacy of oxygenation for conditions such as the following:

- Respiratory distress
- Cardiac disease
- Shock
- Apnea/bradycardia
- Sedation/analgesia

Contraindications and Reasons for Referral to a Specialist

The contraindications to pulse oximetry include those conditions in which the hemoglobin saturation measured by pulse oximetry may be inaccurate and misleading; as such, they are relative contraindications, predicated on an understanding of the limitations of the method by which hemoglobin saturation measurements are generated by pulse oximeters.

As stated previously, pulse oximeters rely on the difference in the absorption of light by oxyhemoglobin and deoxyhemoglobin at two different wavelengths. Any condition in which more than two types of hemoglobin are present in the vascular system may lead to inaccurate and misleading measurements. The presence of significant amounts of carboxyhemoglobin leads to an overestimation of oxygen saturation by pulse oximetry. Methemoglobin may cause overestimation or underestimation of the oxygen saturation, and treatment with methylene blue causes a lowering of the estimated oxygen saturation indicated by pulse oximetry. Actual measurement of both carboxyhemoglobin and methemoglobin, coupled with measurement of oxygen saturation by arterial blood gas determination, allows for more accurate management of children with disorders caused by these hemoglobins.

Sickle hemoglobin affects oxygen saturation measured by pulse oximetry, in general tending to overestimate it. Because the pulse oximeter is somewhat inaccurate, but not in an entirely predictive fashion, measurement of hemoglobin or hematocrit and an arterial blood gas concentration assist in determining how helpful pulse oximetry will be for individual patients with sickle cell disease at a given time.

Another relative contraindication stems from the pulse oximeter's relative insensitivity at both ends of the range of arterial oxygen saturation. Given the shape of the hemoglobin dissociation curve, small changes in oxygen saturation at levels above 90% to 95% can be associated with large changes in the arterial partial pressure of oxygen (Pao_2). Pulse oximeters have not been extensively validated at low oxygen saturation levels because of the obvious danger to volunteers and may be less accurate at saturation levels less than 75%.

Required/Recommended Nursing Skills and Procedures

Probably the most important skill for both physicians and nurses to have is an appreciation and avoidance of the factors that lead to inaccuracy in measuring oxygen saturation by pulse oximetry. The pulse oximeters in use today provide some direct and indirect indications of proper and improper use. The commonly available units have algorithms built in that do not allow the units to operate in the absence of a detectable waveform. Such units also display a waveform or indicate the absence of a satisfactory waveform by producing flashing lights and beeps.

Ensuring appropriate placement of the sensor and observing the unit's displays generally indicates when the numbers that are displayed are technically accurate. Interpreting those numbers depends on the practitioner's skill and knowledge.

Supplies and Equipment

The primary equipment needed is a pulse oximeter. Several models are available, each of which is somewhat different but provides essentially the same information. Some units interface directly with cardiorespiratory monitors, whereas others are stand-alone units. An awareness of the operating characteristics and features of the oximeter in use is critical.

Several different types of oximetry leads are in use, some of which are disposable and some reusable. A major cost difference exists between the two, as well as several usability issues. Again, awareness of the operating characteristics and features of the oximetry leads is critical.

Procedure

Use of a pulse oximeter is relatively straightforward.

1. Attach the oximetry lead to a part of the body that has pulsatile flow. The lead must be placed in a location with as little movement as possible (a challenge in an infant) and where the light emitter and detector portions of the lead can be as directly opposite one another as possible, in order to enhance the signal strength.
2. Attach the lead to the pulse oximeter and turn the device on.

Units typically display the pulse rate, a flashing light to indicate pulse, and a number representing percentage hemoglobin saturation. Some units may display a waveform, with the size of the waveform reflecting the quality of the pulse detected. Most units have alarm functions that can be set at values that are important limits for a given patient. They also have an audible tone or "beep" that can be silenced or made louder; the tone decreases in frequency as the percentage hemoglobin saturation decreases.

Most units currently available monitor themselves in the sense that if a sufficiently strong pulse is not present, they will indicate so by not giving an estimated saturation or by displaying digitally that the signal is insufficient to give a reading. During any monitoring by pulse oximetry, one must ensure that the waveform appears strong and normal and that the pulse rate displayed by the oximeter is the same as that obtained manually or from a cardiac monitor.

Interpretation of Results

For the reasons already discussed, results obtained through the pulse oximetry process must be interpreted cautiously, taking into account the possibilities of technical inaccuracy or malfunction, the presence of abnormal hemoglobins, and the perfusion of the location to which the oximetry probe is attached.

As important as the absolute value is the trend of oxygen saturation over time. If the saturation decreases in the setting of respiratory distress, this may indicate that the patient is tiring, although the P_{CO_2} is a more sensitive sign, given that one can increase the F_{IO_2} as necessary. If the saturation decreases during a sedation event, this may indicate the need to provide supplemental oxygen or even to reverse the sedation if reversible agents have been used.

What the Patient and Family Should Know

Discussing the technique of pulse oximetry with patients and family demystifies the process and allays their fear. Young children may be afraid of the red light at the end of their finger unless one makes a game of it or refers to "E.T." (a character in a movie with a red finger). Appropriate ranges for the oxygen saturation should also be discussed with patients and family, noting that they may see what appear to be low values as a result of temporary loss of signal caused by patient movement and the like. If the family and/or patients are aware of the level of oxygen saturation that may cause concern, they essentially serve as extra sets of eyes to monitor and care for patients.

Possible Complications

No complications result directly from using pulse oximetry. Applying the probe too tightly has a theoretical risk of causing ischemia. Complications, in the sense of undesired outcomes, may occur when the results of pulse oximetry are used without careful consideration of the underlying physiology and pathophysiology.

Aftercare Instructions

No specific aftercare instructions directly related to pulse oximetry are necessary.

Modification for Situations of Limited Resources

Use of nondisposable oximetry probes may reduce the cost of the procedure significantly. Small, handheld oximeters without sophisticated error-checking features are now available at a cost of several hundred dollars. These may be convenient in remote areas, and most are battery powered.

PEAK FLOW MEASUREMENTS AND PULMONARY FUNCTION TESTING

Background and Introduction

Measuring peak expiratory flow rate (PEFR) is one aspect of pulmonary function tests (PFTs) that has been widely recommended for children with asthma. PEFR measures the degree of obstruction to airflow in small airways and can be used not only to judge the severity of an exacerbation of asthma but also to assess progress during both acute and long-term therapy. PEFR is the maximal flow rate that can be generated during a forced expiration that starts at full inspiration. With peak flow meters, which are readily available, PEFR measurement is relatively simple and straightforward.

Using PEFR data is one aspect of monitoring children with asthma, but it should not be relied on as the only monitoring modality. Monitoring of symptoms appears to be as effective as PEFR monitoring for many patients, particularly those with mild asthma. Patients with more severe asthma may benefit from PEFR monitoring as well as symptom monitoring, particularly if self-monitoring is directly linked to a written asthma action plan that leads directly to changes in treatment.

Formal spirometry, or PFTs, are generally the province of subspecialists in pediatric pulmonology or allergy/immunology and are rarely performed by primary care pediatricians. Details of the interpretation of PFTs can be found in several sources.

Relevant Anatomy

PEFR is reflective of changes in small airway diameter and resultant resistance to air flow during expiration.

Indications

PEFR monitoring is primarily recommended for monitoring children with asthma but not for diagnosing asthma. Not all children with asthma may receive additional benefit from PEFR monitoring; further research is needed.

The National Asthma Education and Prevention Program (NEAPP) has developed guidelines for using PEFR monitoring that depend directly on classifying children with asthma into several groups. Patients who fall into one of the two mild groups ("mild intermittent" or "mild persistent") may not benefit from long-term daily peak flow monitoring unless the children, their families, and their pediatricians find it helpful. Patients who fall into one of the two more severe groups ("moderate persistent" or "severe persistent") may benefit from long-term daily peak flow monitoring if it is related to an asthma action plan that is directly linked to the results of the peak flow monitoring program as well as to a symptom monitoring program.

PEFR monitoring may be useful in the following situations for children with asthma:

- Short-term monitoring
  - After changes in chronic maintenance therapy
  - To establish the patient's personal best PEFR
  - To establish a relationship between PEFR changes and exposure to irritants
- Long-term daily monitoring
  - To detect early changes in disease that require changes in treatment
  - To evaluate responses to changes in therapy
  - To provide some assessment of severity for patients who have difficulty perceiving obstruction to airflow
  - To give a quantitative measurement of severity
- Monitoring during an exacerbation
  - To quantify the severity of the exacerbation
  - To evaluate and guide therapy in multiple settings (e.g., home, office, emergency department)

Contraindications

There are no strict contraindications to using PEFR monitoring. Relative contraindications relate to the value of the information gained. If patients and/or their families find daily testing onerous, they are unlikely to continue with the monitoring program. If the families faithfully record PEFR data and their pediatricians ignore the data or fail to provide an asthma action plan that is based on the data obtained, then the process is likely to be useless.

Required/Recommended Nursing Skills and Procedures

The primary required nursing skill, if the nurse is to provide education on using PEFR monitoring, is that of convincing patients and families that PEFR measurements are worthwhile. This skill depends on a thorough knowledge of the rationale for PEFR monitoring, an appreciation of the tremendous commitment required to carry out a monitoring program, and an understanding of the preferences of the pediatrician concerning the use of PEFR data.

Supplies and Equipment

Several PEFR monitoring devices are available on the market. Factors that may be important in the selection of one over another include cost, legibility of numbers, ease of use and cleaning, durability, and portability. What is important is not the specific brand but the knowledge that being able to measure changes in PEFR using a consistent and reproducible technique will provide data that are clinically useful. The actual numbers measured vary with different devices, highlighting the importance of consistently using the same brand and type of PEFR measurement device.

The monitoring devices are sold with instructions that vary in completeness and comprehensibility. Again, crucial to the use of the PEFR meter is understanding how to use it coupled with an asthma action plan that guides changes in self-management or management in the office or emergency department setting. Examples of handouts for use of a peak flow meter, as well as examples of asthma action plans, are included in NEAPP materials.

Procedure

The actual procedure for measuring PEFR is simple and straightforward.

1. Because the measurement involves the maximal flow rate during expiration, starting from full inspiration, ensure that patients understand that the procedure begins with full inspiration.
2. Have patients stand up, if possible.
3. Have patients place their lips around the mouthpiece of the peak flow meter and blow out as hard and fast as possible.

The meter will indicate a peak flow rate by means of a needle, a bar, or some other indicator that is designed to be easy to use.

Although the procedure is simple and straightforward, several factors can affect the results obtained. Primary among those factors is effort because the PEFR is clearly an effort-dependent measurement. Patients should understand that each measurement should be made with as much effort as possible. If maximal effort cannot be ensured reproducibly, then the numbers obtained may be close to useless.

PEFR obtained with these peak flow meters can be compared to national standards for PEFR (Polger), but the most important comparison both short term and long term is comparison with patients' personal-best peak flow. This number should be obtained over a 2- to 3-week period when patients' asthma is under good control. Patients should check their peak flow twice a day, once in the morning and once between noon and 2 P.M.

Once the personal-best peak flow is determined, that number can be used in various situations to provide meaningful clinical data. Long-term PEFR monitoring can provide patients and parents with early warning of exacerbations. A zone system has been recommended to guide patients and parents in using the PEFR numbers obtained during monitoring. The PEFR is measured in the morning, immediately after waking up and before using a bronchodilator. This early morning measurement is recommended because it allows a plan for the day to be instituted, with time to assess responses to changes in medications; measuring PEFR later in the day gives less time to assess responses to changes and less time to consult a pediatrician, if necessary.

A PEFR greater than 80% of personal best indicates that patients' asthma is under good control; this is commonly referred to as the "green zone" in an analogy to a stoplight. A PEFR between 50% and 80% (yellow zone) suggests caution, indicating that patients should take immediate steps to increase the level of treatment of their asthma. Most often, this means immediate use of a short-acting inhaled beta$_2$-agonist.

A PEFR reading of less than 50% of patients' personal best (red zone) indicates a "medical alert." Patients must take a quick-relief medicine (short-acting inhaled beta$_2$-agonist) and call their physician immediately. Alternatively, patients may take the quick-relief medicine and go directly to the hospital emergency department.

PEFR monitoring can be helpful during asthma exacerbations, even if it is not used on a daily long-term basis. Once the personal-best PEFR is determined, a PEFR measured when the patient is experiencing symptoms can provide immediate determination of the severity of the exacerbation (again using greater than 80%, 50% to 80%, and less than 50% to classify mild, moderate, and severe, respectively) and can guide decisions about therapy in the home, the office, and the emergency department.

Interpretation of Results

This topic is covered in the previous section on Procedure.

What the Patient and Family Should Know

The most important thing that patients and family should know is that a system of measuring PEFR, whether short term or long term, represents a significant gain in control of the patient's asthma. This knowledge comes from using the PEFR meter in conjunction with an asthma action plan that can be put into operation quickly, easily, and logically. If a period of PEFR monitoring does not demonstrate value to patients or family, then its use should be reconsidered because there are other ways of monitoring children with asthma. Symptom monitoring makes more sense for children with mild asthma, according to the NEAPP, and for some patients with severe asthma, depending on the preferences of the family and patients.

One group of patients who may benefit significantly from PEFR monitoring includes those who cannot monitor the severity of their disease by symptoms. A particular group of children appear to be insensitive to major changes in peak flow, and this group has been shown to be at increased risk of dying from their asthma. PEFR monitoring in these patients may provide the information that they cannot determine by monitoring their own symptoms. Patients who are in this group, along with their families, should know that PEFR monitoring may represent a very real management tool that may prevent serious morbidity or mortality.

Possible Complications

No recognized complications result directly from PEFR monitoring. Forced expiration may increase airway obstruction, but if this occurs, it is an indication that therapy is not ideal. The management plan may need to be changed, once the acute exacerbation is managed.

The major "complication" relates to incorrect interpretation of the data obtained. Children may cough or sneeze during one expiration, resulting in a PEFR much higher than any others. One determination of PEFR should not be used as a personal-best peak flow; these rates should be based on a series of measurements over 2 to 3 weeks while patients' asthma is under good control. Similarly, lack of cooperation may lead to serious underestimation of peak flow caused by lack of effort. Changes in therapy based on numbers derived from this effort-based measurement depend on maximal effort; lack of maximal effort leads to numbers that may be misleading.

Aftercare Instructions

No aftercare instructions particular to PEFR monitoring are necessary because aftercare represents ongoing care of a chronic condition. The development of an asthma action plan based on patients' symptoms and/or PEFR data, with regular revisions based on changes in symptoms, growth, and season, are the critical aftercare considerations. A patient information sheet is included in Appendix B, Aftercare Instructions, for this section.

Keeping the peak flow meter clean and functional is required. Each peak flow meter comes with instructions concerning care of the device.

Modifications for Situations of Limited Resources

No modifications of PEFR monitoring are required when resources are limited. Peak flow meters are relatively inexpensive and will last over a prolonged period as long as they are cared for appropriately. Appropriate consideration must be given to patient and family preference; the most expensive monitoring device is the one that is never used. If patients and/or family refuse to use a peak flow meter as instructed, then further provision of devices is unlikely to produce any advantage in the management of these children's asthma. Concentrating on other ways of monitoring patients, focusing particularly on symptom monitoring, is more appropriate.

THORACENTESIS

Background and Introduction

Evacuation of air, blood, chylous effusions, pleural effusions, or pus from the intrapleural space for therapeutic or diagnostic purposes is sometimes necessary. At times inserting a chest tube is required because the material is too thick to be drained effectively using a needle or because ongoing drainage of the pleural space is neeeded.

The pleural space is normally a potential space, with very little fluid between the parietal and visceral pleura. Fluid may accumulate in the pleural space as a reaction to a pneumonia, as a result of neoplasm or congenital anomaly, in association with congestive heart failure or low serum albumin levels, or as a result of trauma.

Removing fluid from the pleural space may be required for diagnostic purposes, particularly in instances of pneumonia or when fluid is present with an undetermined origin and neoplasia is in the differential diagnosis. This procedure may also be required for therapeutic purposes when the amount of fluid causes respiratory distress or failure.

Relevant Anatomy

The pleural space lies between the parietal pleural lining of the chest wall and the visceral pleura on the surface of the lung. Normally the space is a potential space, with a thin layer of fluid between the two layers of pleura (Fig. 16-2). Accumulation of fluid within the space can be identified clinically by recognizing decreased breath sounds on the side of the effusion, dullness to percussion on the side of the effusion, and occasionally pain with breathing ("splinting"). Radiological clues to the presence of pleural fluid include blunting of the costophrenic angle on posteroanterior chest radiograph and layering of the fluid when lateral decubitus views are obtained.

It is important to recall that the intercostal vessels and nerve course along the inferior border of the rib. Placement of needles or catheters should occur over the superior border of the rib, avoiding the inferior aspect of the rib above.

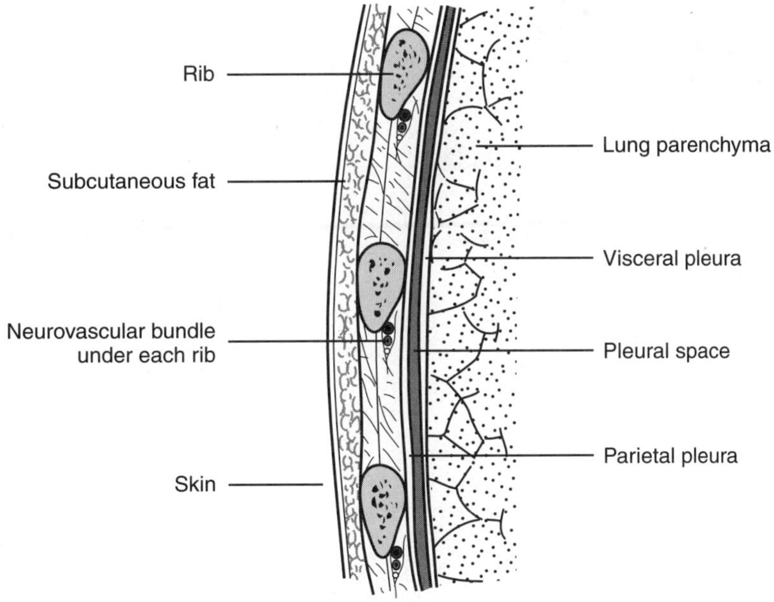

FIG. 16-2. Thoracentesis: normal pleural anatomy.

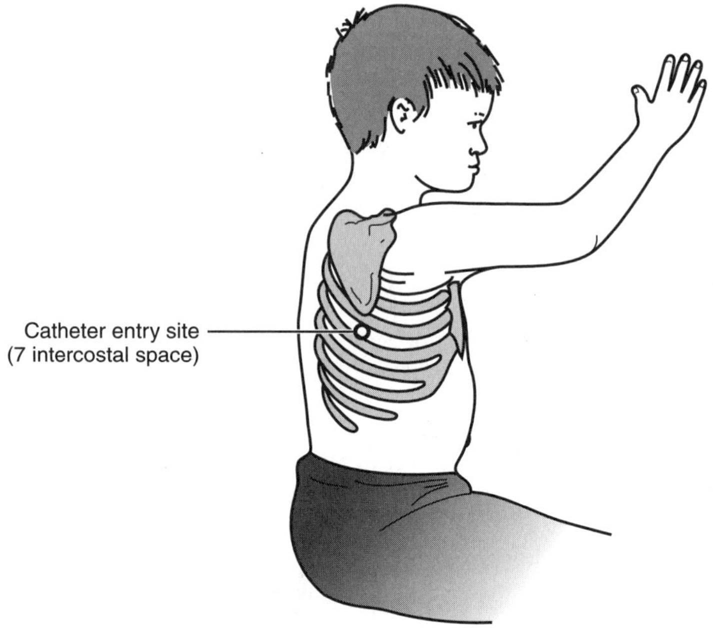

FIG. 16-3. Thoracentesis: seventh intercostal space—site for entry of needle.

The position of the diaphragm varies with the breathing cycle, being highest at the end of expiration. The right hemidiaphragm is normally higher than the left, generally lying at the level of the sixth rib laterally and the eighth rib posteriorly. Accordingly, the seventh intercostal space in either the posterior axillary line or the midscapular line is a safe place to perform the procedure. The seventh intercostal space lies at the point of the scapula when children raise their arm (Fig. 16-3).

Indications

Thoracentesis may be performed for therapeutic or diagnostic indications. Evacuating pus, blood, or fluid that is causing respiratory distress is often required. In such instances, particularly when blood or pus is expected, consider whether placing a chest tube might be a better option than inserting a needle or over-the-needle catheter because the fluid present may be too thick to be aspirated through a relatively small device. When the fluid does not "layer out" on chest radiograph, placement of a chest tube may also be a more appropriate therapeutic maneuver.

Evacuating pleural fluid for diagnostic indications is more straightforward because the fluid is not causing respiratory distress. Common reasons for diagnostic thoracentesis include identifying an organism causing pneumonia with associated effusion, diagnosing neoplasia, or diagnosing relatively rarer causes of pleural effusion associated with chylous effusions.

Contraindications and Reasons for Referral to a Specialist

There are relatively few contraindications to thoracentesis, but there are several reasons one might consult a specialist or consider inserting a chest tube instead of performing a classical thoracentesis. Relative contraindications include conditions of the chest wall that may interfere with a successful procedure or lead to complications (e.g., cellulitis of the chest wall in the location needed for the thoracentesis). Significant respiratory distress, such that children cannot sit or lie still or are breathing so forcefully that chest wall movement may prevent a safe procedure, is another relative contraindication that may be best managed by referral to specialists.

Referring to, or seeking the advice of, specialists is indicated before most thoracenteses when such specialists are available. Specialists in pulmonary medicine and/or pediatric surgery can also be helpful in deciding whether to perform a thoracentesis or insert a chest tube and what laboratory tests ought to be performed on the fluid obtained by either technique. Communicating with the laboratory concerning the tests to be run on the fluid is also advisable if the laboratory does not often test pleural fluid from children.

Required/Recommended Nursing Skills and Procedures

The primary required nursing skill is that of monitoring the cardiorespiratory status of children. Children undergoing thoracentesis may be in mild to moderate respiratory distress. The risk of complications that may worsen the respiratory distress (e.g., pneumothorax) is significant, and close monitoring of vital signs (including pulse oximetry) and clinical condition may allow for early recognition and management of significant problems.

Sedation of children undergoing thoracentesis may be helpful in ensuring that they do not move excessively during the procedure, and the amnesia some agents provide is a distinct advantage; however, sedation of children already in respiratory distress can lead to undesired consequences. Children in respiratory distress are at least Class III ASA (American Society of Anesthesiologists), a level that many practitioners would suggest warrants consultation, and perhaps management, by an anesthesiologist.

Supplies and Equipment

Need to have

- Full cardiorespiratory monitoring equipment (i.e., pulse, blood pressure, respirations, pulse oximetry)
- Local anesthetic
- Needle (18- to 22-gauge)

- Occlusive dressing
- Over-the-needle catheters (18- to 23-gauge)
- Radiograph capability
- Skin preparation equipment (e.g., povidone-iodine solution, sponges, sterile towels)
- Specimen collection tubes for laboratory testing
- Stopcock
- Syringe (15- to 30-ml)

Nice to have

- Evacuated sterile 1-liter bottle
- IV connection tubing
- Prepackaged thoracentesis kit
- Thoracentesis needle

Procedure

1. Confirm the site and side of the thoracentesis.
2. Prepare the patient, the family, and the treatment team.
3. Ensure that appropriate monitoring is in place.
4. Position the child appropriately; in most cases, this will be with the child sitting on a chair or stool leaning over a bed or treatment table with the arm on the appropriate side elevated (see Fig. 16-3).
5. Prepare the site with povidone-iodine solution in a sterile fashion with a wide field.
6. Administer local anesthesia from skin to rib.
7. With the over-the-needle catheter attached to a syringe, enter the skin and push the needle to the rib.
8. "Walk" the point of the needle over the rib, maintaining suction on the syringe (Fig. 16-4, *A*). A slight "pop" or change in resistance may be felt as the pleural cavity is entered; fluid flowing into the syringe indicates entry into the pleural space.
9. After advancing the catheter slightly, withdraw the syringe and needle and cap the catheter with a thumb or finger (Fig. 16-4, *B*).
10. Advance the catheter down, attach a syringe with stopcock and T-connector, and remove enough fluid for the laboratory tests planned and/or until symptomatic relief is obtained (Fig. 16-4, *C*).
11. Reposition the catheter gently if the flow of fluid diminishes.
12. Once sufficient fluid has been obtained, remove the catheter by pulling it out.
13. Apply a sterile occlusive dressing.
14. If a large amount of freely flowing fluid is obtained (more than the syringe can hold), drain additional fluid in order to provide significant relief. This is easily accomplished by connecting a length of IV tubing to the side port of the stopcock and inserting the other end into a prepared, evacuated 1-liter bottle. When the stopcock is opened to the tubing, fluid will be drawn into the bottle

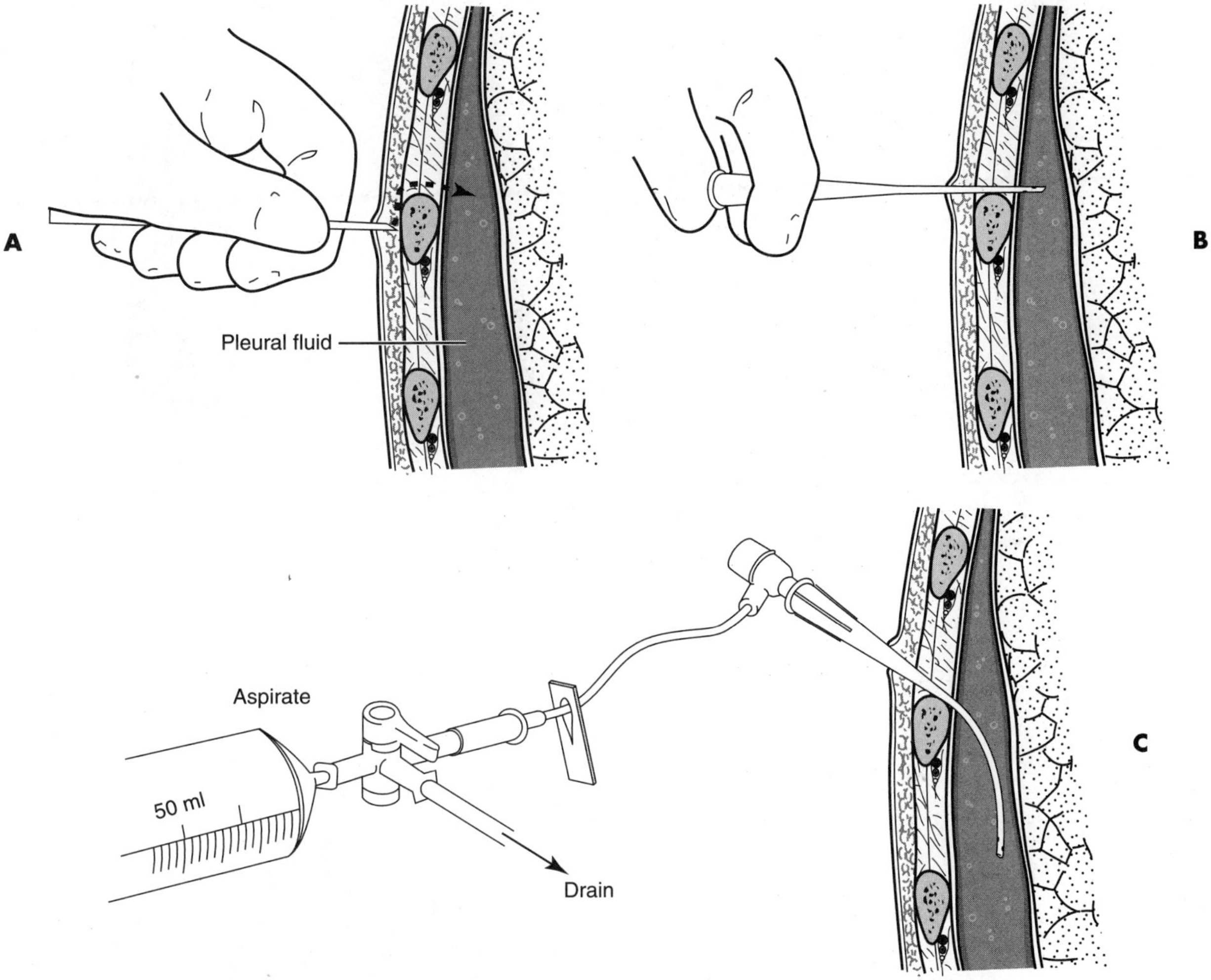

FIG. 16-4. Thoracentesis. **A,** Insertion of needle over rib. **B,** Advance catheter into pleural space; remove needle. **C,** Withdraw fluid for analysis into syringe.

from the pleural space (the bottle should be placed at a level lower than the child's chest) (Fig. 16-5).

15. Obtain a chest radiograph once the procedure is complete to document the presence or absence of a pneumothorax and to evaluate the extent of fluid removed.

Interpretation of Results

Routine studies of fluid removed by thoracentesis include the following:

- Observation of the characteristics of the fluid (i.e., clear, milky, purulent, yellow or red)

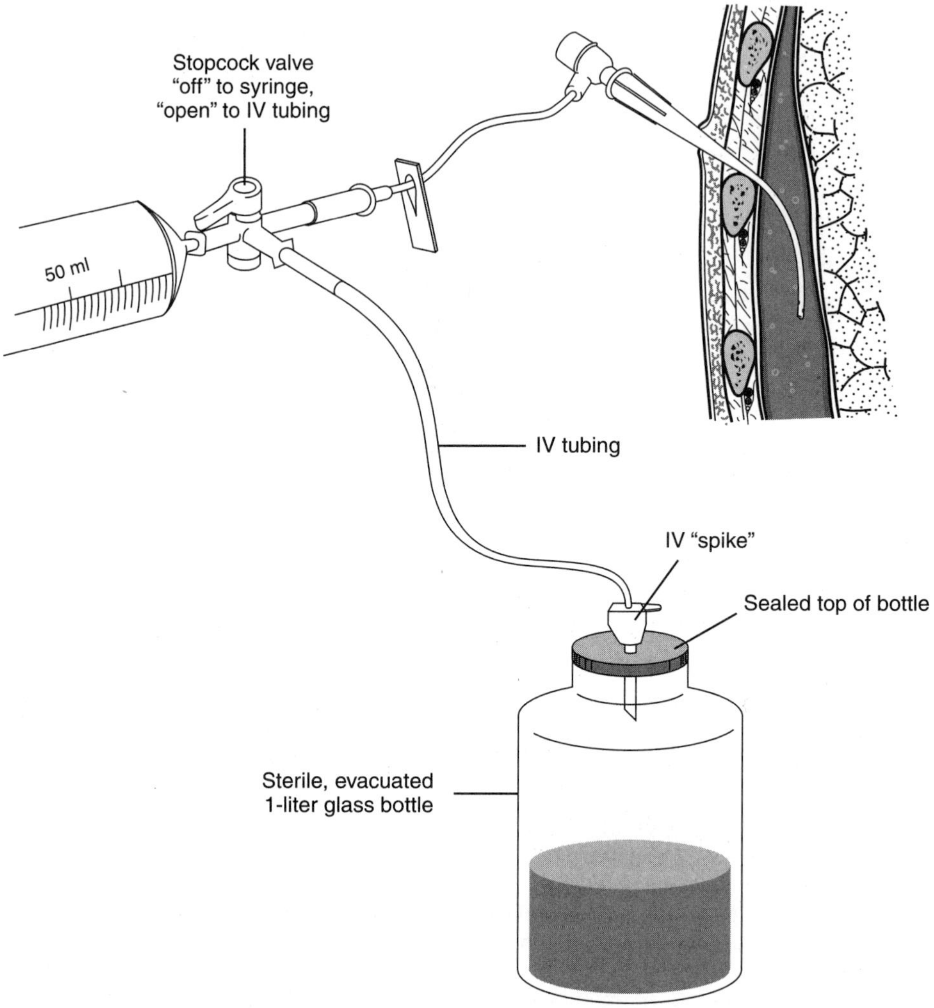

FIG. 16-5. Thoracentesis: drainage apparatus for free-flowing fluid.

- White and red blood cell counts
- Cytological examination
- Hematocrit (in trauma)
- pH
- Glucose
- Gram stain
- Culture
- Acid-fast stain and culture if tuberculosis is suspected
- Lactic dehydrogenase (LDH)

The significant determination to be made is whether the fluid is a transudate or an exudate. A transudate is seen in conditions in which the pleural effusion accumulates as an ultrafiltrate of plasma (e.g., congestive heart failure, nephrotic syndrome, hypoalbuminemia), whereas an exudate, which is seen in infections, neoplasia, inflammatory disorders, and trauma, suggests a loss of vascular integrity.

What the Family and Patient Should Know

Before the procedure, the family (and patients if they are old enough to understand) must understand the basics of the procedure, the indication(s) for the procedure in the particular case, the risks (primarily of pneumothorax), the information that will be derived from study of the fluid obtained, and, when the thoracentesis is expected to be therapeutic, the therapeutic goal.

The risks of the procedure are primarily those of pneumothorax; most authors describe a risk of 11% to 30%. Rare complications include laceration of the intercostal artery and vein, laceration of liver or spleen, and pain at the site of the procedure.

The family and children should understand that patients will be observed closely during a several-hour period after the procedure so that any complications can be recognized early and treated promptly. Pain at the site of the procedure may be evident as the local anesthesia wears off, and appropriate pain management will be provided.

Possible Complications

The primary complication from a thoracentesis is a pneumothorax. Other complications are described previously in the Procedure section.

Aftercare Instructions

Observe children closely, preferably in the hospital or emergency department. After discharge, parents should be instructed to contact their pediatrician immediately if their children have difficulty breathing or develop severe chest pain or cough, cyanosis, or fever. In most cases, immediate return to a hospital is indicated. Acetaminophen generally provides sufficient analgesia. These children should be seen by the pediatrician for a follow-up examination before returning to normal athletic activities.

Modifications for Situations of Limited Resources

Few modifications should be necessary in the setting of limited resources because the equipment is simple and the technique is straightforward. Monitoring can be accomplished with a stethoscope and a watch with a second hand.

TUBE THORACOSTOMY/PLACING A CHEST TUBE

Background and Introduction

Placement of a chest tube (tube thoracostomy) is a procedure by which a flexible tube is inserted into the pleural space and typically left in place for varying periods. The procedure offers certain benefits over simple needle thoracentesis. Because the chest tube is larger than the over-the-needle catheter, thicker fluid and pus can be drained. The tube is longer than the over-the-needle catheter, allowing for placement in the most dependent portion of the pleural space and facilitating drainage of fluid, pus, or blood.

Relevant Anatomy

The pleural space is normally a potential space, with a small amount of liquid separating the parietal and visceral layers. The visceral pleura lines the lung, diaphragm, mediastinum, and lung fissures, while the parietal pleura lines the chest wall. The two layers of pleura meet at the hilum of the lung, forming the pleural sac. The fluid between the two layers serves as a lubricant, allowing the two layers to slide across each other during respiration.

This potential space can be filled with air (pneumothorax), blood (hemothorax), fluid (pleural effusion), chyle (chylothorax), blood and air (hemopneumothorax), or pus (empyema). When the volume of any of these substances is sufficient to displace lung tissue, or to interfere with the normal respiratory cycle, respiratory embarrassment and failure may occur. Such collections can also interfere with cardiac function because they affect both preload and afterload.

Indications

Tube thoracostomy is performed either emergently or semielectively. Emergent tube thoracostomy may be life-saving when a sufficient volume of blood, or blood and air, in the pleural space interferes with either ventilation or respiration. Thoracentesis using over-the-needle catheters is typically not effective for draining large amounts of blood from the pleural space. Transfusion of packed red blood cells, and other blood components if necessary, is recommended either before or during tube thoracostomy for hemothorax because the hemothorax may be tamponading a bleeding vessel; relief of pressure by tube thoracostomy may result in continuing bleeding from an injured blood vessel.

Semielective tube thoracostomy is performed to drain pleural effusions, particularly those that appear loculated, empyemas, chylothoraces, and hemothoraces or hemopneumothoraces that are not immediately life-threatening.

Contraindications and Reasons for Referral to a Specialist

There are no absolute contraindications to emergency tube thoracostomy when it is used as a life-saving measure. Patients with coagulation disorders may require placement of a chest tube, and appropriate weighing of risk and benefit should take place. Correction of coagulation disorders before chest tube insertion is required when possible and when the acuity of the situation permits. Tube thoracostomy is not a substitute for open thoracotomy but may be required before a child is taken to the operating room for definitive management.

Placement of a chest tube semielectively is only contraindicated when the risks outweigh the potential benefits. Unfortunately, those risks and benefits have not been clearly characterized. Referral to a specialist, either a pediatric pulmonologist or a pediatric surgeon, is recommended when possible for children in whom placement of a chest tube is being considered.

Required/Recommended Nursing Skills

Beyond the usual skills of monitoring patients' condition and providing psychosocial support, the primary nursing skill required is that of caring for patients with a chest tube in place. Several unique problems are associated with caring for such patients, not the least of which is maintaining the equipment that generates negative pressure in the pleural space, assisting with drainage of that space. Knowledge of the operating characteristics of the drainage system available and the skills necessary to operate it safely are crucial to the ongoing success of drainage of the pleural space.

Children with chest tubes in place require close monitoring. If the tube malfunctions, immediate action may be required. Cardiopulmonary monitoring, including continuous pulse oximetry, should be used throughout the procedure and for some time after the procedure is completed to ensure stability of patients and the chest tube apparatus.

Supplies and Equipment

Supplies and equipment include the equipment necessary to perform the actual procedure as well as the supplies and equipment necessary to maintain the chest tube once it has been inserted. Institutions that serve children should have chest tubes of various sizes available for use in children. A suggested guideline for choice of chest tube size is presented in Table 16-1.

TABLE 16-1
Chest tube size recommended guidelines

Age	Chest tube size (Fr)
Premature	8-12
Newborn	10-14
5 kg	10-16
10 kg	16-24
15 kg	16-24
20 kg	20-28
30 kg	28-32
Adolescent	32-42
Adult	32-42

Other equipment necessary will typically already be in place on a "chest tube tray," a prepackaged and sterilized set of instruments and other supplies necessary for the procedure. Critical equipment on that tray includes the following:

- Curved Kelly clamps
- Gauze and sponges
- Needle holder
- Syringes and needles
- Scalpels with No. 11 and No. 15 blades
- Sterile basin or cups
- Sterile drapes
- Sutures
- Suture scissors

Other equipment that may be necessary includes:

- Drainage equipment, including adaptors and tubing
- Lidocaine
- Petroleum jelly–soaked gauze
- Povidone-iodine solution
- Sterile gloves
- Tape

The drainage system can be confusing if one is not familiar with the rationale behind the design of the system. The chest tube, when left open to the environment, allows for entry of air into the pleural space with inspiration. If the distal end of the tube is placed under water, air or fluid can be expelled from the pleural space during expiration, while air is prevented from returning to the pleural space during inspiration by the water seal. The current drainage systems all operate with this principle in mind but provide a space for collection of fluid, a water seal to prevent return of air to the pleural space, and a connection that makes continuous suction possible.

Procedure

1. Prepare patients and family for the procedure; child life personnel may be helpful.
2. If children are awake and alert, administer sedation/analgesia, if necessary. The extent of sedation/analgesia depends on patients' condition and psychosocial support, the time of the last oral intake, and the presence of other medical or surgical conditions that affect the delivery of sedation/analgesia. In the semielective setting, an opioid and a benzodiazepine (e.g., fentanyl and midazolam) are often beneficial. Consideration can also be given to ketamine, with the addition of an anticholinergic such as atropine to counteract the increase in airway secretions.
3. Place patients lying on the side opposite the insertion site (at the level of the nipple, usually the fifth intercostal space, in the midaxillary line), with the ipsilateral arm over the head and secured so that it will not fall into the field once the procedure starts.
4. Once the patient is secured, monitored, and comfortable, palpate the selected site and prepare it as for any sterile procedure.

5. Infiltrate the chosen site with a local anesthetic at the skin and subcutaneous levels.
6. "Walk" the needle up over the rib, avoiding the neurovascular bundle at the inferior margin of the rib, and instill local anesthetic over the rib to the pleural surface.
7. Once the local anesthesia has taken effect, make a small skin incision (0.5 to 1.5 cm) one intercostal space below the desired intercostal space. This allows for tunneling of the tube subcutaneously, resulting in a tube that is more stable and less likely to become dislodged (Fig. 16-6, *A*).
8. Using the curved Kelly clamp, carry out blunt dissection through the incision. Insert the tip of the Kelly clamp into the incision and direct it superiorly to the rib surface.
9. Advance the clamp up the rib and into the intercostal space, avoiding the inferior aspect of the rib above and the neurovascular bundle there (Fig. 16-6, *B*).
10. With pressure, advance the tip of the Kelly clamp through the soft tissue into the pleural space; a "pop" or sudden loss of resistance will be felt as the tip enters the pleural space.
11. Stop advancing the Kelly clamp, and spread the tips of the clamp to enlarge the hole slightly (Fig. 16-6, *C*).
12. If children are large enough, place your finger through the incision and into the pleural space; insert the chest tube, using your finger as a guide.
13. In small children, seize the chest tube with the jaws of the Kelly clamp and advance it through the incision into the pleural space (Fig. 16-6, *D*).
14. Insert the chest tube at least until all of the holes in the end of the chest tube are in the pleural space. If the intent is to evacuate a pneumothorax, direct the tip of the tube anteriorly and superiorly. If the intent is to evacuate fluid, pus, or blood, direct the tip of the tube posteriorly and superiorly.
15. Attach the chest tube to the drainage system, with one person directed to hold the tube at the level of the skin so that it does not come out.
16. Suture the tube into place. A purse-string suture around the tube can keep it in place and allow for easy closure of the incision once the tube is removed. To use this technique, place a suture in the skin close to the tube. Tie the suture, wrap the ends around the tube, and tie it again securely.
17. Place sterile petroleum jelly–soaked gauze over the tube at the skin junction and place a dressing.
18. Assess the function of the drainage system both by observing bubbles or fluid drainage through the tube and apparatus and by a postprocedure chest radiograph.

Interpretation of Results

Fluid obtained from the insertion of a chest tube can be sent to the laboratory for several tests (see the previous discussion on thoracentesis).

Relief of respiratory distress, stabilization of vital signs, resolution of fluid or air collections evident on chest radiograph, and bubbles in the drainage apparatus can all be interpreted as results indicating success at placing the chest tube;

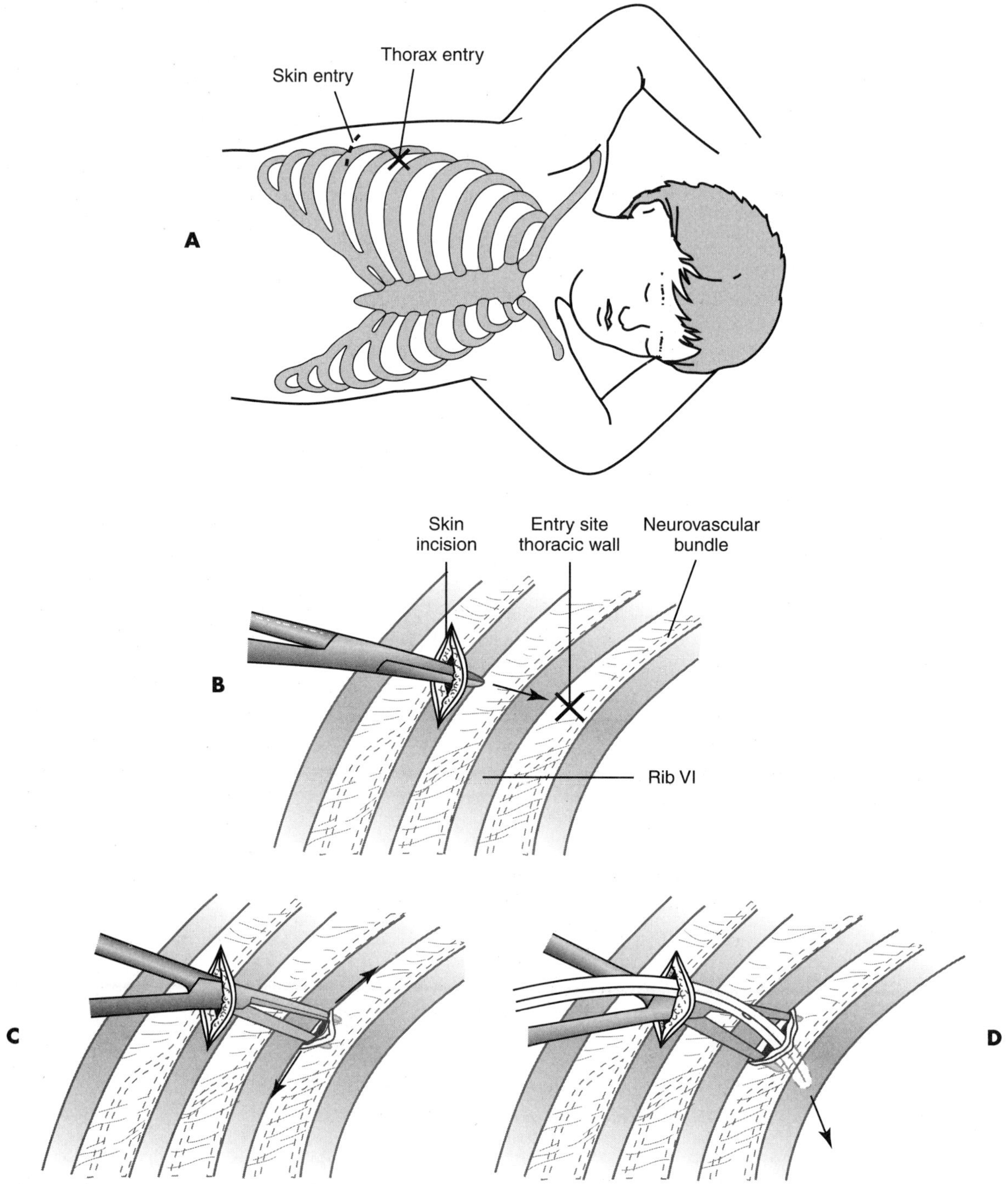

FIG. 16-6. Thoracostomy. **A,** Skin incision site. **B,** Tunnel over rib to pleura. **C,** Penetrate pleura, widen hole with Kelly clamp. **D,** Advance tube with clamp.

however, if the chest tube continues to drain large amounts of blood in the trauma setting, significant injury to the great vessels must be presumed. Immediate movement to the operating room is generally required.

What the Patient and Family Should Know

Patients and family should be told why the chest tube is necessary, the steps of the insertion procedure, the expected benefits, and the possible risks and complications. The age and developmental level of children influence the manner in which details of the procedure are explained to them. The family's developmental level and stress level must be taken into account when explaining the details of the procedure to them.

The family and patients must be informed that placing a chest tube requires hospitalization once the tube is in place. They should also understand that removing the chest tube depends on the patient's response to therapy, and the exact date and time for removal cannot be predicted in advance. Building a therapeutic alliance with patients and family early on makes the remainder of the hospital stay much easier.

Patients and family should also be told that patients will feel some pain, both during the actual procedure and afterward. They should be reassured that the pain can be managed. In addition, sedation/analgesia during the procedure may provide not only anxiolysis and analgesia but some degree of amnesia.

Patients and family should be told whether laboratory specimens will be collected during the procedure and what they may show if they are collected. They should also be informed about possible complications of the procedure and given some estimate of the frequency of those complications. If sedation/analgesia is used, a separate discussion of the techniques, agents, benefits, and risks of sedation and analgesia should be held.

Patients and family should be given some sense of the alternatives to tube thoracostomy. These choices might include doing nothing or performing a thoracoscopy in the operating room.

Possible Complications

Complications of chest tube insertion can occur anywhere along the track created for the tube or in the areas that the tube occupies while in use; there are also some slightly distant complications. The anatomy of the intercostal space, with the neurovascular bundle coursing along the inferior margin of the rib, suggests that injury to this bundle can cause nerve, vein, or arterial damage. Careful attention to placement of the incision, blunt dissection with the Kelly clamp, and careful blunt dissection with the finger can all help avoid these complications.

Entry into the pleural space is forceful; lung tissue directly under the tip of the Kelly clamp can be injured, and pulmonary contusions and bleeding can be seen after the procedure. Forceful insertion can also damage the diaphragm, the heart, the liver, the stomach, and the spleen. Injury to abdominal organs may be a result of particularly forceful expiration during insertion, when the diaphragm can rise to the level of the procedure. Previous lung surgery with volume loss or diaphragmatic paralysis, or abdominal distention with elevation of the hemidiaphragm, may also make injury to abdominal contents more likely. Performing the procedure with children in a sitting position may help minimize chances of these complications if any of these risk factors are present.

Pneumothorax after chest tube placement should be easily treated because the chest tube is presumably in the right place and functional. If a postprocedure chest radiograph shows a persistent pneumothorax, then reassessment of (1) chest tube placement; (2) the possibility of any leaks in the chest tube, the connecting tubing, or the drainage apparatus; or (3) nonfunctioning suction equipment, must be done. A chest tube with any of the holes outside the pleural space will render the system nonfunctional and may cause subcutaneous emphysema.

These complications are rare when the procedure is performed by trained personnel and with the appropriate supplies, equipment, and monitoring capabilities. No population-based studies provide estimates of the rate of complications after chest tube placement.

Aftercare Instructions

Aftercare instructions for this procedure are limited by the fact that aftercare is provided in a hospital setting. By the time patients with a chest tube are ready to go home, aftercare instructions are generally limited to instructions concerning pain management. Otherwise, specific aftercare instructions are directed at the underlying disease or injury that prompted placing the chest tube in the first place.

Modifications for Situations of Limited Resources

The equipment necessary for tube thoracostomy is relatively basic and should be widely available. The drainage apparatus can be put together using bottles and corks, as long as the rationale for using the apparatus is appreciated.

REPLACING TRACHEOSTOMY TUBES

Background and Introduction

Children have tracheostomy tubes for one of three reasons: (1) they have airway obstruction proximal to the site of the tracheostomy; (2) they require frequent instillation of saline and medication into the airway and frequent suctioning ("pulmonary toilet"); or (3) they require prolonged assisted ventilation. They typically present needing acute care related to their tracheostomy because they are in respiratory distress, which may or may not be directly related to the tracheostomy, or because the tracheostomy has come out and the parents have been unable to reinsert it.

Children who need their tracheostomy tube replaced may or may not have respiratory distress. A calm, knowledgable response goes a long way toward ensuring that patients do not worsen and that the problem is resolved as quickly as possible.

Relevant Anatomy

Performing a tracheostomy, and subsequent healing, essentially creates a tracheocutaneous fistula, the walls of the tract being formed during the immediate postoperative period. In general, pediatricians are presented with children who have a "mature" tracheostomy, one in whom the tract is well-developed and not easily breached (Fig. 16-7, *A*). The distal end of the tracheostomy cannula sits in the trachea and can cause injury to the trachea itself, particularly if it is too long or is inserted with significant force.

The tracheostomy cannula typically has an outer cannula, which is designed to remain in the patient at all times; an inner cannula, which can be removed for cleaning; and an obturator for insertion, although soft tracheostomy tubes may not have an obturator.

Indications

The indications for replacing a tracheostomy tube emergently include accidental decannulation and respiratory distress caused by an obstructed cannula that cannot be overcome by suctioning. If the tracheostomy tube becomes dislodged, the stoma may become tighter in a relatively short period. Replacement as soon as possible is recommended, but if no respiratory distress is present, the procedure

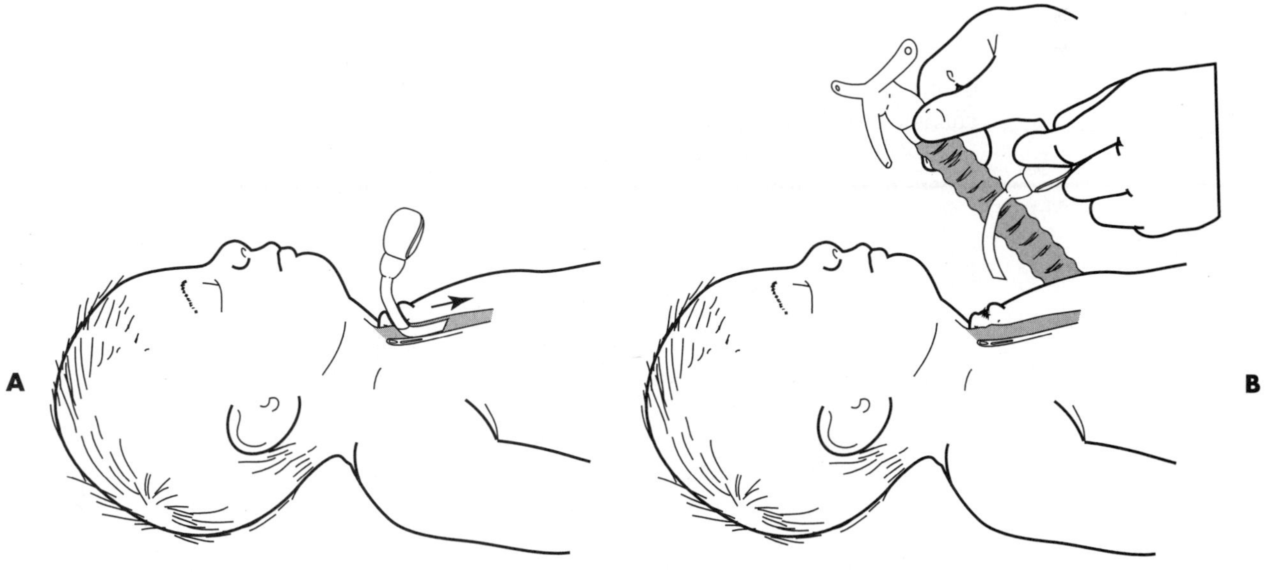

FIG. 16-7. Tracheostomy tube replacement.

can be semielective, taking a few minutes to review such issues as size of the tracheostomy cannula, the original indications for the tracheostomy, and any problems with prior replacements or insertions, such as difficult anatomy caused by stenosis or mass, or bleeding during insertion.

Contraindications and Reasons for Referral to a Specialist

Because parents can replace tubes at home, children who require changing of a tracheostomy tube by a practitioner may have a problem that suggests the need to seek consultation from a specialist. If parents or practitioners have experienced previous problems with insertion, particularly related to physical difficulty with reinsertion, bleeding, or previous creation of a false channel between skin and trachea, then advice and assistance from an otolaryngologist may be advisable. Appropriate alternatives if immediate respiratory assistance is required include the use of an endotracheal tube through the tracheostomy stoma, oral endotracheal intubation, or bag-valve-mask ventilation with a finger occluding the tracheostomy stoma. Such measures may be helpful while awaiting the arrival of a specialist.

Required/Recommended Nursing Skills and Procedures

The most essential nursing skill is that of calming the patient. The calmer the patient, the lower the oxygen need, the less muscle tension, and ultimately the easier the procedure. Skills at bag-valve-mask ventilation or provision of high-concentration oxygen by face mask or tracheostomy mask are also necessary.

Supplies and Equipment

Required equipment includes equipment needed to support ventilation or assume control of the airway, as well as the equipment and supplies needed to actually change or reinsert the tracheostomy tube.

The following supplies are required for airway control:

- Bag-valve-mask
- Endotracheal tubes of the correct size for the child and smaller and larger sizes
- Gloves
- Laryngoscope
- Oxygen
- Suction and suction catheters, including rigid, large-volume suction tips

The following supplies are required for the actual tracheostomy tube insertion:

- Scissors
- Sterile saline for cleaning the site if necessary, as well as for lubricating the tracheostomy tube before insertion
- Tracheostomy cannulae of the correct size; typically, this includes the size the child has had, as well as one or two sizes smaller
- Tracheostomy tube ties (twill tape)

Procedure

1. Prepare children for the procedure.
2. Enlist the aid of parents, nurses, and child life workers to calm children (and the parents, if necessary), explaining, if possible, that their relaxation will help make the procedure easier.
3. Provide 100% oxygen for children, particularly if they are in any distress.
4. Lie children down supine, with a small towel roll under the upper back and shoulder. The towel keeps the head extended on the neck, offering the best view of the tracheostomy site and clearing the area of any excessive tissue that might block access.
5. If the tracheostomy tube is in place, attempt to suction it by instilling several milliliters of sterile saline through the tube and suctioning gently.
6. If respiratory distress is not relieved by suctioning, proceed to change the tube.
7. Cut the tracheostomy tube ties, holding the old tube in place, and gently remove the old tube. Be ready to suction as necessary.
8. Insert a new tracheostomy tube of the same size through the stoma, with the tube passing through the stoma and the tip proceeding caudad toward the carina (Fig. 16-7, *B*).
9. Tie the tube in place with twill tape. Pass one end of the tape through the eyelet on the flange of the tube. Slide both ends of the tape around the back of the head or neck and pass one end of tape through the eyelet on the other flange of the tube. Tie ends of the tape with a square knot.
10. Check to make sure that the tracheostomy tube is in place by listening for breath sounds bilaterally and making sure that ventilation is adequate.
11. Obtain a chest radiograph to indicate proper placement, especially the location of the distal tip of the tube, if concern exists that the tube is not in proper position.

What the Family Should Know

The families of children with tracheostomy tubes should be well-versed in how to change the tube, both routinely and semiemergently. They should know when to call for assistance and when and how to summon emergency aid (e.g., calling "911," notifying rescue services of the presence of a child with a tracheostomy in the home), and they should have 24-hour access to someone who is knowledgable in the care of children with tracheostomies. Sites on the Internet are helpful to families with such children (e.g., www.twinenterprises.com/trach).

Possible Complications

The primary complication of replacing a tracheostomy tube is pneumomediastinum and/or pneumothorax caused by forcible insertion of the tube and penetration into the subcutaneous tissue surrounding the tracheostomy stoma. This complication can be prevented by avoiding force when reinserting the tube.

The tube should fit into the tracheal stoma easily and follow the natural curvature of the airway easily and without force.

A rare complication is bleeding from trauma to the trachea itself or to an area of stricture or granuloma, but such bleeding is usually inconsequential.

Aftercare Instructions

After replacement of a tracheostomy tube, the general instructions followed by the family for the care of the tube should be reinforced. No specific instructions are necessary as a result of a simple change of a tracheostomy tube.

Modifications for Situations of Limited Resources

In general, no modifications in areas of limited resources are necessary because the procedure is straightforward and easily taught to family members and other lay personnel.

SUGGESTED READINGS

Alkrinawi S, Chernick V: Pleural infections in children, *Semin Respir Infect* 11:148, 1996.

Bazeman WP, Myers RA, Barish RA: Confirmation of the pulse oximetry gap in carbon monoxide poisoning, *Ann Emerg Med,* 30:608, 1997.

Carlson DW et al: Insertion of a chest tube. In Fleisher GR, Ludwig S, Henretig FM, editors: *Textbook of pediatric emergency medicine,* ed 4, Philadelphia, 2000, Lippincott Williams & Wilkins.

Chan W et al: Empyema thoracis in children: a 26-year review of the Montreal Children's Hospital experience, *J Pediatr Surg* 32:870, 1997.

Chameides L, Hazinski MF, editors: *Pediatric advanced life support,* Dallas, 1997, American Heart Association.

Chiang LK, Dunn AE: Cardiology. In Siberry GK, Iannone R, editors: *The Harriet Lane handbook,* St Louis, 2000, Mosby.

Murray CB, Loughlin GM: Making the most of pulse oximetry, *Contemp Pediatrics* 12:45, 1995.

Mower WR et al: Pulse oximetry as a fifth pediatric vital sign, *Pediatrics* 99:681, 1997.

Park MK, Gunteroth WG: *How to read pediatric ECGs,* ed 3, St Louis, 1992, Mosby.

Rowe PC: Chest tube insertion. In McMillan JA et al, editors: *Oski's pediatrics: principles and practice,* ed 3, Philadelphia, 1999, Lippincott Williams & Wilkins.

Zeitlin PL: Pleural effusions and empyema. In Loughlin GM, Eigen H, editors: *Respiratory disease in children,* Baltimore, 1994, Williams & Wilkins.

CHAPTER 17

Gastrointestinal Procedures

Christina M.S. Johns

INTRODUCTION

Many gastrointestinal (GI) procedures appear intimidating to practitioners because they seem unpleasant and invasive, yet understanding certain basic procedures for diagnosis and management can save time and money. Most of these procedures can be performed simply and effectively in an office or treatment room setting. Some GI procedures are true emergencies (such as gastrostomy-tube replacement) for which timely intervention is crucial to good outcome, whereas others (like oral rehydration therapy) require patience and persistence to achieve maximum effect.

NASOGASTRIC/FEEDING TUBE INSERTION

Background and Introduction

Placement of nasogastric (NG) or orogastric (OG) tubes requires little time and effort when performed correctly. Tubes rarely make their way down the trachea, and they can be helpful in decompressing a distended stomach or delivering feedings and rehydration fluids to infants. Larger tubes are used for GI decontamination and control of bleeding.

Relevant Anatomy

The floor of the nasal passage forms the bony hard palate, and the nasopharynx communicates directly with the oropharynx and thus both the trachea and the esophagus. The esophagus lies posterior to the trachea, which is protected by the epiglottis. In conscious patients, the presence of a foreign body, such as a plastic tube, in the oropharynx produces a powerful gag reflex that protects the airway. With the head flexed forward on the neck, the trachea is further protected anatomically, and the esophageal opening comes to lie more or less directly under the posterior nasopharynx. These structural features are helpful in passing a tube through the nose and into the esophagus.

Indications

Indications for placement of NG tubes include presence of a toxin in the stomach that requires gastric emptying or instillation of activated charcoal, persistent GI bleeding, abdominal distension with bilious emesis (potential abdominal obstruction), introduction of radiographic contrast for imaging studies, and direct gastric feeding or medication administration.

The decision whether to place NG or OG tubes depends on several factors. First, NG tubes must not be placed in trauma patients for whom there is concern about the integrity of the cribriform plate because the potential exists to introduce the tube into the cranial vault. Second, in older children, NG tubes are usually better tolerated than OG tubes, but in small infants with small nares OG tubes are easier to place and are well tolerated. When the intent is to remove pill fragments from the stomach, OG tubes are likely to be necessary to adequately remove them.

Contraindications and Reasons for Referral to a Specialist

There are no absolute contraindications to placing a gastric tube except for placing NG tubes in head trauma patients as discussed previously. Introduction of NG tubes may also result in bleeding, and if coagulopathy is present or suspected, OG tubes are preferred. Older, uncooperative patients may tend to bite on OG tubes, thereby occluding them.

Required/Recommended Nursing Skills

Nurses who will be involved in placement of NG or OG tubes should be trained in the procedure and the use of suction and oxygen delivery systems, as well as in the care of young and anxious children.

Supplies and Equipment

- Bag and mask, appropriately sized
- Lubricating gel
- NG tube: either Salem sump (double-lumen radiopaque) or Levin tube (single-lumen nonradiopaque), sized appropriately to fit a diameter just smaller than the naris, or feeding tube (for simple liquid feedings, the smallest-sized tube should be used for patient comfort)
- OG tube: large-bore (24 Fr or larger) blunt-ended tube with side holes
- Oral airway or other bite block for use with OG tubes
- Oxygen
- Suction (Yankauer and flexible catheters)

- Syringe (60-ml) with catheter tip
- Tape or skin adhesive

Procedure

NG tubes

1. After explaining the procedure to children (if possible) and parents, place children on a cardiorespiratory monitor with pulse oximetry.
2. Ensure appropriate airway control (if necessary).
3. Measure the approximate length of advancement of the tube by measuring the distance from the tip of the nose around the left ear to just below the left costal margin.
4. Wrap a small piece of tape around the tube at the appropriate length to mark how far the tube must be advanced.
5. Position children sitting upright or at a 45-degree angle, with the head in midline.
6. If any concern exists about impaired airway protective reflexes, intubate patients before tube placement to avoid aspiration of gastric contents.
7. Suction the oropharynx and spray the nose with a nasal decongestant (such as neosynephrine 0.25%) to shrink the mucosa on the turbinates.
8. Spray the posterior oropharynx with a topical anesthetic spray, if desired. Tubes will occasionally coil in the posterior oropharynx, and placing the tube in icy water before insertion may help to stiffen the tube for easier advancement.
9. Using a generous amount of lubricated gel on the end of the tube, advance the tube into the naris straight back, not angled, in the direction of the occiput or back of the head. Avoid the tendency to pass the tube upward; pressure should be applied in a downward direction toward the hypopharynx.
10. If impedance is encountered, try the other naris or obtain a smaller tube. The tube should advance without difficulty to the premeasured mark.
11. Encourage older children or adolescents to swallow repeatedly (aided by small sips of water) to facilitate advancing the tube. Placement may be further facilitated in cooperative children by having the neck in full flexion, which also protects the trachea.
12. Apply the syringe to the end of the tube in an attempt to aspirate gastric contents.
13. Fill the syringe with air and inject the air rapidly into the tube while auscultating over the stomach.
14. Confirm proper tube placement (Fig. 17-1) by the sound of air entering the stomach. Chest radiograph may also be used to confirm placement.
15. Once placement is confirmed, secure the tube to the adhesive-prepared cheek with tape or a skin adhesive, coiling and taping any loose tubing to prevent children from pulling the tube out.
16. If patients cough or gag excessively, remove the tube immediately, but crying

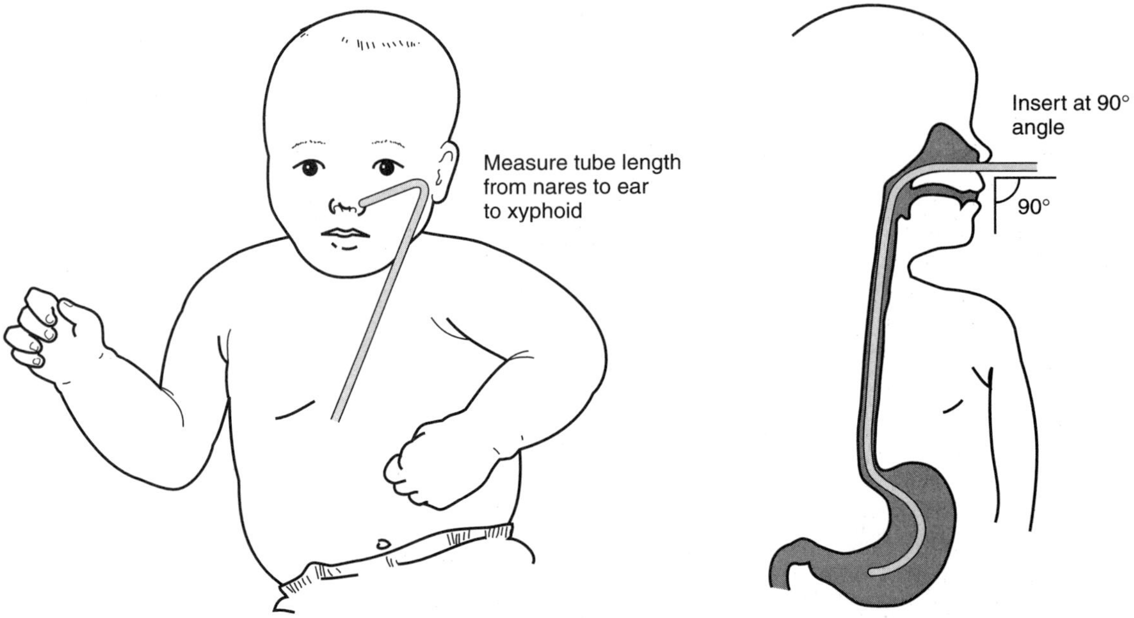

FIG. 17-1. Nasogastric tube placement.

or the ability to talk is an encouraging sign that the trachea has not been entered.

Excessive force should never be used in this procedure because the nasal mucosa and adenoidal and tonsillar tissues bleed copiously and easily with minimal trauma. Excessive force could also potentially result in developing a false tract along the hypopharynx. Consequently, gentle, steady pressure is all that is required to successfully pass NG tubes.

OG tubes

OG tube placement is done with patients in a similar upright or partially upright position, or may be accomplished by having patients lie in a left decubitus position, which is especially useful when the goal is gastric emptying in the case of toxic ingestions.

1. Explain the procedure to patients and/or parents.
2. Have patients bite on a large oral airway covered with adhesive tape. This step prevents patients from biting the tube and provides a useful distraction from the inevitable discomfort.
3. Have a large-bore suction catheter ready because some vomiting is almost inevitable during this procedure.
4. Apply anesthetic spray to the upper part of the oropharynx only.
5. Lubricate the tube generously with surgical lubricant.
6. Adequately restrain patients with several assistants.

7. Standing directly in front of patients, place the tube into the mouth and firmly advance it by pushing posteriorly and caudad, following the natural curve of the tongue. In awake patients, accidental passage of the large-bore tube into the trachea is nearly impossible. The reflux of stomach contents up the tube confirms proper placement.
8. Use extreme care to prevent patients from reaching up and pulling the tube out.
9. After the OG tube is placed and its position confirmed, perform lavage with saline solution and instill activated charcoal and cathartic.
10. When removing the tube, have the patient sit upright, have a large, clean towel ready to assist with cleaning the mouth and face, and gently but firmly withdraw the tube. Emesis may occur at this point.

What the Patient and Family Should Know

Placement of either NG or OG tubes is generally uncomfortable. The exception is when a very small, flexible tube is placed for feeding or fluid instillation only, when the procedure is only mildly noxious. Otherwise, patients should understand that the procedure will be uncomfortable, that they will feel like gagging, and that the discomfort will end almost as soon as the tube is properly secured. Asking patients to help by swallowing the tube is helpful. The family and patients should understand that a small amount of blood is often seen at the nose or mouth after the procedure. The length of time that the tube will need to remain in place should be clearly communicated.

Possible Complications

The most important complication is inadvertent introduction of the tube into the trachea, which can be avoided by having patients flex their neck and by withdrawing the tube at once if patients' ability to vocalize or breathe appears compromised. Vomiting and potential aspiration are other complications that can be avoided by proper positioning of patients and provision of adequate suction and attentiveness to patients. Minor complications include small amounts of bleeding of the nasal or oral mucosa.

Aftercare Instructions

No special instructions are required beyond pointing out that children may experience a sore throat for one or more days.

Modifications for Situations of Limited Resources

If central suction is not available, a bedside suction pump may be used. Where no electrical power is available, simple manual suction by using a large-bore syringe works well.

GASTROSTOMY TUBE REINSERTION

Background and Introduction

A percutaneous endoscopic gastrostomy (PEG) or gastrostomy tube (G-tube) that has fallen or been pulled out is truly an emergency because the longer it stays out, the more difficult it is to reinsert. The stoma through which the tube is inserted begins to close immediately upon removal of the tube. PEGs or G-tubes are inserted for multiple reasons: (1) children who have gastroesophageal reflux and/or who vomit frequently; (2) children who need extra nutritional support; and (3) children who have a dysfunctional swallow.

It is always prudent to insert either a replacement tube or a temporary Foley catheter in whatever size will fit into the stoma immediately on recognition of a displaced G-tube because this will ease further replacement, even if dilation of the stoma site is ultimately required. If this is done in a timely manner, replacement of the correct size and type of G-tube can be achieved in the emergency department without difficulty. Many practitioners provide families with a spare tube or Foley catheter of the appropriate size so that such a tube can be immediately inserted at home if the tube comes out.

Relevant Anatomy

The G-tube, regardless of how it was originally placed, essentially maintains an open gastrocutaneous fistula. The stomach wall is attached to the abdominal wall, and a healing track develops, with the tube simply maintaining patency of the fistula.

Indications

G-tubes may require replacement if they become clogged by formula deposits; if the tubing kinks, cracks, or breaks; or if they are accidentally or intentionally pulled out. It cannot be underscored enough that time is of the essence in replacing a G-tube that is completely out because the stoma will begin to close within minutes and replacement will then be more painful and difficult.

Contraindications and Reasons for Referral to a Specialist

Presence of frank peritoneal signs constitutes an absolute contraindication to replacement of the tube and warrants immediate surgical evaluation. Recent (within 6 weeks) placement of the stoma, particularly if it was surgically performed, makes consultation with the surgeon or physician who originally placed the tube a prudent idea. Tracks that have not fully matured may be at greater risk of perforation or false-track development. Similarly, frank evidence of infection of the skin at the tube site merits consultation, although in most cases the correct maneuver is to replace the tube to prevent closure of the stoma, followed by referral.

Required/Recommended Nursing Skills

Nurses who will assist with this procedure should be skilled pediatric nurses familiar with the procedure and with techniques for comforting children.

Supplies and Equipment

- Adhesive dressing
- Cotton-tipped and Dacron-tipped swabs for dilation
- Lubricating gel
- Replacement tube (either exact size and type of tube or Foley catheter of similar diameter); it is prudent to have a selection of smaller tubes available if the stoma have begun to close significantly
- Syringes: one (usually 5-ml) to fill up the balloon at the end of the tube and one (usually catheter-tipped) to aspirate gastric contents once tube is placed (20 to 60 ml)
- Tape

Procedure

1. Before replacing the tube, as with any procedure, check the equipment to ensure that it is functioning properly. Inflate the balloon on the end of the tube to be sure that no holes exist.
2. If a malfunctioning tube is currently in the stoma, leave it in place until the last possible moment before inserting the new tube.
3. Apply lubricant liberally to the end of the new tube and place children in the supine position.
4. Consider sedation for children who are unable to lie still; however, in most cases, the presence of an assistant to help restrain children is all that is required.
5. If children are able to follow commands, ask them to inhale deeply and then hold their breath.
6. Deflate the balloon in the old tube and remove the tube easily with gentle traction.
7. Apply lubricant liberally to the stoma site.
8. With the new tube aimed perpendicular to the body, apply gentle pressure and pass the tube into the stomach.
9. Inflate the balloon and aspirate gastric contents from the end of the tube.
10. As a double-check, instill air (approximately 10 ml) into the tube while listening with a stethoscope; a sound of rumbling or rushing confirms placement.

If the tube has come out and has been out for more than approximately 1 hour, it will be more difficult to replace. If the tube was originally placed within the preceding 2 weeks, it is advisable not to attempt to replace it because healing of the peritoneum and gastric wall may not be complete, and an attempt to replace the tube may result in a false lumen being created into the peritoneum. In this case, the surgeon or gastroenterologist who initially placed the tube should be consulted for further management.

It is best to use the same type of tube as the one that was most recently in place; however, if this is not possible because of size or availability, then either a Foley catheter or another similar type of tube can be used as a temporary agent until the original type and size can be found. A smaller-size Foley catheter is often the only tube that fits into the shrinking stoma.

1. After inserting the smaller catheter and waiting several minutes for the stoma to dilate, insert the next largest size tube that fits, using gentle, firm pressure and plenty of lubricant.
2. Successively remove and insert larger tubes (holding the tip perpendicular to the skin) until the appropriate size tube is inserted. On occasion, the stoma will have become so far closed that only a Dacron- or cotton-tipped swab can be placed as the initial dilating instrument, followed by the smallest (5- or 8-Fr) tubes available.
3. Instruct cooperative children to hold their breath while removing any remnants of the old or malfunctioning tube.
4. Once any tube is inserted, check for proper placement by first attempting to aspirate gastric contents and then auscultate over the stomach while instilling 10 to 20 ml of air.
5. Once placement is confirmed, close the distal port and dress and secure the tube.

In general, it is not necessary to obtain a contrast study to determine adequate placement; this should only be necessary if suspicion of incorrect placement exists.

For a clogged tube, various remedies can be used, but all involve instilling liquid into the tube and allowing it to drain out repeatedly. The most preferable type of liquid appears to be debatable, but warm water is the most commonly advocated. Some practitioners believe that carbonated soda, specifically diet soda, is the best agent.

What the Patient and Family Should Know

In most cases, family members are familiar with the process of removing and replacing G-tubes. For those experiencing the procedure for the first time, or when unforeseen complications have occurred, patients and family should understand that the procedure causes some discomfort but is not painful if performed properly. Younger children may be anxious and uncooperative and rarely may require an anxiolytic agent such as midazolam. Small amounts of blood may be seen after replacement, especially if the stoma has been allowed to begin to close.

Fever, vomiting, or abdominal pain after tube replacement are abnormal and require immediate reevaluation to rule out false tracks and resulting peritonitis. It is a good idea to send families home with a spare tube, or a Foley catheter of appropriate size, so that when the existing tube is inadvertently removed, a new one can be immediately inserted to hold open the stoma. When a family can successfully do this, an unnecessary trip to an emergency department can often be avoided, and definitive care can be deferred until a clinic or physician's office is open.

Possible Complications

Complications are few with replacement of tubes in well-healed stomata. The most dangerous complication is inadvertently placing the tube into the peritoneum by creating a false track between the abdominal wall and the stomach. This complication results in feedings and medications being delivered directly into the peritoneal space, with the almost inevitable development of peritonitis. This complication is extremely rare in mature sites but is of sufficient concern in newer (less than 2-week-old) stomata to merit consultation with a surgeon or gastroenterologist.

Aftercare Instructions

Routine dressing of the gastrostomy site should be done by the family. Family members should be warned about the implications of fever, abdominal pain, or vomiting after tube replacement and should be instructed to return or call the physician if these symptoms develop.

ORAL REHYDRATION

Background and Introduction

One of the most common presenting complaints of children is vomiting and diarrhea, or symptoms of gastroenteritis and dehydration. Gastroenteritis can be caused by a variety of viral and bacterial pathogens, but they all produce the same result: diarrhea because of increased GI fluid losses relative to absorption. Hypovolemic shock is the most severe complication of dehydration. It occurs when circulating volume is diminished and end organs and tissues have poor perfusion. Electrolyte disturbance is another complication, along with acid-base abnormalities because of poor tissue perfusion.

Given the number and severity of complications related to dehydration, many practitioners are surprised that rehydration of a child with significant volume loss can be accomplished without an intravenous (IV) line or fluids. With patience and perseverance, a family and staff educated on the appropriate use of oral rehydration therapy can be quite effective at restoring the lost circulating volume, as well as at correcting the unusual electrolyte and acid-base disturbance.

Relevant Anatomy (and Physiology)

Fluid and electrolyte absorption occurs primarily at the brush border of the villi of the small intestine, where several molecular mechanisms exist to promote fluid absorption. The most important of these mechanisms for rehydration is the "co-transport" system, which relies on the presence of small carbohydrate or amino acid molecules in combination with sodium to produce rapid absorption of water.

Oral rehydration solutions are made of balanced mixtures of carbohydrates and sodium and capitalize on the co-transport system for their function. Although patients who exhibit signs of shock should have IV fluids during their initial fluid resuscitation, early intervention with oral rehydration therapy (ORT) can be begun in alert children of any age with mild or moderate dehydration.

Indications

Detectable dehydration from diarrhea or diarrhea and vomiting is the most important indication for ORT. Children with fluid losses from other sources (e.g., increased insensible losses, decreased oral intake) may be candidates for ORT but only after the cause of dehydration has been well-established.

Contraindications and Reasons for Referral to a Specialist

Absolute contraindications to ORT are shock, impaired airway protective reflexes, and the suspicion of intestinal obstruction or surgically acute abdomen, in which case prompt consultation with a surgeon, placement of peripheral IV lines, and orders for nothing by mouth are indicated. It is commonly thought that vomiting is a contraindication to ORT, but this belief is false. Most children vomit less than half of the total volume they receive by mouth, but simple persistence, with the use of frequent, very small volumes of fluid, usually overcomes vomiting within 1 hour. Children with vomiting alone (without diarrhea), however, should be approached with caution because the differential diagnosis in such cases includes many abdominal and extraabdominal emergencies that require further evaluation. Occasionally, children or parents may be simply too exhausted to participate in effective ORT.

Enteral rehydration can also be achieved by inserting NG or OG feeding tubes and delivering oral rehydration solution continuously via an infusion pump, as outlined in the Procedure section. The only requirement for this procedure is that patients must have intact airway reflexes. A final relative contraindication occurs when children have oral ulcers such as are encountered with herpetic gingivostomatitis, for whom swallowing is extremely painful.

Required/Recommended Nursing Skills

ORT is only likely to be successful if all members of the health care team understand and support its use. Nursing skills, in addition to familiarity with the techniques involved, include patience and a strong motivation to teach families to care for their children. Accuracy at assessing degrees of dehydration is also important.

Supplies and Equipment

- Clock with a second hand
- Cup
- Flexible feeding tube (5- or 8-Fr, if needed)
- Kangaroo pump
- Oral rehydration solution: either Pedialyte, World Health Organization oral rehydration solution, Rehydralyte, or Infalyte. (Note that fluids with high concentrations of sugars such as fruit juices and soft drinks exacerbate diarrhea as a result of an increased osmotic load in the gut and should NOT be used.)
- Small bottle with nipple
- Syringe, 5-ml

Procedure

In order to properly perform ORT, it is important to understand the degrees of dehydration to help guide the management of fluid replacement. Table 17-1 shows the degrees of dehydration with their associated clinical signs and symptoms and recommended fluid therapy.

The most basic principle of ORT is that small but frequent amounts of fluids must be given to ensure success. Although it is difficult to volume-restrict thirsty infants or children, allowing vomiting patients to drink large volumes all at once often results in repeated episodes of vomiting, yielding frustration all around. It is

TABLE 17-1
Degrees of dehydration and recommended fluid therapy

Degree of dehydration	Signs	Rehydration phase (first 4 hours, repeat until rehydrated)	Maintenance phase (until illness resolves)
Mild	Increased thirst, slightly dry mucous membranes	Oral rehydration solution (ORS), 50 to 60 ml/kg	Breast feeding, undiluted lactose-free formula, half-strength cow's milk or lactose-containing formula Other age-appropriate feedings low in simple sugars and high in complex carbohydrate
Moderate	Sunken eyes/fontanelle, loss of skin turgor, dry mucous membranes	ORS 80 to 100 ml/kg	Same as above
Severe	Signs of moderate dehydration plus one or more of the following: rapid thready pulse, cyanosis, rapid breathing, delayed capillary refill, lethargy, coma	IV/IO isotonic fluids (0.9% normal saline or Ringer's lactate), 40 ml/kg/hr until pulse and state of consciousness return to normal, then 50 to 100 ml/kg of ORS based on remaining degree of dehydration	Same as above

critical to review with parents exact instructions of how much fluid to give and how often. For example, in a 10-kg infant, giving 5 ml of oral rehydration solution every minute results in 300 ml/hr (30 ml/kg), usually resulting in complete replacement of fluid losses in under 4 hours and with minimal vomiting.

In order to calculate the total volume of fluid to be given for rehydration, body weight is multiplied by the degree of dehydration, expressed as a percentage. For example, a 10-kg infant who is 8% dehydrated has an approximate fluid deficit of 800 ml (10 kg × 0.08 = 0.8 L or 800 ml). The goal is to replace the total fluid deficit within 4 hours. If possible, this is done under intermittent observation by staff. Children and parents should be able to see a clock with a second hand and be placed in a quiet area where they can be most comfortable. It is important to remind parents that children may vomit, and if this happens, the amount of emesis can be estimated as a fluid loss but ORT should continue. Children routinely swallow more fluid than they vomit, and despite perceptions to the contrary, they only rarely "throw everything up."

Children should be reassessed after 15 minutes to determine the quantity of fluids consumed as well as further losses and to encourage parents. In most situations, parents (and occasionally staff) are surprised at the amount of fluid taken in and tolerated without emesis. At this point, it is important to discuss and emphasize that parents continue this process at home until children are clearly tolerating this fluid and may be advanced to higher volumes, again slowly. From there, children's diet is advanced to bland foods with large amounts of complex carbohydrates and small amounts of simple sugars, such as potatoes, rice, toast, saltine crackers, and bananas. It should be stressed that early return to normal diet is important in reducing the duration and severity of diarrheal illness. Fried foods and highly acidic foods should be avoided until the acute illness is over.

ORT can be difficult if children are "unwilling participants." Some parents have success by using a 5-ml syringe and instilling the fluid into the mouth, but there are occasions when children are too tired to drink or for other reasons will not tolerate swallowing the fluid by mouth. In such instances, placing an NG tube and infusing an oral rehydration solution continuously may be beneficial. A slow rate can be infused at the beginning and then advanced according to the level of tolerance of fluids. A good guideline to start is 20 to 30 ml/kg per hour. It is important to remember not to use this technique in children whose mental status is truly questionable and whose protective airway reflexes might not be intact.

Interpretation of Results

Careful observation of children during the early parts of the rehydration phase help determine whether rehydration is proceeding as planned. Fairly rapid resolution of the signs and symptoms of dehydration is expected, with near-disappearance of these symptoms within about 4 hours, assuming that initial calculations were correct and adequate amounts of fluids are given. Failure to observe these changes should suggest that either a different pathological process is underway or that rehydration efforts are inadequate. IV rehydration should be started once a definite treatment failure has been identified.

Possible Complications

Few complications are associated with ORT. It is a safe, economical, and effective procedure that is used all over the world. The most important factor is the correct diagnosis of simple gastroenteritis because continued enteral intake may be contraindicated in conditions that may require subsequent surgical intervention. Some patients may become acutely glucose intolerant and may have large, explosive stools that start soon after commencing ORT; these patients usually require IV hydration until they are improved enough to return to normal feedings.

HERNIA REDUCTION

Background and Introduction

Several different types of hernias occur in children, many of which resolve spontaneously without any intervention. Hernias occur when a viscus that is normally contained in a cavity protrudes through the wall or confines of that cavity.

Relevant Anatomy

The most common type of hernia is the indirect inguinal hernia, but other types include the direct inguinal hernia, the femoral hernia, and the abdominal hernia. Hernias all have the potential to become incarcerated or be trapped in the space through which they have protruded. The result is strangulation and vascular compromise, leading to necrosis of the viscera. Although incarceration of most types of hernias is relatively rare, indirect inguinal hernias need to be reduced on a relatively frequent basis to avoid strangulation and necrosis. This section concentrates on the inguinal hernia and methods for its detection and reduction.

Indications

The diagnosis of an inguinal hernia can be complicated in some children. In general, inguinal hernias develop more commonly in premature babies (9% vs. 5% in full-term infants), occur more often in males than females (8.5 to 1), and are more likely to be right-sided than left-sided or bilateral. They usually present in the first year of life. Inguinal hernias are most often detected by the presence of a groin or scrotal mass, usually when straining or crying. These hernias are usually reducible, either spontaneously or with gentle manual pressure.

An incarcerated hernia is usually painful and children appear fussy and may vomit. The parents may note that the groin or scrotum is tense, discolored, or swollen. Although a previously undiagnosed hernia rarely presents for the first time as an incarcerated hernia, it may occur. More commonly, patients awaiting elective repair of their inguinal hernias present with acute incarceration. It is important to act quickly if incarceration is suspected because an unreduced inguinal hernia can lead to abdominal distension and bowel obstruction, and ultimately strangulated bowel can become necrotic.

Contraindications and Reasons for Referral to a Specialist

Reduction of inguinal hernias can be safely and effectively accomplished in the office or emergency department with proper technique and awareness of situations in which it is not appropriate to undertake manual reduction, such as patients with large, discolored, obviously strangulated hernias. Associated signs and symptoms of strangulation include fever and leukocytosis. In these instances, prompt surgical intervention is necessary to eliminate further compromise to the herniated structure.

In patients who appear toxic, are passing bloody stools, or have discolored, entrapped viscera, a pediatric surgeon should be consulted before attempting manual reduction. Although it was previously thought that it is impossible to reduce necrotic bowel manually, cases of successful manual procedures have been reported, although they are usually better left to a pediatric surgeon.

Supplies and Equipment

For the procedure itself, no specific equipment or supplies are needed. If using sedation, the following supplies will be needed:

- Bag-valve-mask
- Cardiorespiratory monitor
- IV supplies
- Oxygen
- Sedation/analgesic medication(s)
- Suction

Procedure

It is worthwhile to attempt the manual reduction without sedation at first, although crying children make the procedure much more difficult.

1. Apply pressure with both hands along the inguinal canal, expressing the contents of the displaced bowel back up into the abdomen (Fig. 17-2).
2. Reduce the bowel itself by constant, continuous pressure on the distal-most part of the hernia for approximately 5 minutes.
3. Gently but firmly press the thumb and forefinger of one hand around the neck of the hernia at the inguinal ring to compress it and reduce edema, while using the other hand to gently "milk" the hernia sac proximally toward the ring. Often, a sudden crepitant sensation is felt, heralding the successful reduction of the hernia.
4. Maintain pressure over the inguinal ring for several minutes after reduction to ensure that the hernia remains reduced and children cease crying.

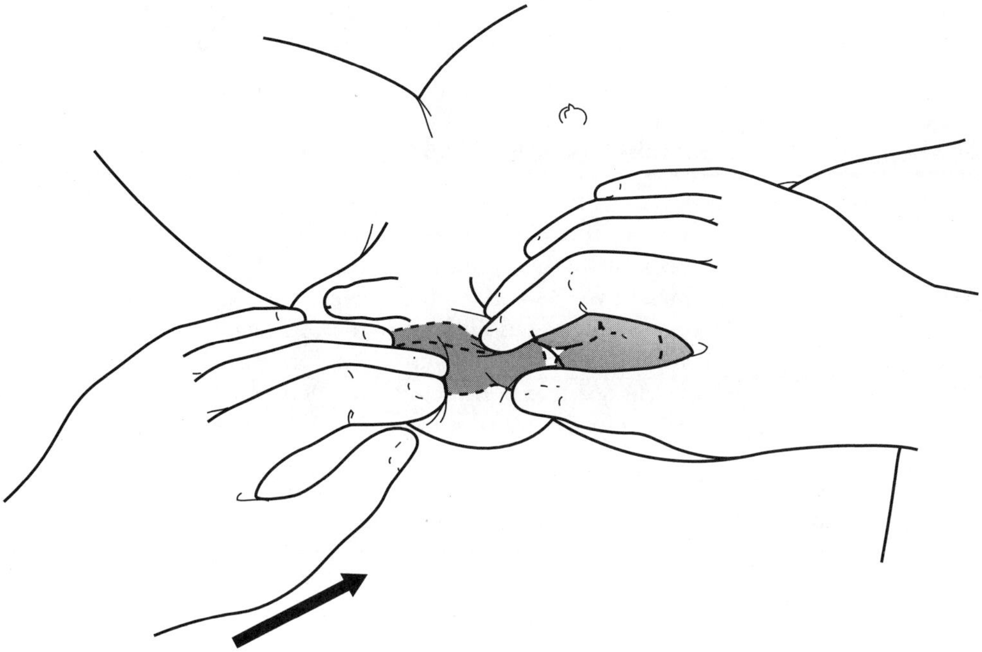

FIG. 17-2. Inguinal hernia reduction.

5. If simple reduction is unsuccessful, administer sedation and/or analgesia (morphine IV/IM or fentanyl/midazolam IV are good choices for anxiolysis and pain relief). Additionally, some practitioners advocate the Trendelenberg position and ice packs over the hernia area before repeating the procedure.

Once the hernia has been reduced, many practitioners advocate hospitalization and observation because many inguinal hernias that have been incarcerated once will become so again. On the other hand, an easily reduced hernia in the setting of observant parents and readily available primary care can be easily managed on an elective basis. In general, the longer the duration of symptoms at the time of presentation, the less likely a successful manual reduction will occur. Further, it is more difficult to reduce inguinal hernias in younger patients.

What the Patient and Family Should Know

Before the procedure, the hernia should be explained to the family (and to children if they are old enough to understand). Some discomfort and pain are associated with reduction, although once reduced, pain should dissipate immediately. Parents should be told to expect the procedure to take up to 15 minutes. Gentle, steady pressure is the key to successful reductions, and every effort to calm children should be made. On occasion, some sedation or analgesia is necessary, and this procedure should also be explained to parents.

Possible Complications

There are no complications of hernia reduction itself, but inadequate or incomplete reduction does occur, with potentially destructive consequences. It is important to be certain that the hernia has been fully reduced and that no residual bowel is left in the inguinal canal. Bowel left in the hernia sac can become incarcerated and strangulate, causing necrosis and further intraabdominal complications. It can also compromise the vascular supply to the testis, which can result in permanent damage from ischemia and testicular atrophy. After hernia reduction in boys, palpate and document the presence of the testis in the scrotal sac.

For girls, it is important to consider the ovary as a source of the hernia, which can occur when the incarcerated hernia is irreducible. This condition is a true emergency because increased risk for future torsion with strangulation exists if the hernia is left untreated or electively surgically reduced at a later time. Urgent surgical reduction is warranted.

Aftercare Instructions

After reduction of an inguinal hernia, pain should vanish almost immediately, but acetaminophen may be offered to children who still appear to be in distress. Patients may return to normal diet and activity immediately. Parents should be warned that the hernia is likely to reappear, particularly with increases in intraabdominal pressure, such as with cough or straining. Parents may be shown how to gently push the hernia sac back up the canal as soon as it appears to reduce the chances of incarceration. Although surgical follow-up care can usually be arranged electively, it should be scheduled to occur within 1 week of the initial visit. Parents should watch for evidence of abdominal obstruction or strangulation, such as vomiting, abdominal pain, fever, or discoloration of the inguinal area, and they should be instructed to return for immediate evaluation if these symptoms occur.

RECTAL PROLAPSE

Background and Introduction

The occurrence of rectal prolapse, in which rectal mucosa protrudes through the anus, is most commonly seen in children less than 3 years old. It is often associated with other conditions, including cystic fibrosis, chronic constipation, and some anatomic abnormalities that predispose the upper part of the rectum to be displaced downward and out through the anus. Chronic constipation or any situation that causes hardening of the stool, malnutrition, and muscle weakness are all associated with rectal prolapse. Because of the intrinsic weakness of the perineal musculature in infants and young toddlers, rectal prolapse may occasionally occur in otherwise normal patients at this age.

Relevant Anatomy

Initially, the upper part of the rectum prolapses internally through to the lower part of the rectum; then as the prolapsing upper rectum continues to extend downward, it eventually protrudes through the anus. The prolapse may be partial, with some of the upper part of the rectum prolapsing through to the exterior, or it may be complete, with all of the rectum prolapsing through.

Indications

Rectal prolapse is occasionally an incidental finding, and children with rectal prolapse are typically not ill or toxic appearing, although parents are generally very anxious about the condition. Often, a prolapsed rectum will reduce spontaneously. If it does not, it is important to reduce the prolapse manually. Although it may be possible to reduce the rectal prolapse without sedation, using sedation to relax children will make the process easier because any crying or resistance increases intraabdominal pressure and lowers the chances of a successful reduction.

It is important to be certain of the diagnosis. Occasionally, hemorrhoids or a prolapsed rectal polyp may look similar to rectal prolapse, although typically the whole rectal mucosa is not involved in the prolapse in such cases. Intussuception with prolapse is different in that the child is usually ill appearing, and it is impossible to pass a finger between the anal sphincter and the prolapsed bowel. Intussuception is the most serious of these disorders and must be diagnosed and managed as rapidly as possible.

Contraindications and Reasons for Referral to a Specialist

There are no absolute contraindications to attempted reduction of a rectal prolapse. Inability to perform adequate reduction after several attempts is a strong indication for referral, usually to a pediatric surgeon. Repeated episodes of prolapse in children, especially after the toddler years, should mandate further evaluation by a gastroenterologist.

Supplies and Equipment

- Gauze
- Gloves (nonsterile)
- Lubricant
- Sedation equipment as required (includes CR monitor, airway equipment, medicines)

- Sterile saline
- Tape

Procedure

1. Place relaxed and/or sedated patients in the knee-chest position prone, or supine with knees and hips flexed on the examining table or in a parent's lap.
2. Using the fingers of gloved hands, apply gentle but firm pressure circumferentially around the base of the prolapsed mucosa.
3. Place a saline-soaked sterile gauze over the exposed mucosa while using the thumbs to gently press inward on the tissue. The mucosa may glide more easily if a lubricated finger is placed into the rectum as a guide (Fig. 17-3).
4. Once the rectal mucosa has been reduced, apply a pressure dressing with tape to keep the mucosa reduced between bowel movements.
5. If the tissue has been prolapsed for a significant amount of time, it may be edematous and require some manual compression before reduction. During the reduction, pain and some mucosal bleeding can occur.

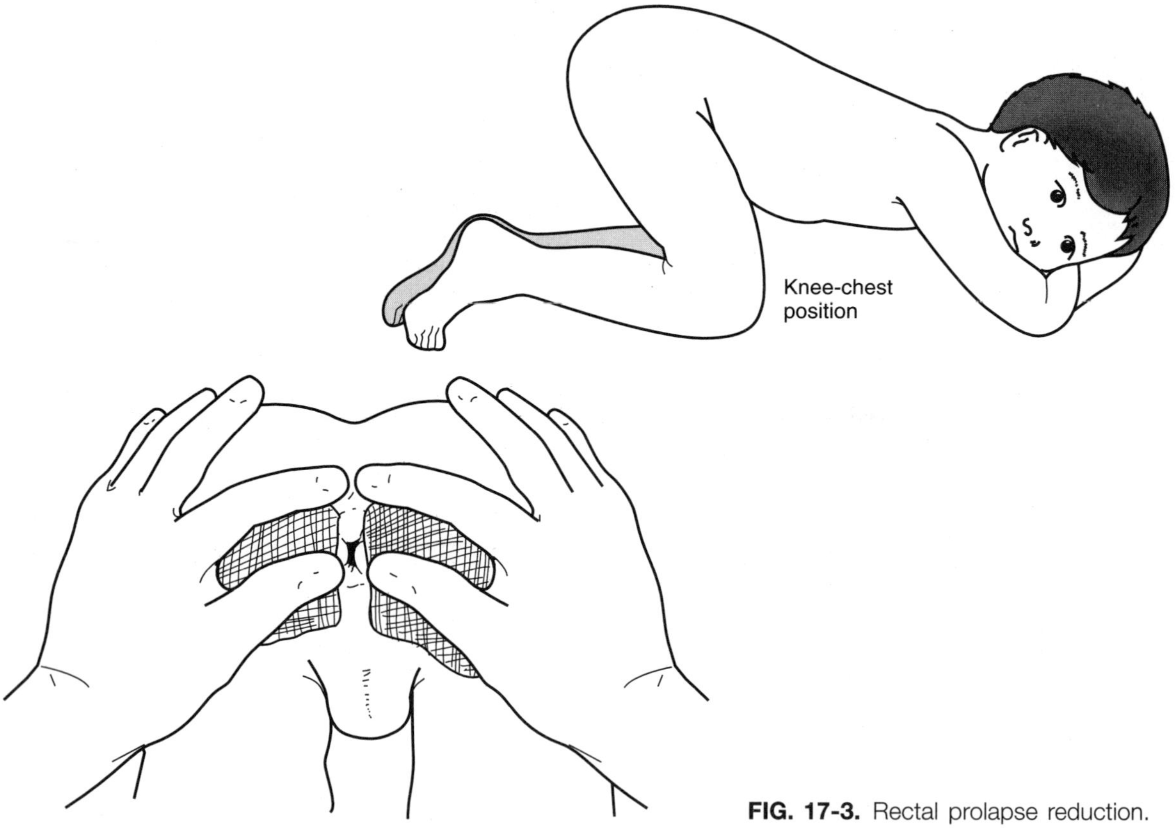

FIG. 17-3. Rectal prolapse reduction.

It is worthwhile to demonstrate the reduction to the parents because the rectal prolapse may recur, and they may be able to perform the reduction themselves. Rectal prolapses do not usually become incarcerated, and children usually outgrow them. In the event that attempts at manual reduction are unsuccessful, surgical consultation and intervention are necessary. Children who have recurrent rectal prolapse may also require ultimate surgical correction and should be referred to a pediatric surgeon.

What the Patient and Family Should Know

Family members should be informed about the procedure and warned about the possibility of small amounts of rectal bleeding. Children should be reassured and asked to cooperate as much as possible. For children who are especially anxious or unable to cooperate, consideration should be given to administering sedation in order to facilitate the procedure.

Possible Complications

No particular complications are associated with successful reduction of a rectal prolapse. Failure to reduce the prolapsed tissue represents a small risk of progressive ischemia and, in such cases, immediate referral is mandatory. Misdiagnosis of a more serious condition, such as advanced intussusception, can lead to disastrous outcomes.

Aftercare Instructions

Once the prolapsed tissue has been reduced, consideration must be given to the underlying cause and a bowel regimen must be begun. Children with chronic constipation should be started on stool softeners and motility agents. Children in whom cystic fibrosis is suspected should be first diagnosed and then, if the sweat chloride test is positive, started on pancreatic enzyme supplements.

Modifications for Situations of Limited Resources

This simple procedure requires no special equipment or supplies. It can be performed exactly as described, even without lubricant or gauze.

SUGGESTED READINGS

Corman ML: Rectal prolapse in children, *Dis Colon Rectum* 28:535, 1985.

Davies N, Najmaldin A, Burge DM: Irreducible inguinal hernia in children below 2 years of age, *Br J Surg* 77:1291, 1990.

Fleisher GR, Ludwig S, editors: *Textbook of pediatric emergency medicine,* ed 4, Baltimore, 2000, Lippincott Williams and Wilkins.

Gauderer MWL: Percutaneous endoscopic gastrostomy: a 10-year experience with 220 children, *J Pediatr Surg* 26:288, 1991.

Gauderer MWL, Ponsky JL, Izant RJ: Gastrostomy without laparotomy: a percutaneous endoscopic technique, *J Pediatr Surg* 15:872, 1980.

Goepp JG, Santosham M: Oral rehydration therapy. In Oski FA, McMillan J, editors: *Principles and practice of pediatrics supplement,* ed 2, Philadelphia, 1994, JB Lippincott.

Grosfeld JL: Current concepts in inguinal hernia in infants and children, *World J Surg* 13:506, 1989.

Hafner CD, Wylie JH, Brush BE: Complications of gastrointestinal intubation, *Arch Surg* 83:147, 1961.

Henretig FM, King C, editors: *Textbook of pediatric emergency procedures,* Baltimore, 1997, Williams and Wilkins.

Korula J, Harma C: A simple and inexpensive method of removal or replacement of gastrostomy tubes, *JAMA* 265:1426, 1991.

Ramanujam PS, Venkatesh KS: Management of acute incarcerated rectal prolapse, *Dis Colon Rectum* 35:1154, 1992.

Sader AA: New way to stabilize nasogastric tubes, *Am J Surg* 130:102, 1975.

Stringer MD et al: Irreducible inguinal hernia, *Br J Surg* 78:504, 1991.

Stylianos S, Jacir NN, Harris BH: Incarceration of inguinal hernia in infants prior to elective repair, *J Pediatr* 23:582, 1993.

Wyllie GG: The injection treatment of rectal prolapse, *J Pediatr Surg* 14:62, 1979.

Zempsky WT: The cause of rectal prolapse in children, *Am J Dis Child* 142:338, 1988.

CHAPTER 18

Genitourinary Procedures

Ann M. Lenane

PELVIC EXAMINATION

Background and Introduction

This examination is performed for an adolescent girl who is sexually active or who requires a pelvic examination to evaluate a gynecologic problem. In the primary care pediatric setting, the pelvic examination is usually part of a complete physical examination.

Supplies

- Appropriate-size speculum
- Cervical brush and wooden stick, for a Papanicolaou smear
- Cotton-tipped swabs, large (scopettes)
- Glass slides, two (one for a potassium hydroxide [KOH] preparation and one for a wet preparation)
- Gloves
- Light source appropriate for the type of speculum being used
- Lubricant
- Swabs, four (one for each specimen: gonorrhea culture, chlamydia culture, a wet preparation, and a KOH preparation)

Procedure

The pelvic examination on the adolescent patient is often a new and unfamiliar procedure for the patient. Therefore for the first part of this proceeding, the practitioner should describe the examination to the patient, reassuring her that it will not be painful and offering ample opportunity for her to express fears and concerns. An appropriate family member, friend, or a medical staff member should be in the room at the time of the examination to act as a chaperone and to offer support. If the support person is a medical staff member, she may assist the practitioner with some of the procedures; however, with some advance preparation, the examination may be done without assistance.

1. Provide the patient with a gown and sheet and request that she disrobe from the waist down.
2. Leave the room and assemble the supplies needed for the examination on a wheeled tray, with all swabs opened for easy access during the examination.
3. Drape the tray, transport it into the room, and place it at the foot of the examination table.
4. Ask the patient to lie supine on the examination table, with the sheet covering her from the waist down and a pillow at her head for comfort.
5. Show the patient where to place her feet in the stirrups and how to slide her buttocks down to the end of the table where the examination is to be done.
6. Tell the patient to let her knees fall apart so that the external genitalia may be visualized.
7. Thoroughly examine the external genitalia for any signs of cysts, genital warts, or discharge. This part of the examination also allows the patient to relax and the practitioner to check that the light is in a proper position for the internal part of the examination.
8. Show the speculum to the patient, explaining how it will be inserted.
9. Warm the speculum with tepid water, keep it closed, and insert it into the vagina. The easiest way to insert it is at an angle. If a clock's face is used to identify specific positions, the pubic symphysis is at 12 o'clock and the anus is at 6 o'clock. The handle of the speculum should be at halfway between 6 and 9 o'clock.
10. Apply downward pressure during insertion.
11. As the speculum is being inserted into the vagina, turn it so that the handle is in correct position at 6 o'clock.
12. Slowly open the speculum in order to visualize the cervix. It may need to be moved slightly in order to have the cervix at the open end of the speculum. Lock the speculum into position.
13. If the open speculum is uncomfortable for the patient, slowly close it, pull it out, and redirect it toward the cervix.
14. If the patient's cervix is difficult to find and to see, perform a bimanual examination, using only water or saline on the gloves as a lubricant, to locate the position of the cervix. Then, insert the speculum more easily, open it so that the entire cervix is seen, and lock it into position. At this point, the speculum should be resting without any support in the vagina so that the examination may continue.
15. If discharge is present in the vagina and the cervix cannot be seen, use a scopette to clear the discharge.
16. Take cultures by inserting each of the appropriate swabs, one each for gonorrhea and chlamydia, into the cervical os and rotating it, then, using the

same swab, also taking some of the fluid from the vaginal pool at the base of the cervix.

17. To obtain the wet preparation, repeat this procedure with an additional swab, then insert the swab into a small test tube of saline, which is used to make a slide.
18. Alternatively, place the contents of the swab directly on a slide. Later, in the laboratory, saline may be put on the slide, before placing a cover slip over the specimen.
19. For the KOH preparation, insert the swab into the cervical os and sample any discharge at the base of the cervix. This swab may then be used to prepare a slide, and later in the laboratory, KOH may be applied.
20. Perform the Papanicolaou smear, using a Papanicolaou smear brush inserted into the cervical os and rotated. If using a wooden stick, place the rounded end at the cervical os, then rotate it around the os to collect the cells. Place this specimen on a slide and then either spray it with, or insert it into, the appropriate fixative.
21. After these specimens are taken, slowly close and simultaneously remove the speculum, taking care not to catch the cervix, which can be very uncomfortable for the patient.
22. To begin the bimanual examination, use either the index, or index and middle, finger(s), depending on the size of the patient's vagina.
23. After applying lubricant to the glove, insert the fingers of the dominant hand, palm up, into the vagina to feel the end of the cervix. Any cervical motion tenderness should be noted because this may indicate infection.
24. Place the other hand on the patient's abdomen to feel the top of the uterus, the adnexa, and both ovaries. Any tenderness in this area should also be noted because this may further indicate infection. Once these structures have been palpated, the pelvic examination is complete.
25. If a rectal examination is needed, first change gloves to avoid contaminating the rectum with vaginal contents.
26. Tell the patient that she may remove her legs from the stirrups and slide back up the table. She should also be provided with a wipe to remove the lubricant from the external genitalia.
27. Cover the cultures and slides on the table, remove them from the room, and allow the patient to change into her clothing in privacy.
28. Place the swabs for the gonorrhea and chlamydia cultures in an appropriate transport medium, depending on the laboratory requirements.
29. Examine the slide for wet mount by placing saline and then a cover slip on the slide and looking for clue cells, as well as trichomonas.
30. For the KOH preparation, place KOH on the slide, allowing a few seconds for it to mix with the slide contents, and perform a "whiff test." A fishy odor indicates bacterial vaginosis. If a yeast infection is suspected, check the slide under a microscope for hyphae.
31. Send the specimen for the Papanicolaou smear to the laboratory, according to the protocol of the laboratory or hospital.

VAGINAL FOREIGN BODIES

Adolescent Patients

The following procedure is used not only for removing the most common vaginal foreign body in adolescent girls, a lodged tampon, but also as an outpatient procedure to remove most other vaginal foreign bodies.

The foreign body can often be seen and removed by having the patient lie in stirrups on the examination table, as if she were having a pelvic examination. This position alone may push the vaginal foreign body into a position where it can be seen with a thorough external examination. If the object cannot be seen in this way, the next step is to insert a speculum partially into the vagina and open it in order to see the foreign body. A clear plastic speculum works best if one is available. Once the foreign body is seen, it can be removed with a small hemostat. If the object cannot be seen in this fashion, the next step is to perform a bimanual examination to attempt to palpate and manually remove the foreign body. If this technique is also unsuccessful, the patient should be evaluated by a gynecologist to determine the need for an examination under anesthesia.

Prepubertal Children

The presence of a vaginal foreign body in a prepubertal child is considered a risk indicator for child sexual abuse. Children with vaginal foreign bodies should therefore undergo careful evaluation, including a sensitive and thorough history.

If a vaginal foreign body is suspected in a prepubertal child, it may be seen by having the child lie on an examination table, with her feet in the stirrups in a pelvic examination position, or in the frogleg position used to examine young children (Fig. 18-1). Exerting gentle downward and outward traction on the lower part of the labia minora will open the hymen so that the distal vagina can be seen. If the foreign body can be seen in this manner, it may be removed with a small hemostat. If this procedure is unsuccessful, it may be repeated, using the knee-chest position (Fig. 18-2). If this technique fails, several more invasive alternatives, each of which may require sedation of the patient, can be tried.

The first and best-tolerated approach is to attempt to flush the foreign body out. Because the most common vaginal foreign body in a young child is toilet paper, this approach is often successful. A small, lubricated, straight catheter, nasogastric tube, or the plastic portion of an intravenous catheter is passed into the vagina until it no longer moves forward, even with gentle pressure. Warm saline may then be gently flushed through the catheter in order to irrigate the vagina. This procedure often dislodges a foreign body, such as toilet paper.

An alternative approach is to use a small, plastic test tube, with the rounded or slightly pointed and rounded bottom (such as is used for centrifugation of urine) and the light that is used for a plastic speculum. The practitioner first lubricates the test tube and places the light inside it. The test tube is then inserted into the hymenal opening, exerting gentle downward and outward traction on the lower labia minora, in order to open the hymen. Then, the practitioner can identify the

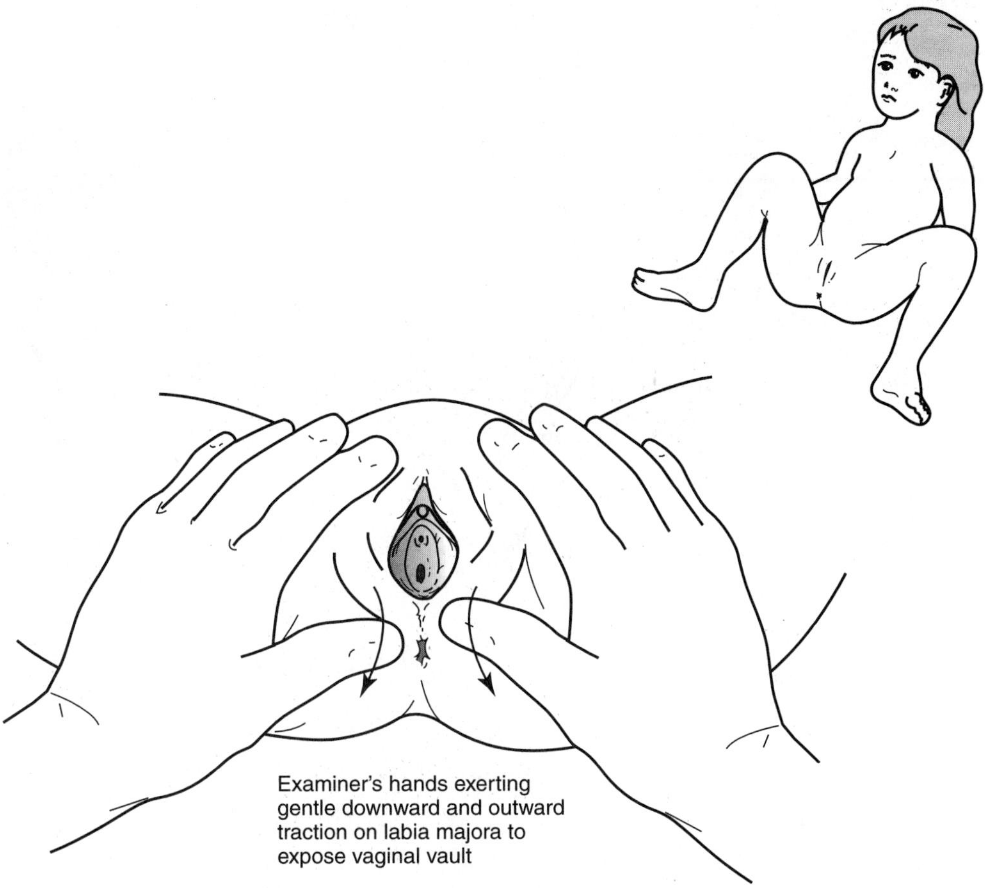

FIG. 18-1. Pelvic examination position, frogleg.

foreign body and more easily plan its removal. The nonsedated patient usually does not tolerate this procedure, so sedation is likely to be necessary for its success.

A third approach is to use a very small pediatric speculum. The patient is placed either on the pelvic table, using stirrups, or in the frogleg position. Gentle downward and outward traction is exerted on the lower labia minora in order to expose the hymenal opening. Meanwhile, the speculum is warmed with tepid water and may be lubricated because this procedure is not intended for obtaining cultures or cytology specimens. The practitioner then inserts the speculum through the hymen in order to expose the vagina and to see the foreign body. This procedure, which is very rarely tolerated in the awake patient, is generally performed under conscious sedation or general anesthesia.

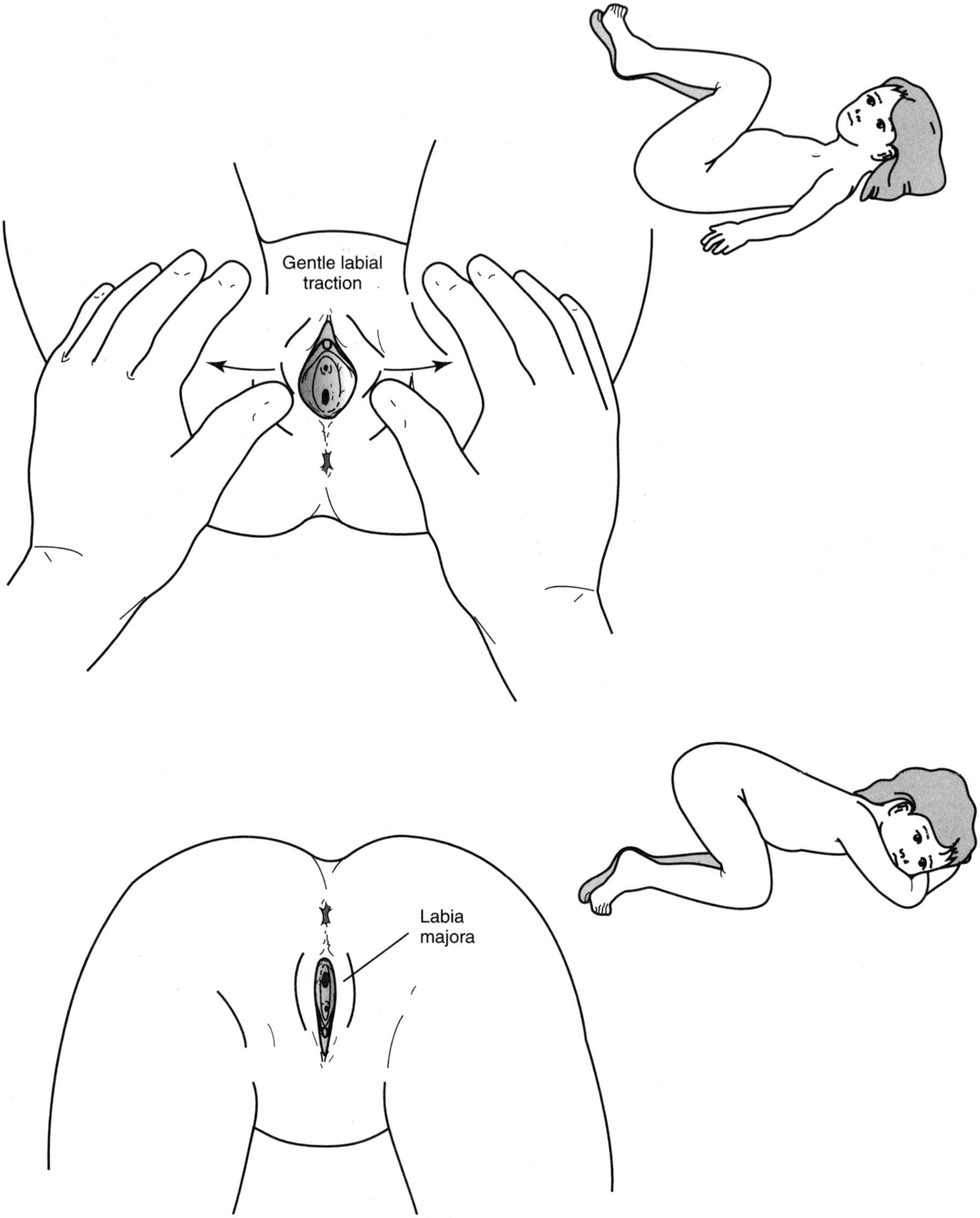

FIG. 18-2. Knee-chest position.

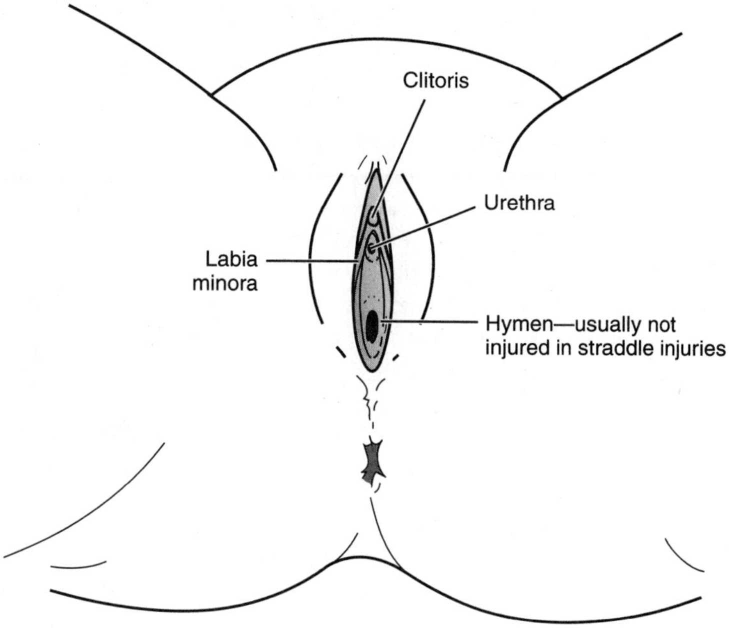

FIG. 18-3. External female genitalia.

GENITAL TRAUMA

The most common type of genital trauma in girls is usually caused by straddle injuries. Because of the nature of a straddle injury, the injured structures are generally the more anterior areas: the labia minora, clitoris, and urethra (Fig. 18-3). Most often, bleeding is brief and self-limited, and healing is rapid; however, occasionally, a child presents with active bleeding from trauma to the genital area.

In cases of genital trauma, the evaluation begins with a history of the event causing the injury. It should also include questions about the possible presence of a foreign body as part of the injury, the amount of bleeding that occurred, the time of the injury, and any measures the patient or family may have taken to treat the injury and halt the bleeding.

The next step is a physical examination, with an investigation of the abdomen to determine the possibility of internal injury. A thorough general physical examination is performed before proceeding to the genital examination to accustom the child to the idea of being at the physician's office. Subsequently, the external genitalia may be gently examined. It may take a few minutes and a great deal of patience to convince a child to permit this procedure. It is useful to have a support person stand at the head of the bed, using distraction devices, such as books or toys. The child should be placed in supine, frogleg position, or on a pelvic table with stirrups. Younger children tolerate the frogleg position better, whereas older children are sometimes more comfortable in stirrups. A light should be focused on the genital area, and gauze pads and saline should be easily accessible to stop any bleeding.

If bleeding is continuous and its source is identified, the practitioner can apply a wet dressing with gentle pressure on the area for about 10 minutes, or as long as the child will tolerate. If bleeding persists after this, the situation cannot be managed in the office setting, and the lesion may require surgical repair. The child should be sent to a pediatric urologist or pediatric gynecologist, who can perform the repair in an emergency department or in an operating room setting, with the child under sedation or general anesthesia.

If the bleeding has ceased, surgical repair may be unnecessary, and the child can be managed in the office setting. It is also critical to ensure that she is able to void. If the child feels uncomfortable voiding in the office, the practitioner may send her home. The parents should be advised to encourage the child to drink enough fluids to keep the urine diluted and to call the practitioner within 4 hours if the child has not voided. Occasionally, children fare better by being told that they may sit in a tub of lukewarm water and void into the tub. This is often more comfortable when injury to the genital area has occurred.

The home management plan includes frequent tub soaks and loose clothing, with reassessment if bleeding recurs. If the child cannot void in 4 hours or if bleeding recurs and does not stop with several minutes of pressure, the child should return to be seen in a medical setting. Such a referral should be to an emergency department where a pediatric urologist or gynecologist may be consulted if necessary.

All straddle injuries raise the suspicion of sexual abuse or assault. It is important to make certain that the injury fits the history provided and that no social concerns are present. If the hymen itself has been injured in what was described as a typical straddle injury, the practitioner should consider the possibility of sexual assault. Please refer to the section on The Sexual Abuse Examination for further details.

SUSPECTED SEXUAL ABUSE

Overview

This section is not meant to replace any policies, protocols, or guidelines that may already be part of a child sexual abuse management plan. If a child sexual abuse expert is available to evaluate children at the time of presentation, or is available for telephone consultation, that person's expertise should be utilized as part of the management of children who present for sexual abuse evaluation. This section is intended to supply practitioners with information necessary to perform an initial examination for child sexual abuse.

The evaluation of child sexual abuse can be divided according to the algorithm in Fig. 18-4. If the most recent episode of abuse occurred within 72 hours of the medical evaluation, then an evidence collection kit may be indicated; the kit will not be necessary if the time since the event is greater than 72 hours. The decision to use an evidence collection kit depends on the nature of the abuse, as well as

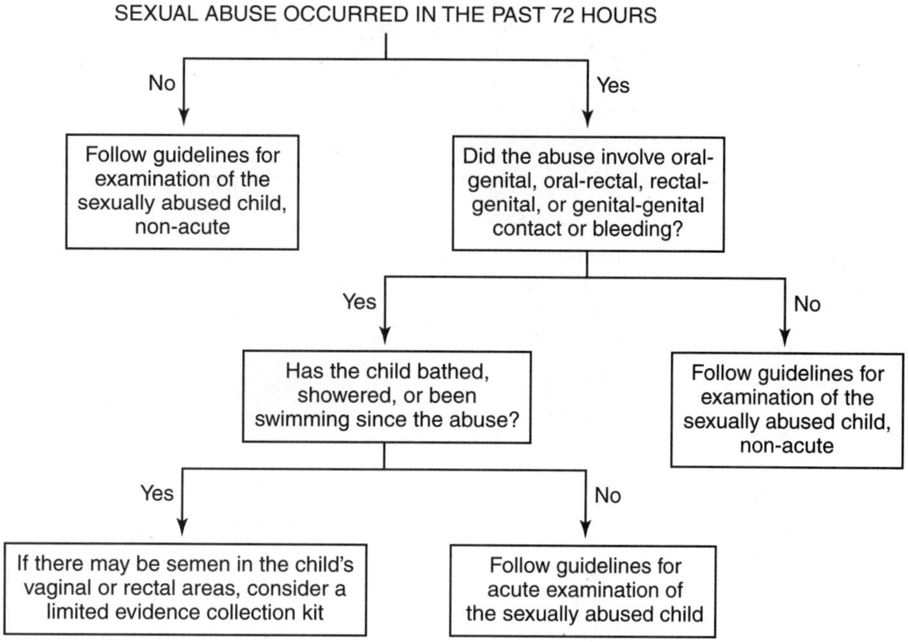

FIG. 18-4. Emergency evaluation of child sexual abuse flowchart for evidence collection.

BOX 18-1 SEXUAL ABUSE: WHO NEEDS CULTURES?

All pubertal children and all adolescents
Children with genital discharge (by examination or history)
Children with genital or rectal bleeding (by examination or history)
Children with a history of sexual contact (i.e., genital-genital, oral-genital, oral-rectal, or genital-rectal contact) with the perpetrator
Children with a household member who has a history of a sexually transmitted disease
Cases of risk of sexual contact between child and perpetrator, in which the child cannot provide the history (e.g., because of age or developmental stage)

whether or not children have bathed, showered, or been swimming since the most recent episode of abuse.

Other relevant issues that depend on the history of the abuse include the necessity of testing for sexually transmitted diseases (STDs), human immunodeficiency virus (HIV), pregnancy, and the need for prophylaxis for STDs, HIV, and prevention of pregnancy. The guidelines for taking cultures for STDs are in Box 18-1. The guidelines for testing and HIV prophylaxis are shown in Box 18-2. Prophylaxis regimens for STDs, HIV, and pregnancy have changed frequently in the past few years. Current recommendations are in Boxes 18-3 and 18-4, but consult the most recent Centers for Disease Control guidelines about STD and HIV issues for relevant updates.

BOX 18-2 HIV SCREENING/PROPHYLAXIS

Screening

Performed at the time of initial evaluation or during the patient's follow-up visit
If there was significant exposure of a mucosal surface (mouth, vagina, rectum) of the victim to blood, saliva, or semen of the perpetrator
If there was any trauma, tissue damage, or bleeding during the assault
Repeated screening required at 1, 3, 6, and 12 months

Prophylaxis

If screening is indicated, and the assault occurred within 36 hours of the assault, HIV prophylaxis is also indicated.
The first dose should be given as soon as possible and within 36 hours of the assault.
Currently, a 30-day schedule is recommended.

The medications used for HIV prophylaxis vary from one institution to another. Consult the HIV or infectious disease department at your institution for recommendations.

BOX 18-3 PREGNANCY PROPHYLAXIS

Indications

Sexual assault occurred within 72 hours of the evaluation
Genital-genital contact occurred, with known or possible ejaculation
The victim does not use hormonal contraceptives, and a barrier method was not used

Contraindications

Positive pregnancy test
Migraine headache, with neurologic symptoms at the time of evaluation
History of thrombophlebitis
Unprotected intercourse greater than 72 hours, but less than 5 days, before the evaluation

Medication

Combination oral contraception tablets, usually with estrogen and progesterone components

Instructions to Patient

Take one dose at the time of evaluation and repeat in 12 hours (e.g., Ovral, 2 tablets every 12 hr for 2 doses; or Lo-Ovral, 4 tablets every 12 hr for 2 doses)

Antiemetic

Nausea and cramps are common side effects. It is advisable to have the patient take an anti-emetic, such as Phenergan (12.5 to 25 mg) with each dose.

BOX 18-4 STD PROPHYLAXIS (ADULT DOSES)

One of the following:
- Ceftriaxone, 125 mg, IM, single dose
- Cefixime, 40 mg po, single dose
- Ciprofloxacin, 500 mg po, single dose
- Ofloxacin, 400 mg po, single dose

Plus one of the following:
- Azithromycin, 1 gram po, single dose
- Doxycycline, 100 mg po bid, for 7 days
- Plus Metronidazole, 2 grams po, single dose

To determine the type and extent of evaluation necessary, a history must be taken from a responsible adult. If a social worker, child protective worker, or law enforcement officer has already taken a history, the practitioner should try to review that information, which may save time and avoid multiple interviews of family members. Significant information obtained on history includes whether genital-genital, oral-genital, oral-rectal, or rectal-genital contacts occurred between the perpetrator and the child. It is also important to know if bleeding or ejaculation occurred, and the best estimated time of the latest contact between the child and the perpetrator.

Ideally, responsible adults should provide this history, with children absent from the room. Overhearing other descriptions of the incident may alter children's memory of the event, making future interviews with them unreliable. In some cases, adults, with children present, cannot provide details about the nature of the abuse. If children are 12 years or older and developmentally appropriate, they may also be interviewed for the necessary information. If this is done, interview children alone, without any of their caretakers present because these people may interfere with children's ability to speak freely about the abuse. One should avoid multiple interviews and interviewing young children (under 12), unless one has been trained in interviewing children. The interview is not an emergency and can be done at a later time.

Once the essential information has been obtained, children should have a complete physical examination and be allowed to choose which adult(s) may be present. This examination should include a detailed look at the genital and rectal areas, a thorough look at the skin for any bruising and bite marks, and a very precise head, eyes, ears, nose, and throat (HEENT) examination, looking for any oral lesions.

Prepubertal Children

Young children may not cooperate well with the genital and anal examinations. Therefore all required materials should be arranged and at the practitioner's fingertips before the examination. Culture swabs should be available and ready to take cultures for gonorrhea and chlamydia from the genital and anal areas, as well as extra swabs to make a wet mount and a KOH preparation, if indicated. The light source should be placed at the foot of the bed. A supportive adult should be stationed at the head of the bed to elicit children's cooperation, by using distractions, such as books or handheld toys.

The most comfortable examination position for young children is the frogleg position, which exposes the external genitalia for examination (see Fig. 18-1). Clothing is first removed from the waist down, and a gown or sheet is furnished to cover children, if desired. When children are lying supine and relaxed, with feet flat on the bed and the knees bent, the practitioner should instruct them to let their legs fall apart at the knees, so that they look like a frog's legs.

The anal area may also be examined in this position or in the knee-chest position (see Fig. 18-2). In young children, the anal examination is often better tolerated than the genital one, so it may be advisable to do the external anal examination first. This procedure may be done by spreading the buttocks apart and examining the anal area for tone, as well as for any fissures, scars, swelling, bruising, and asymmetry of the anal rugae. An internal rectal examination is usually not necessary.

In female children, the genitalia should be viewed by exerting gentle downward and outward traction on the lower labia, in order to expose the hymen. It is customary to use the face of a clock to describe and document the position of any lesions or abnormalities noticed on the genital or rectal examinations. Thus 12 o'clock would be at the symphysis pubis, and 6 o'clock would be at the rectum (a diagram of the external female genitalia is given in Fig. 18-3). In some cases, the hymen will not open spontaneously, and thus it will be difficult to see. Relaxation techniques, such as having children talk about a favorite activity, taking some deep breaths, or sometimes a Valsalva maneuver, such as having children cough, may assist in opening the hymen.

Another successful technique is to dribble a few drops of warm water or saline on the hymen, causing it to open. If these techniques fail, children may be placed on their stomachs in a knee-chest position (see Fig. 18-2). In this case, they lie with their head turned to one side on the examination table and push their buttocks up. The practitioner exerts gentle outward and upward traction to separate the labia, and the hymen can usually be seen. Children do not tolerate this position for very long, but it often allows the practitioner to visualize the posterior portion of the hymen, as well as the posterior forchette, if these cannot be seen in the frogleg position.

Another technique, which is best done in the frogleg or pelvic table position, allows one to examine the edges of the hymen. The practitioner first lubricates a minitip swab with nonbacteriostatic water or saline, places it into the middle of the hymen, and passes it around the hymenal edge to detect any irregularities or scars. This procedure is often uncomfortable for young children. If cultures need to be taken, this procedure should be done as part of taking the final cultures, because children may not tolerate any further examination.

If cultures are indicated for young children, they should be acquired first from the anal area and then from the genital area, with two culture swabs obtained from both areas. For each procedure, the two swabs may be held together and done simultaneously, which is particularly advisable for young and/or uncooperative children. For rectal cultures, the culture swabs should be lubricated with nonbacteriostatic saline and gently inserted about 1 cm into the rectum.

An internal rectal examination is usually not necessary in prepubertal children. The exception to this rule is children with abnormal anal tone on external examination. This finding, in the absence of stool in the rectal vault, may support a history of anal penetration. Therefore it is necessary to perform a digital rectal examination, or to use "test tube proctoscopy," to determine if stool is present in the vault. Test tube proctoscopy is performed by using a small test tube with a rounded bottom and a pelvic light, or otoscope light. The end of the tube is lubricated and passed slowly into the rectum, and when the pelvic light shines into the tube, the distal rectum can be visualized. Cooperation from children is essential for this procedure. If this is not possible, and children require an internal rectal examination to check for stool, then a digital examination should be done because this technique is safer. If children have active rectal bleeding at the time of the evaluation, a pediatric gastroenterologist or surgeon should be consulted.

Because genital cultures from the end of the cervix do not need to be obtained from prepubertal girls, the practitioner only needs to insert the culture swab about 1 cm into the hymen. The procedure is best tolerated using a minitip swab, which is also lubricated with nonbacteriostatic saline or water. The practitioner should avoid touching the outside edge of the hymen when the cultures are taken because this contact can be uncomfortable for young girls. If discharge is present from the genital area, a wet mount and KOH preparation should also be obtained, according to the procedure described in the Pelvic Examination section.

Speculum examination of the prepubertal child is not necessary because the hymen is not large enough to introduce a speculum without sedation or anesthesia. Any significant findings can be seen on an external genital examination. The exceptions to this case are children with vaginal bleeding. In this situation, a physician who is experienced in pediatric gynecology should perform the procedure with children under sedation or anesthesia. If an evidence collection kit is indicated, this procedure should be performed as described in the following Acute Sexual Assault section.

Pubertal Female Children

Please refer to the Pelvic Examination section.

Male Children

Once the general physical examination of male children is complete, the next step is the genital/anal portion of the examination. As with female children, the light source and culture swabs should be prepared and available before the procedures begin. Male children should be allowed to put on a gown or cover up with a sheet and requested to disrobe from the waist down. They may sit or lie on the examination table, with a support person at the head of the table, offering reassurance and distraction, as described for female children. The external genitalia should be examined, and any abnormalities should be noted. Any urethral bleeding warrants consultation with a pediatric urologist.

The practitioner may select one of several techniques for the anal examination. One procedure is done by having children bend their knees up in supine position, so that the anal area can be visualized by gently spreading the buttocks apart. Children can also lie in the left lateral decubitus position, prone position, or knee-chest position (see Fig. 18-2). The anal area should then be thoroughly evaluated for any lesions, such as scars, bruises, fissures, abnormal tone, or asymmetry of the rugae. If cultures are indicated, they should be taken from the rectal area first, and then from the urethra. Minitip swabs are necessary for the urethral cultures, and each swab is inserted at least one-half to one centimeter into the urethra, if children will tolerate this action.

HIV/Hepatitis Testing

If the sexual abuse involved any direct contact of children's oral, genital, or rectal areas with semen or blood from the perpetrator, children should be tested for Hepatitis B and HIV. A serological test for syphilis may also be performed at this time. Policies and protocols for testing for hepatitis, HIV, and syphilis vary significantly from one facility to another. If the local medical center has specific guidelines for these issues, they should be followed. If HIV testing is done, children will need to have follow-up testing, usually recommended at 1 month, 3 months, 6 months, and 12 months after the exposure. The timing of these tests, therefore, depends on the timing of the exposure. Please see the following Acute Sexual Assault section for guidelines regarding prophylaxis for Hepatitis B and HIV.

SEXUAL ASSAULT: THE ACUTE EXAMINATION

Overview

If the sexual assault occurred within 72 hours of the medical evaluation and, because of the nature of the assault, may have left any bodily fluids, such as saliva, semen, or blood, from the perpetrator on or inside the victim, an evidence collection kit should be obtained. These kits are usually standard kits that the practitioner's office and forensic laboratory in the community have selected and provided to the hospital for this purpose.

The kit usually contains forms that need to be filled out by the examining practitioner, including a consent form. An instruction sheet also describes which forms need to be completed, which forms should go into, and remain outside of, the kit, as well as instructions for collecting medical evidence. In all cases, collection of evidence requires the victim's consent (depending on the victim's age). The collection of each specific piece of evidence is done at the discretion of the practitioner, and only relevant evidence needs to be obtained. This section includes general advice on collecting each specimen; however, the practitioner is required to follow the specific instructions for the kit used by the institution.

Because this kit is sealed and given to a law enforcement officer, the specimens contained therein cannot be used for cultures that may need to be part of the medical evaluation. These cultures should be obtained during the appropriate portion of evidence collection and kept separate for the necessary medical testing.

The evidence collection kit provides for approximately 10 to 15 pieces of evidence that should be gathered. Because this collection can be a lengthy process, the practitioner should review the kit's contents and organize them so that the evidence collection proceeds as quickly as possible. This preparation will not only minimize the discomfort for older children, but it will also get crucial evidence during the very small window of cooperation in young children.

Once the practitioner has begun to collect evidence, none of the contents of the collection kit should leave the practitioner's sight until the kit is sealed and turned over to a law enforcement officer. If the practitioner needs to leave the room, another medical staff member should guard the contents of the kit to prevent any tampering with evidence. If practitioners have never used a medical collection kit, they should review the contents of a kit (not the one to be used for the patient) before the evidence collection procedure. Once familiar with the kit, practitioners can then determine which portions need to be collected on the particular child.

Brief Review of the Medical Collection Kit

The kit contains a consent form for the victim or parent to sign, instructions for the practitioner, and often instructions for the patient as well. There may also be forms for the practitioner to use in order to document the history and the medical examination. Most kits include a body diagram and a diagram of the genital and rectal areas for documentation.

The kit usually contains materials for collecting specific types of evidence. Because of the high sensitivity of modern tissue and bodily fluid identification technology, practitioners must use extreme care to avoid contamination of physical evidence with their own tissue. Two kinds of evidence are collected from the mouth. Swabs are used for evidence that the perpetrator may have left inside the oral cavity, and filter paper is provided for a saliva sample. Swabs are provided for collecting any dried secretions that may be found on the patient, as well as an envelope for any other debris remaining on the patient.

For collecting specific debris from the fingernails, an envelope and pointed sticks are provided so that children or an adult can scrape underneath the nails for this piece of evidence. Envelopes are also provided for collecting pulled hairs from the head and the pubic area. Swabs for collecting evidence from the genital and rectal areas are provided, as well as a test tube(s) or filter paper for collecting a blood sample from the victim. There may also be a bag for the victim's underwear, which is usually the only piece of the victim's clothing that must be placed inside the kit. If other clothing is collected for evidence, it should be placed in a paper bag, which is then sealed with the victim's name and initialed by the person who collected the evidence.

When sealing the envelopes in the kit, the practitioner should use tape or labels and must never introduce any saliva by licking the envelopes. The practitioner should also wear gloves when handling specimens to avoid introducing any skin into the samples. Upon completion of the kit, the practitioner should also seal and initial it, then turn it over to a law enforcement officer. The details of using the items in the kit are discussed in the next section.

Supplies and Equipment

The following list of items, in addition to the kit, should be available in the examination room during the evidence collection period:

- A large piece of paper, such as examination table paper, or a sheet, for the child to stand on while undressing
- Camera (if available)
- Equipment needed for obtaining the blood sample

- Examination gloves
- Examination gown and sheet for the patient
- Glass slides for collection of wet mounts and KOH preps (two for the genital and one for the rectal)
- Light for the pelvic examination
- Speculum (depending on the child's age)
- Swabs for obtaining cultures, wet mounts, and KOH preps (four for genital specimens and three for rectal specimens)
- Tape, or several labels, stamped with the patient's name, used for sealing the evidence collection kit and labeling cultures

History and Physical Examination

As with the nonacute sexual assault examination, the history should be obtained from a family member. If a protective worker or law enforcement officer has given a history, it should also be secured and read before the medical examination, if possible. While discussing the history, the practitioner should also talk about the need for testing and prophylaxis for STDs, including hepatitis and HIV, as described as follows. If HIV testing is part of the emergency evaluation, the consent form should be signed. Both the consent form and the materials to collect the specimens should be in the examination room so that a second venipuncture is not necessary. The appropriate history taking is the same as described in the previous Sexual Abuse section.

The examination begins, as in the setting of nonacute abuse, with rapport building, followed by a general physical examination. During the HEENT examination, oral specimens for the evidence collection kit may be obtained while children are still dressed. Patients should not have anything to eat or drink for 30 minutes before the collection of the saliva sample. If children have eaten just before the procedure, this sample should be collected at the end of the examination. The HEENT examination should consist of a thorough inspection of the head and neck for any signs of trauma. It should also include inspection of the mouth, along with the frenulum and the soft palate, for any signs of trauma.

During the rest of the examination, any debris that is found on children, as well as any dried secretions, are collected as part of the medical evidence kit. Children should stand on a piece of examination table paper, or a sheet, if paper is not available. Any debris that falls from children should be gathered up and put into the appropriate debris envelopes of the collection kit. After children undress, the skin can be examined for dried secretions, which are collected with the appropriate swabs for the collection kit. Any bruises or markings on the skin, as well as the areas that contained any specimen evidence, should be noted as part of the documentation.

At this point, children can put on a gown and sit on the examination table for the rest of the evaluation. Their underwear should be placed in the appropriate bag and sealed. If children become agitated at seeing their clothing removed, leave the clothing in sight and seal it up later in order to maintain rapport and allow the examination to continue. If children were wearing the same clothing during the assault, with possible evidence on it, each piece should be sealed in a separate paper bag and submitted with the evidence collection kit. In this case, the hospital is obliged to provide clothing for children to wear home after the examination. If that is impossible, and children are not going to be admitted to the hospital, they may wear the original clothing home (minus the underwear). A law enforcement officer can meet the family at the home and collect the clothing later.

During the general physical examination, the hands and nails should be checked. If evidence might exist underneath the fingernails, children should be assisted in collecting that evidence, using the appropriate portion of the kit. Usually, the kit provides a piece of filter paper to be placed under each hand, which is labeled as such, and two sticks, one for each hand, to scrape underneath the nails. Once the sticks have been used to scrape the nails over the paper, they are placed inside the paper, which is folded, sealed, and labeled in an appropriate envelope.

After the general physical examination is completed, the anal and genital areas should be inspected. Because young children generally tolerate the anal examination better, it may be done first. The swabs should be prepared for both evidence and culture collections by being moistened with nonbacteriostatic saline before obtaining the specimens. This preparation usually makes the specimen collection more tolerable. An additional slide is necessary to make a wet mount to detect any sperm if the history of the assault suggests that semen may be present in the rectum. The culture should be obtained as described in the previous examination section, with children either in supine, prone, or lateral decubitus position. Any abnormalities during the rectal examination should also be noted, and a hemoccult specimen can be taken by using one of the cotton-tipped swabs. After obtaining the specimens, it is not necessary to perform a digital examination. The anal examination should be followed by the genital examination.

Before positioning children for the genital examination, the swabs should be moistened with nonbacteriostatic saline in order to make the procedure more comfortable. Female children should be placed in the knee-chest or the better-tolerated frogleg position, so that they can see both the practitioner and the support person. The genital examination should begin with a thorough examination of the external genitalia and then the more internal structures of the labia minora, urethra, and hymen (see Fig. 18-3). The practitioner exerts downward and outward traction on the labia if children are in the supine position. Any abnormalities, particularly abrasions, bruising, bleeding, or any foreign material, should be noted. Any dried secretions that were not noted on the general examination should be swabbed and put into one of the evidence collection envelopes for the genital examination. It is important to document the site from which the swab was obtained in the evidence collection kit.

Once the external genitalia have been examined, the swabs for evidence collection, as well as for culture, wet mount, and KOH preparation, can be acquired. The wet mount should be used to investigate for sperm and trichomonas. In prepubertal children, the genital swabs are collected by inserting them inside the hymen. In pubertal children, a speculum examination should be attempted, although it may not be tolerated because of children's anxiety and the nature of the trauma. If this is the case, the swabs should be obtained in the same manner as for prepubertal children, by inserting them through the hymen and into the vagina. The hymen is very sensitive, and specimen collection may be irritating for young children. If possible, the practitioner should obtain specimens from the distal vagina, without touching the hymen.

The other types of evidence that may be required are pulled or clipped head hairs and pulled or clipped pubic hairs. Specific instructions for collecting these specimens are included in the particular kit used. This part of the evidence collection process is particularly unpleasant for patients, and it is not essential that it be performed during the acute evidence collection period. These specimens are collected for comparison with hair from the perpetrator.

The other part of evidence collection involves taking a tube or filter paper sample of the victim's blood, which is also used as a comparison analysis in case any of the perpetrator's blood is found in the evidence collection. As with collecting hair samples, this process is uncomfortable for patients and can be done at a later date. If obvious blood is detected as part of the medical evidence during the collection, the blood sample should be taken as part of the acute evaluation. Also, if HIV testing, hepatitis testing, and/or a rapid plasma reagin are to be done as part of the medical evaluation, they can be obtained from a single venipuncture.

Once all of these samples are taken, labeled, air-dried, and sealed, they, along with the tubes used, should be placed into the evidence collection kit. Because this procedure is lengthy, it is advisable to review the instructions from the kit before sealing it, to ensure that all of the necessary specimens have been obtained. Slides used by the practitioner for clinical evaluation should not be included in the evidence collection kit. Any paperwork from the kit should be completed first and then returned to the kit. Every item should be carefully checked before the kit is sealed. Then the practitioner can take the sealed kit, as well as the medical specimens for cultures and microscopic analysis, outside the room and allow children to dress. Practitioners must keep the kit within their sight until it is turned over to a law enforcement officer. In many institutions, the kit is placed in a lockbox until a law enforcement officer can pick it up. Appropriate institutional policies should be followed in order to maintain the chain of evidence.

Treatment

After the evidence collection kit has been secured and patients have dressed, the following issues must be considered:

- *Patient safety:* Immediate medical or psychosocial needs must be addressed.
- *Pregnancy prophylaxis* (if appropriate)
- *STD prophylaxis:* This is not indicated in prepubertal children because the incidence of acquiring an STD from sexual assault is less than 5%. Prophylaxis may be appropriate for adolescents, particularly if concerns exist about compliance with the follow-up regimen.
- *HIV:* If testing or prophylaxis is indicated, patients usually need a follow-up visit within a few days of the assault to check that they are correctly taking the medications and to arrange the necessary retesting.

- *Counseling:* Many rape crisis centers and child abuse programs can help arrange acute and long-term counseling.
- *Medical follow-up:* If the assault placed children at risk for contracting an STD, cultures should be repeated in 7 to 10 days. If the assault involved physical trauma, pertinent follow-up care should be arranged.

SUGGESTED READINGS

AIDS Institute, New York State Department of Health: *HIV prophylaxis following sexual assault: guidelines for adults and adolescents,* 2000.

American Academy of Pediatrics Committee on Child Abuse and Neglect: Guidelines for the evaluation of sexual abuse of children: subject review, *Pediatrics* 103:186, 1999.

Centers for Disease Control and Prevention: 1998 guidelines for treatment of sexually transmitted diseases, *MMWR* 47:53, 1998.

Emans SJH, Goldstein OP: *Pediatric and adolescent gynecology,* ed 3, Boston, 1990, Little, Brown.

Herman-Giddens M: Vaginal foreign bodies and child sexual abuse, *Arch Pediatr Adolesc Med* 148:195, 1994.

Peter G, editor: *Redbook: report of the Committee on Infectious Diseases,* ed 24, Elk Grove Village, IL, 1997, American Academy of Pediatrics.

Siegel RM et al: The prevalence of sexually transmitted diseases in children and adolescents evaluated for sexual abuse in Cincinnati: rationale for limited STD testing in prepubertal girls, *Pediatrics* 96:1090, 1995.

CHAPTER 19

Toxicological Emergencies

Lynne M. Palmisciano
James G. Linakis

BACKGROUND AND INTRODUCTION

The following four modes of therapy are used to treat toxicological emergencies:

1. *Supportive care* is the cornerstone of treatment for all patients.
2. *Decontamination* limits further absorption of the toxin. Methods for decontamination include irrigation of the skin or eyes, gastric emptying, adsorption of toxin to activated charcoal and whole bowel irrigation. Gastric emptying can be accomplished by inducing emesis with syrup of ipecac or by gastric lavage.
3. The *elimination* of some toxins can be enhanced using alkalinization or hemodialysis.
4. For a very few toxic exposures, specific *antidotes* are available.

Each toxic exposure must be evaluated individually. General principles include doing no further harm and not becoming a second victim. Some substances are absorbed so rapidly that decontamination is not feasible. Certain categories of toxins do not adsorb to activated charcoal. Only a relatively few compounds are candidates for enhanced elimination and antidote therapy. The regional poison center can assist the practitioner in determining appropriate treatment options for a given patient.

CUTANEOUS DECONTAMINATION

Indications and Contraindications

All cases of dermal exposure should be decontaminated to restrict further cutaneous absorption, limit additional local tissue damage, and prevent exposure of practitioners. The primary goal is to dilute the substance so that the amount absorbed is in a nontoxic range. This decontamination should begin as soon as possible after the exposure.

There are no absolute contraindications for cutaneous or ocular decontamination. Inability to treat patients without exposing the practitioner constitutes a relative contraindication. Immediate life-saving procedures may limit the extent of decontamination performed in some cases. Penetrating eye trauma is not a contraindication to decontamination; however, care must be taken not to increase intraocular pressure by irrigation.

Certain chemical exposures, such as elemental sodium, lithium, or phosphorus, require specific decontamination procedures. The regional poison center can advise in these circumstances.

Supplies and Equipment

Need to have

- Bags for patient clothing and belongings
- Large quantity of water or saline, warm but not hot
- Mild soap
- Protective gowns, gloves, goggles, and masks

Nice to have

- Collecting system for drainage
- Low-pressure shower head

Procedure

1. Have all practitioners wear gloves, masks, eye protection, and impermeable gowns.
2. Take patients to a predesignated decontamination site, preferably with a separate collection system for fluid drainage.
3. Have patients remove contaminated clothing and jewelry and place these items in biohazard bags.
4. Brush excess particulate debris from patients' skin before irrigation. Similarly, adherent liquids can be blotted off the skin.
5. Rinse the skin with lukewarm water under low pressure. A low-pressure showerhead, hose, or bucket may be utilized. Hot water is avoided because it may induce vasodilation and further absorption. Irrigation with cold fluid may lead to hypothermia.
6. After thorough rinsing, wash patients with a mild soap to remove any remaining material. Carefully inspect areas prone to collection of debris, such as skin folds, the umbilicus, hair, and nails.
7. Dry patients gently to avoid abrading the skin.

Complications

The primary complications associated with dermal decontamination are hypothermia and contamination of practitioners. Overly vigorous decontamination with high-pressure irrigation or hot fluids can increase absorption of toxin.

OCULAR DECONTAMINATION

Indications and Contraindications

If any concern exists about ocular contamination, irrigation should begin immediately. This process should be initiated at home or by emergency medical services, if possible. Any history compatible with ocular exposure or symptoms such as burning, redness, itching, or pain warrant ocular decontamination by irrigation.

Supplies and Equipment

Need to have

- Emesis basin or bucket
- Gloves
- Intravenous (IV) tubing
- Normal saline, room temperature
- pH paper or urine dipstick with pH values

Nice to have

- Eyelid retractor
- Fluorescein strips
- Morgan lens
- Papoose board or similar restraint
- Topical anesthetic, 0.5% proparacaine
- Wood's lamp

Procedure

1. Don appropriate safety apparel.
2. If patients are wearing contact lenses, remove them.
3. If pH paper is readily available, obtain an initial pH measurement. Many urine dipsticks measure midrange pH and can substitute for pH paper.
4. Have patients lie on their side with the affected eye down.
5. If patients have significant pain, administer topical anesthetic drops to facilitate adequate irrigation. Because cessation of pain is often used to guide adequacy of therapy, anesthesia should be used with caution.
6. If a Morgan lens is used, anesthetic drops also must be used. This device is a large contact lens with a central port for irrigation. Some practitioners believe that this device allows pooling of chemicals beneath the lens and that it should be used only after direct irrigation is completed. Irrigation should commence as early as possible.
7. Connect IV tubing to a bag of room-temperature saline.
8. Place the end of the tubing at the inner canthus and allow the fluid to flush across the eye. Place an emesis basin under the dependent side of the face to collect the drainage.

9. Continue irrigation for a minimum of 20 minutes. Redirect the stream of saline at various angles to achieve clearance of materials from all portions of the eye.
10. Recheck the pH. Irrigation should stop only when a normal pH of 7.4 is reached. Perform repeat measures of pH at 10 and 20 minutes after irrigation to evaluate for reequilibration.
11. After irrigation is complete, instill fluorescein and inspect the eye for corneal abrasions using a Wood's lamp. Record visual acuity at this time.

The practitioner may advise parents on methods for performing irrigation in their homes. With cooperative children, hold their head under the regular faucet tap and let the water flush over the eye. If the emergency medical services system is called, apparatus similar to the ones described previously should be available.

Possible Complications

Irrigation may result in small corneal or conjunctival abrasions. If irrigation fluids are administered under pressure, corneal damage may occur. Avoiding the use of fluids under pressure is particularly important in cases with potential penetrating trauma to the globe. Most of the damage seen with ocular exposures comes from the initial injury. Failure to adequately irrigate the eye can result in ongoing damage.

GASTRIC EMPTYING

Indications and Contraindications

Syrup of ipecac is indicated as a means of gastric evacuation in the period immediately after a potentially toxic ingestion (up to 10 minutes). This treatment may be used by lay people with the guidance of medical personnel (e.g., physician, telephone triage nurse, or poison center staff). In most cases, ipecac should not be used in the physician's office or emergency department.

Gastric lavage requires personnel trained in gastric intubation with assistants capable of safely restraining patients and managing the airway in case of aspiration. This procedure may be accomplished in an office setting or, in some cases, by paramedics. Lavage should be completed within 30 to 60 minutes after the ingestion.

Because ipecac induces emesis and gastric lavage can produce emesis, their use is contraindicated in situations in which aspiration poses a significant risk. This includes patients with airway compromise or the potential for rapid deterioration in airway control because of central nervous system depression, respiratory failure, or seizures. Gastric emptying is contraindicated in cases of known caustic or hydrocarbon ingestions because of the high risk of aspiration and resulting chemical pneumonitis. Delayed presentation (greater than 1 hour after the ingestion) is also a contraindication because of the significantly reduced efficacy of delay in gastric emptying.

Consultation with a toxicologist or poison center can help determine the utility of gastric emptying at the time of presentation. In patients with an underlying medical condition, contact with the primary care provider or a specific specialist may help determine special considerations for that patient. If the family is at home and does not have ipecac available, involving local emergency medical service providers may be beneficial because many stock syrup of ipecac.

Supplies and Equipment

- Emesis basin
- Protective clothing
- Syrup of ipecac
- Teaspoon measure
- Water

Additional materials for gastric lavage:

- Cardiac monitor
- Lubricant, water-soluble such as Surgilube
- Orogastric tube (24- to 50-Fr depending on patient size)
- Oxygen and mask
- Papoose board or similar restraint
- Specimen container
- Suction
- Syringe (wide-tipped)
- Tape measure
- Warmed saline for lavage (1 to 2 L)

Procedure

Syrup of ipecac is administered orally under advisement of a regional poison center. For children under 6 months of age, the decision to treat with ipecac should be made on a case-by-case basis in conjunction with a toxicologist. For infants 6 to 12 months old, the dose of ipecac is 10 ml (2 teaspoons); for children 1 to 12 years, it is 15 ml (3 teaspoons); and for adults, it is 30 ml (6 teaspoons or 1 ounce). Older children should be given a glass of clear liquid to drink after administration of syrup of ipecac. Generally, a single dose is given, but a single repeat dose may be given if no result has occurred in 20 minutes.

In certain circumstances, gastric lavage may be performed in the prehospital setting as a method of gastric emptying.

1. Have the practitioner and assistants don protective equipment such as goggles, gloves, and fluid-impermeable gowns.
2. Have an assistant restrain children during insertion of the lavage tube. A papoose board or rolled sheet may be helpful.
3. Follow the procedure for inserting an orogastric tube as described in Chapter 13. The size of tube used varies with patient size, ranging from 24- to 50-Fr.

4. After confirming gastric intubation by air insufflation or aspiration of stomach contents, empty the stomach.
5. Gently infuse sterile saline by syringe in approximately 100-ml aliquots. Equal aliquots of fluid should be aspirated by syringe.
6. Continue this procedure until the returning fluid is clear. Contents recovered immediately after tube placement may be sent for toxicological evaluation.

Complications

The use of ipecac or gastric lavage may result in vomiting, and both hold the potential for aspiration. Therefore suction equipment should be readily available when these procedures are performed. Additional complications of gastric lavage include malposition of the orogastric tube (including, rarely, intubation of the trachea) or trauma to the esophagus or stomach. Overly vigorous instillation of lavage fluid can force the substance beyond the pylorus, making it unavailable for recovery by lavage.

ACTIVATED CHARCOAL

Indications and Contraindications

Activated charcoal is most effective in cases in which the ingested toxin is readily adsorbed by activated charcoal. Consideration must be given to the accuracy of the ingestion history, including the time of ingestion and the possibility of multiple ingestions. For potentially lethal ingestions, many toxicologists recommend the use of activated charcoal even when patients present 12 to 24 hours after ingestion.

Activated charcoal is also used to enhance the elimination of certain toxins. With ingestions involving toxins that undergo significant enterohepatic recirculation, activated charcoal may be effective in eliminating toxin beyond its initial absorption. In these cases, multiple-dose activated charcoal (MDAC) is often indicated. Regional poison control centers can advise the practitioner about the role of MDAC in any specific case.

The absolute contraindications to the use of activated charcoal are few. Patients without stable airways or at risk of rapid loss of airway control should not receive activated charcoal until definitive airway control is obtained. Patients with caustic ingestions requiring endoscopy should not receive charcoal because it will impair visualization during the procedure and because caustics are not adsorbed by charcoal. A relative contraindication includes states in which emesis and/or aspiration may significantly worsen the patient's condition because activated charcoal administration may increase the occurrence of aspiration.

Toxicological emergencies often do not allow the time necessary for referral to a specialist, but consultation with a specialist may be helpful. Regional poison control centers may be able to provide instruction directly and can assist in accessing other resources. Specific circumstances requiring specialty care include caustic ingestions that will require endoscopy, ingestions of dialyzable substances, and any patients requiring intensive or prolonged monitoring.

Supplies and Equipment

Need to have

- Activated charcoal (with or without added cathartics)
- Emesis basin
- Oxygen supply with blow-by or mask
- Suction

Nice to have

- Covered container with straw (optional)
- Equipment for nasogastric intubation, 10- to 14-Fr catheter (optional)
- Fruit juice or syrup (optional)
- Magnesium citrate, sorbitol, or other cathartic (optional)
- Water-resistant gowns for patient, parent, physician, and assistant (optional)

Procedure

Activated charcoal is provided as a slurry, either in plain water or mixed with sorbitol or magnesium citrate as a cathartic. In a best-case scenario, patients will drink the activated charcoal, making the procedure very easy. An attempt to administer charcoal orally should be made in most cases. The initial dose is 1 g/kg up to a maximum of 50 to 60 g. Many toddlers and some older children will not drink the charcoal suspension despite one's best efforts. If the charcoal is not consumed within 10 minutes, the practitioner should proceed with nasogastric intubation to administer the charcoal.

Universal precautions should be used. For further details, please refer to the section on nasogastric intubation in Chapter 13. Charcoal is infused via the nasogastric tube over approximately 5 to 10 minutes. Charcoal should be infused by gentle pressure on the syringe; force should not be required. Care must be taken to prevent clogging of the tube, and flushing may be necessary. Unless repeated doses of charcoal are anticipated, the tube is removed when the procedure is completed.

Complications

The most common complications of activated charcoal administration are vomiting and aspiration. Severe aspiration pneumonitis and fatalities have been reported after large aspirations of charcoal. Therefore any patients with an unstable or potentially unstable airway should undergo endotracheal intubation before charcoal administration. A cuffed endotracheal tube will not completely prevent patients from aspirating charcoal but can minimize the amount aspirated.

Administration of activated charcoal can lead to constipation; this complicaton can be prevented by the coadministration of a cathartic. With MDAC, bowel obstruction has been reported.

WHOLE-BOWEL IRRIGATION

Indications and Contraindications

Whole-bowel irrigation should be considered for life-threatening ingestions that are not well managed by other methods of gastrointestinal decontamination. These situations include substances not well adsorbed to activated charcoal, quantities of toxin overwhelming the adsorptive ability of charcoal, sustained-release preparations, and some foreign bodies.

Known gastrointestinal pathology, such as obstruction, ileus, perforation, or hemorrhage, are contraindications to the use of whole-bowel irrigation. The quantity of fluid instilled necessitates gastric intubation in even the most cooperative patients. The inability to safely perform this procedure is a relative contraindication to its use. If the airway is not stable or if the potential exists for rapid deterioration of airway protective reflexes, definitive airway control should be established before initiating gastric intubation.

Supplies and Equipment

Need to have

- Commode or close proximity to bathroom
- Nasogastric tube, 10- to 14-Fr
- Polyethylene glycol electrolyte lavage fluid (e.g., GoLytely, CoLyte)

Nice to have

- IV pole (optional)
- Large (60-ml) syringe (optional)
- Reservoir bag (optional)

Procedure

1. Observe universal precautions.
2. Place a nasogastric tube as described in Chapter 13.
3. To prevent aspiration, have patients sit upright or elevate the head of the bed to at least 45 degrees.
4. Instill the lavage solution at a rate of 0.5 L/hr in children less than 6 years old, 1 L/hr in children 6 to 12 years old, and 1.5 to 2 L/hr in children older than 12 years.
5. Connect a reservoir bag of the kind used for tube feedings directly to the nasogastric tube. Suspend the bag above patients on an IV pole or similar device.

6. Allow fluid drainage to occur by gravity.
7. Whole-bowel irrigation continues until the rectal effluent is clear. Ancillary data used to determine the endpoint may include clearance of radiopaque foreign bodies from abdominal radiographs.

Complications

The currently recommended polyethylene glycol electrolyte lavage solutions are not associated with fluid and electrolyte shifts. Potential complications of administration of these fluids include emesis with aspiration and perforation of bowel.

NATURAL TOXINS

Background and Introduction

Sources of exposure to environmental toxins include venomous snakes, jellyfish, spiders, and stinging insects. Although such exposures vary by geographic location, the growing popularity of exotic animals as pets has increased the prevalence of envenomations outside of indigenous areas.

Pediatric patients are at increased risk for poisonous bites and often experience a more complicated course after envenomation. Because the amount of venom administered relative to body size is greater in smaller individuals, children experience more morbidity than do adults.

Snakebites

Relevant anatomy and physiology

Two families of venomous snakes are indigenous to North America: the crotalids (rattlesnakes and pit vipers) and the elapids (coral snakes). These two families produce distinct venoms. In addition to significant local tissue damage, crotalid venom damages capillary endothelium, has cardiotoxic and neurotoxic properties, and produces a disseminated intravascular coagulopathy (DIC)–like syndrome. In contrast, elapid venom is primarily a systemic neurotoxin.

Snake identification may be a helpful component of the history; however, treatment decisions should be guided by patients' condition, not by the type of snakebite. Several morphologic characteristics are shared by most venomous crotalids indigenous to the United States, including a triangular-shaped head, presence of fangs and venom pits, elliptical pupils, and a single row of caudal plates (Fig. 19-1). For identification of elapids, the mnemonic device "red on yellow, kills a fellow; red on black, venom lack" may be useful. The colors describe the pattern of rings on the coral snake (Fig. 19-2). These guidelines must be followed with caution because exceptions exist, especially among species imported to North America.

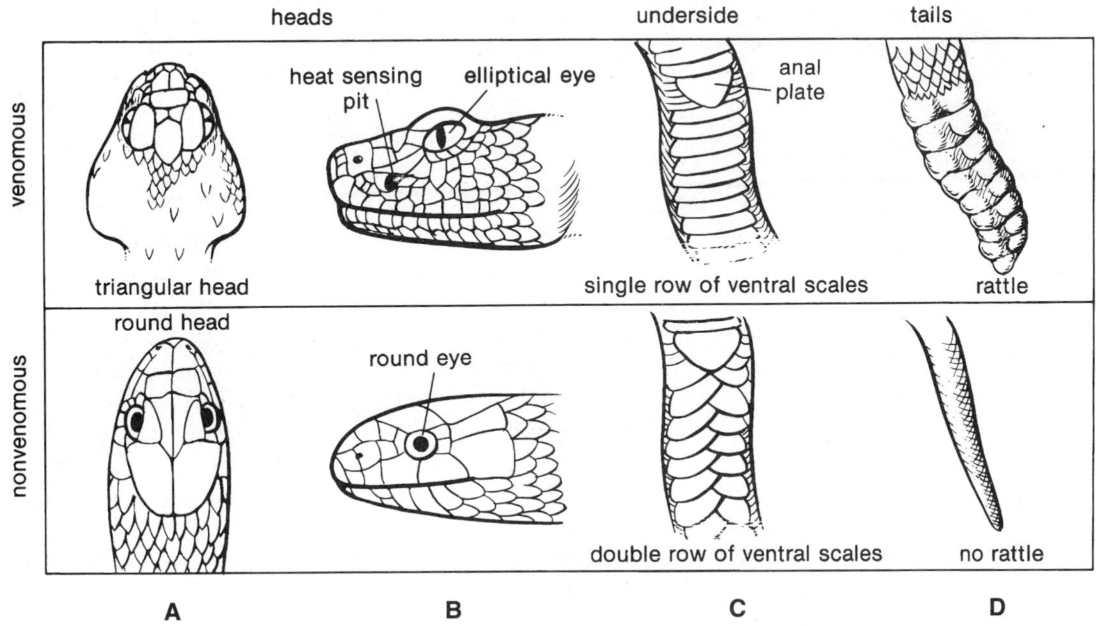

FIG. 19-1. Identification of venomous pit vipers. **A,** Triangular head. **B,** Elliptic eyes. **C,** Single row of ventral scales leading up to the anal plate. **D,** Rattles on tail (baby rattlesnakes have only "buttons," but are still quite venomous). *(From Auerbach PS:* Wilderness medicine, *ed 2, St Louis, 1995, Mosby.)*

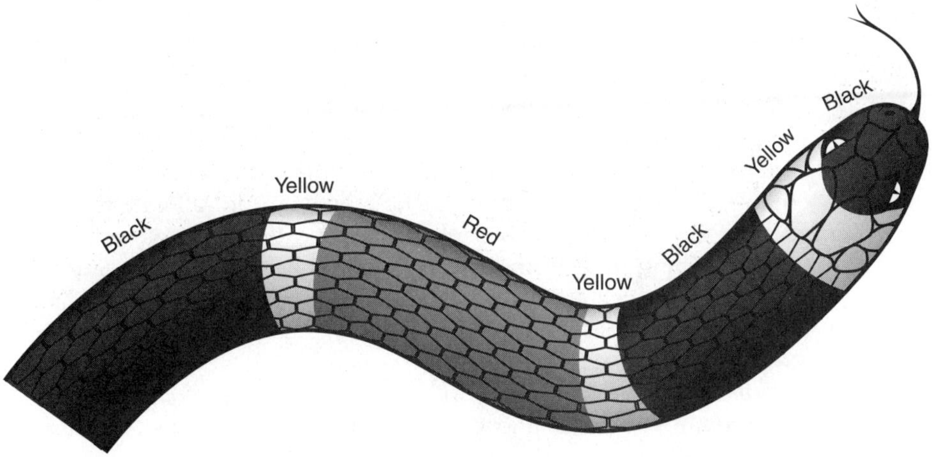

FIG. 19-2. Colors of the coral snake.

It is not uncommon for family or friends of snakebite victims to bring the snake, or its head, to the emergency department in an effort to help identify the snake. Treat all snakes as though they are alive, and use extreme caution in opening containers and examining snakes in order to avoid becoming a second victim.

Indications

Relatively few snakebites require antivenin therapy. For all snakebites, general supportive care and prevention of further morbidity are the mainstays of treatment. All patients with potential envenomations should be evaluated in a hospital setting. Stabilization may be initiated in the prehospital setting but should not delay transport to definitive care.

Crotalid antivenin is used in cases of severe crotalid envenomations or in patients exhibiting rapid progression of symptoms. Severe reactions include signs of systemic toxicity such as respiratory compromise, tachycardia, coagulopathy, and changes in mental status. In the case of extremity bites, if pain, ecchymosis, and swelling involve the entire limb, antivenin therapy is indicated. In less severe envenomations, proximal progression of these signs at a rate greater than 0.5 cm/hr is an indication for antivenin therapy. Substantial regional variation exists in the use of crotalid antivenin, so consultation with local experts is recommended.

Because elapid venoms are neurotoxic with the potential for respiratory muscle paralysis, decisions to treat must be based on historical information and physical assessment rather than on symptom progression. Definitive identification of a venomous coral snake or onset of any symptoms, including paresthesias, motor weakness, vomiting, blurred vision, and drowsiness, should prompt immediate therapy.

Contraindications and reasons for referral to a specialist

All victims of potentially venomous snakebites should be evaluated in a hospital setting. The regional poison center can assist the practitioner in contacting local experts regarding decisions to initiate antivenin therapy and in locating antivenin. In cases of envenomation with exotic species, staff from a local zoo may be of assistance.

Because antivenin is derived from horse serum, there is a high incidence of hypersensitivity reactions. Antivenin should never be used in a setting that is not equipped to manage an anaphylactic reaction. Prior allergic reaction to antivenin or other equine products is a relative contraindication, but in the case of a severe life-threatening envenomation, its use is often recommended. Concomitant administration of antihistamines, steroids, and an epinephrine infusion may be used in this setting.

Supplies and equipment

- Antivenin (For doses and kinds of antivenin to be used, always consult with a regional poison control center)
- Blood pressure cuff or wide constricting band (controversial)
- Commercially available venom extractor (controversial)

- Splinting materials
- Stretcher or litter
- Tetanus vaccine

Procedure

The initial therapy of venomous snakebites should be directed at attempts to limit the systemic absorption of toxin. Considerable controversy exists regarding the efficacy of various methods, and few have been evaluated in controlled clinical trials. Conservative recommendations include immobilizing the affected extremity at the level of the heart and limiting patient activity (nonambulatory, if possible). Because of the risk of vascular collapse, IV access should be established early. Attempts should be made to identify the type of snake involved but not at the expense of rapid, supportive patient care.

Some authorities recommend applying a constricting band on the extremity proximal to the site of the bite. If applied, the band should be adjusted to produce considerably less pressure than a venous tourniquet; its goal is simply to reduce lymphatic flow in the extremity.

Incision and suction have a limited role in treating venomous snakebites and are not recommended in most instances for which definitive care is readily available. A commercially available plunger system that extracts venom may be useful in remote locations.

Therapies that have been shown to *increase* morbidity include arterial tourniquets and ice immersion because of the resultant tissue ischemia. Therefore both strategies are contraindicated.

Complications

When using equine-derived antivenin, allergic reactions ranging from serum sickness to anaphylaxis may occur. Constricting bands can impede blood flow to the affected limb, leading to tissue ischemia. Rapid release of tourniquets results in a bolus of toxin entering the systemic circulation. Attempts at suction and drainage of venom can increase local tissue damage as well as expose the rescuer to the venom.

Marine Envenomation

Relevant anatomy and physiology

The Portuguese man-of-war, sea anemones, and the box jellyfish are examples of coelenterates that possess venoms poisonous to humans. These toxins contain proteolytic enzymes, inflammatory mediators, and phosphodiesterases, which are introduced into the subcutaneous tissue of human skin. Contact with the toxins produces local tissue injury and results in the release of endogenous mediators of inflammation such as histamine, which may have systemic effects.

Indications

The initial step in the treatment of coelenterate (jellyfish) stings is to identify patients. Patients may report the sting, or a witness may observe victims in an infested area. Tentacles may be observed adhering to victims. In other cases, urticaria resulting from the sting may be observed. In areas of the world where lethal coelenterates are endemic, identification of nematocysts (stinging cells) is helpful. This is accomplished by removing nematocysts from the lesions by scraping with a scalpel or applying transparent tape. Species identification is not usually necessary in the United States.

Contraindications and reasons for referral to a specialist

Anyone with a jellyfish sting should receive basic first aid unless the rescuer cannot safely approach victims without being stung. Patients exhibiting signs of systemic toxicity, including allergic reactions and cardiovascular instability, should be rapidly transported to an emergency department. Patients in severe pain requiring narcotics should undergo further evaluation. When treating young children or patients with underlying medical conditions, there should be a low threshold for referral to the emergency department for further evaluation.

Supplies and Equipment

- Forceps
- Gloves
- Razor, knife, etc.
- Seawater
- Shaving cream or baking soda paste
- Tetanus vaccine
- Vinegar

Procedure

1. Remove patients from contact with the jellyfish without exposing the rescuer to envenomation. Gloves (consider double pairs) and gowns may provide added protection. Tentacles may be pulled off victims using a heavy towel.
2. Rinse the wound with seawater to remove additional nematocysts. Fresh water should not be used, nor should the wound be rubbed or wiped because these treatments can result in further discharge of nematocysts attached to the skin.
3. Wash the affected area with 5% acetic acid (vinegar) to inactivate the remaining nematocysts. This procedure applies to all North American species except the Chesapeake Bay sea nettle. The nematocysts from these coelenterates are inactivated using baking soda rather than acidic compounds.
4. If tentacles remain adherent to the skin at this point, apply shaving cream or a baking soda paste and scrape the area with a razor, dull knife, or credit card. Forceps may also be used, if available.

Patients with minor stings may not require evaluation in the emergency department. Any patients continuing to have pain after initial treatment should be evaluated further. Tetanus prophylaxis is necessary if patient vaccination is not current. Pruritis may be treated with topical or oral antihistamines. Local wound care is advised; however, prophylactic antibiotics are not recommended.

Complications
Any attempt to manipulate the tentacles may result in nematocyst firing. Envenomation of the rescuer is a significant risk. Even after removal of nematocysts, local tissue injury may occur.

Spider Bites

Relevant anatomy and physiology
Although almost all species of spiders are venomous, few are capable of injecting venom through human skin. In North America, the two types of spiders responsible for much of the human morbidity are the black widow and the brown recluse. Black widow spider venom is a potent neurotoxin causing release of acetylcholine at the neuromuscular junction. The brown recluse venom contains several cytotoxic enzymes producing progressive tissue necrosis.

Indications
The onset of systemic symptoms, including severe muscle spasm, tachycardia, hypertension, and vomiting, after a black widow spider bite can begin within 20 minutes of the bite. The initial presentation may be of abdominal or chest pain. The bite itself may be difficult to locate, so the practitioner must have a high index of suspicion in patients with compatible histories and physical findings. For severe cases, an equine-derived antivenin is available.

Most patients with brown recluse spider bites are unaware of the actual bite and usually present only several days later, when the initial small, red papule has evolved to a vesicle or even further to the early stages of necrosis. Treatment of the local necrosis is indicated, as well as careful observation of progression of the affected area and evaluation for systemic signs such as hemolysis.

Contraindications and reasons for referral to a specialist
Most patients exhibiting toxicity from black widow spider bites require hospital care because of the high doses of narcotics and benzodiazepines required for pain relief. Antivenin therapy requires monitoring in a hospital setting. Sensitivity to equine-derived products is a relative contraindication that should be managed as described previously for snake antivenin. Late presentation and pregnancy are not contraindications to the use of black widow spider antivenin.

Patients requiring surgical debridement or with signs of hemolysis after brown recluse spider bites should be evaluated in a hospital setting. The decision to use experimental therapies, such as dapsone, hyperbaric oxygen, or antivenin, should be made in conjunction with local experts. The regional poison center can help to identify these experts.

Supplies and equipment
- Antibacterial wound cleaner (hand soap or commercial product)
- Morphine or meperidine (for black widow bite)
- Tetanus vaccine

In more remote settings, additional treatment for black widow bites includes benzodiazepines (diazepam).

Procedure

The muscle spasms associated with black widow spider bites may begin within 30 minutes of the bite. Treatment is supportive, with narcotics (usually morphine or meperidine) for analgesia and benzodiazepines (usually diazepam) for muscle relaxation. Calcium is no longer recommended for treating muscle spasms.

The brown recluse spider bite requires routine wound care and tetanus prophylaxis. Empiric antibiotic therapy is not recommended. Complicated cases may require wound debridement and transfusions for hemolytic anemia. Other therapies have not been evaluated in large, randomized trials but may be appropriate in cases of bites to the face or other cosmetically significant areas. Local experts should be consulted in these cases.

Antivenin is commercially available for severe cases of black widow spider bites. Experimental use of antivenin has been reported for brown recluse bites. These antivenins are derived from horse serum and pose a significant risk for anaphylaxis.

Complications

Complications such as respiratory depression associated with high doses of narcotics may be seen in black widow bites. Aggressive debridement may increase the scarring seen with brown recluse bites.

HEAT-RELATED ILLNESS

Heat-related illnesses comprise a spectrum of disease ranging from mildly symptomatic to life-threatening. Although geographic and seasonal variations exist, any person can be affected. Infants, the elderly, and patients with underlying medical problems are particularly at risk.

Both hypothermia and hyperthermia may result from accidental exposures to extreme temperatures or as a result of chronic illnesses that prevent patients from adapting to temperature variations. Physiological responses to changes in ambient temperature are not as well developed in infants.

Hypothermia

Relevant anatomy

Cold exposure produces a range of illness from mild to severe hypothermia. Hypothermia is a lowering of core body temperature below 35° C (95° F). In mild hypothermia (34° C to 35° C or 93° F to 95° F), patients exhibit shivering and peripheral vasoconstriction. With moderate hypothermia (30° C to 34° C or 86° F to 93° F), additional symptoms of poor coordination, disorientation, and paresthesias may be seen. As the core temperature drops below 32° C (90° F), the body's homeostatic mechanisms fail, producing bradycardia, decreased cardiac output, decreased respiratory rate, and progressive decline in central nervous system function. Severe hypothermia is defined as a core temperature below

30° C (86° F). These patients are comatose with severe impairments in vital signs, which may progress to apnea and asystole.

Indications for rewarming

The degree of rewarming used depends on the extent of illness. For mild hypothermia, this includes transferring patients to a warm environment, removing wet clothing, and applying warm blankets. For moderate hypothermia (core temperatures of 30° C to 34° C or 86° F to 93° F), more intense warming is indicated, utilizing warmed IV fluids and warmed, humidified oxygen. Such relatively noninvasive methods are referred to as "passive" rewarming. More invasive (active) methods of rewarming include infusing heated fluids into the bladder, peritoneum, and thoracic cavity. Severely hypothermic patients may be placed on cardiopulmonary bypass.

Contraindications and reasons for referral to a specialist

Severely hypothermic patients require active rewarming. At these temperatures, body functions slow to a minimum. Because this physiological state can offer some survival advantage, attempts to passively rewarm patients with core temperatures below 30° C (86° F) should be avoided. If patients are asystolic, cardiopulmonary resuscitation is initiated and, if apneic, intubation and ventilation is indicated. These patients require transport to a regional trauma center capable of active rewarming.

Supplies and equipment

Need to have

- Thermometer (rectal or tympanic) able to record low-range temperatures
- Warm blankets
- Warm room

Nice to have

- Blood pressure cuff
- Cardiac monitor
- Face mask
- Hot packs (to wrap around IV or oxygen tubing)
- IV catheters
- IV fluids (Lactated ringer's or normal saline)
- Microwave
- Oxygen humidifier
- Oxygen tank
- Pressure bag (or blood pressure cuff around IV bag)
- Radiant heater

Procedure

1. Remove patients from the cold environment and remove all wet clothing.
2. Measure the core body temperature using a thermometer capable of recording low-range temperatures.

3. Apply warm blankets or insulating blankets to maintain heat produced by the body.
4. For stable patients with core temperatures higher than 30° C (86° F), use passive rewarming techniques such as applying bags of warmed fluids to the head and trunk. Avoid application to the extremities, however, to prevent peripheral vasodilation and subsequent shunting of cooler blood into the central circulation.
5. Deliver heated, humidified oxygen by face mask and infuse warmed IV fluids heated to 40° C to 43° C (104° F to 109° F) using a microwave oven or incubator. Measure the temperature of the fluid in the bag or tubing using a tympanic thermometer.
6. Infuse fluids at rapid rates using short tubing to avoid cooling of the fluid before it reaches patients. In this relatively warmer group of patients, rewarming may be accomplished as rapidly as is practicable.

The approach to stabilization of severely hypothermic patients (less than 30° C or 86° F) is significantly different from that used in less severely affected patients. Active rewarming is indicated in this group of patients with colder core temperatures at presentation. Active rewarming should occur at a rate of 1° C to 3° C per hour and should be continued until the core temperature is in the normal range. Patients should be connected to a cardiac monitor, when available, with vital signs recorded frequently. Repeated or continuous measures of the core temperature should be followed. Severely hypothermic patients requiring invasive methods of rewarming should be transported directly to a pediatric trauma center.

Complications

Passive methods of rewarming are generally very safe. Active rewarming may lead to peripheral vasodilation and a drop in core temperature. Use of superheated oxygen (more than 50° C) may lead to airway burns, and overheated fluids can cause burns or cellular damage. When aggressive, active rewarming is used in severely hypothermic patients outside of a critical care setting, the survival advantage associated with this state of low metabolic activity is lost. Warming these patients may induce cardiac dysrhythmias such as fibrillation.

Modifications for conditions of limited resources

To maximize the retention of heat produced by the body, plastic bags or insulating blankets may be wrapped around patients. Sleeping bags may be used to warm patients, and rescuers may use skin-to-skin contact to rewarm victims.

Hyperthermia

Relevant anatomy

The spectrum of illness seen with elevated core body temperature ranges from minor skin rashes to life-threatening heatstroke. Physical activity increases heat production regardless of ambient temperature.

Heat-related illnesses requiring treatment include heat cramps, heat exhaustion, and heatstroke. *Heat cramps* are seen in individuals performing strenuous activity in hot environments. These patients have some degree of dehydration, with a minimal rise in body temperature and preserved mental status. *Heat exhaustion* involves a constellation of symptoms including nausea, vomiting, anorexia, thirst, headache, and lethargy. Patients may be irritable, but mental status is otherwise preserved. Core temperature is elevated but remains below 40° C (104° F).

Heatstroke occurs when the body temperature rises above 40° C (104° F), at which point the normal homeostatic negative feedback system fails, and mechanisms for heat retention and increased heat production are inappropriately called into play. Disturbances in central nervous system function are the hallmark of heatstroke. These symptoms include irrational behavior, headaches, ataxia, seizures, and coma. At this stage, patients' skin may be dry, having lost the ability to dissipate heat by sweating. Lacking the normal mechanism to regulate temperature, the core temperature rises rapidly, leading to cellular injury.

Indications for cooling

All patients affected by heat-related illness need to be cooled. For milder symptoms (heat rash, heat edema, and heat cramps), removal from the hot environment and fluid replacement (passive cooling) may suffice. More aggressive attempts at cooling (active cooling) are indicated for patients exhibiting signs of heat exhaustion and heatstroke.

Contraindications and reasons for referral to a specialist

There are no absolute contraindications to passive cooling. Certain methods, such as cooling blankets that may induce shivering, thereby increasing heat production, should be avoided. Patients with heat exhaustion require observation for several hours and basic laboratory analyses. This care may be accomplished in several settings, including primary care offices and aid stations. Heatstroke victims need to be transferred to a facility capable of intensive care monitoring.

Supplies and equipment

Need to have

- Fan
- Ice packs
- Salt-containing fluid for oral rehydration (such as sports drinks)
- Spray bottle

Nice to have

- Blood pressure cuff
- Cardiac monitor with waterproof leads
- Hammock or slotted-bottom litter
- IV catheters
- IV fluids (Lactated ringer's or normal saline)
- Thermometer (rectal or tympanic)

Procedure

1. Transfer patients to a cooler environment and remove excess clothing.
2. For stable patients with heat cramps or mild heat exhaustion, initiate oral rehydration with salt-containing fluids. Patients experiencing nausea or

vomiting require fluid repletion using IV salt-containing fluids (0.9% saline initially, as boluses of 20 ml/kg).

3. Monitor peripheral blood count, electrolytes, glucose, and urinalysis.
4. If no complications arise, release patients after a period of observation with demonstrated improvement.

Techniques for passive cooling exploit the body's normal mechanisms for heat dissipation. Fans are used to maximize heat transfer by convection. When a fine spray of tepid water is repeatedly applied to patients' skin, heat is dissipated by convection and evaporation. The goal is to keep the skin moist but not to immerse patients in cold water. A hammock or slotted-bottom litter may be useful. Ice packs may be applied directly to the skin of the axilla and groin to transfer heat by conduction. Care should be taken to avoid inducing shivering, which will increase the body's heat production. The core temperature should be monitored throughout the cooling procedure, and cooling should be terminated at 39° C (102° F) to avoid subsequent hypothermia.

Complications

The major complication of cooling hyperthermic patients is overshoot hypothermia. Efforts to cool patients should stop at 39° C (102° F).

SUGGESTED READINGS

Givens T, Holloway M, Watson S: Pulmonary aspiration of activated charcoal: a complication of its misuse in overdose management, *Pediatr Emerg Care* 8:137, 1992.

Gouldboume KB, Cisek JE: Small-bowel obstruction secondary to activated charcoal and adhesions, *Ann Emerg Med* 24:108, 1994.

Harsh HH: Aspiration of activated charcoal, *N Engl J Med* 414:318, 1986.

Watson WA, Cremes KF, Chapman JA: Gastrointestinal obstruction associated with multiple dose activated charcoal, *J Emerg Med* 4:401, 1986.

Wright RO et al: Use of infrared thermometry to measure lavage and IV fluid temperature, *Am J Emerg Med* 13:281, 1995.

CHAPTER 20

Triage, Stabilization, and Transport

Mohamed Badawy
Colleen O. Davis

BACKGROUND AND INTRODUCTION

Parents typically bring their children to the pediatrician's office for routine care, mild to moderate illnesses, or minor injuries. Occasionally, however, seriously ill or injured children present to the physician's office. Primary care pediatricians and their staff members are often unprepared to manage these medical emergencies. In addition to treating their patients' urgent medical needs, office practitioners must coordinate rapid and safe transportation for sick patients.

Although emergency medical services (EMS) crews are readily available to most office practitioners in the United States, these services are often underutilized. Children with possible life-threatening illnesses are often sent from the physician's office to the emergency department via family automobile. Physicians who choose to use family automobile instead of EMS express concerns about lengthy EMS response time, cost of EMS transportation, and the quality of the medics' pediatric training. Additionally, some physicians are not fully aware of the EMS resources available to them. When asked to explain their transport decisions, an alarming 10% of primary care physicians responded that they simply forgot to consider calling EMS.

Patients with life-threatening illnesses may deteriorate in the office or en route to the emergency department. Once a serious condition is identified, appropriate medical care should be provided without interruption. Office-based pediatricians and their staff should be trained to identify patients with serious illnesses, activate the EMS system, and stabilize patients until the EMS crew arrives. This chapter

NOTE: The editors strongly recommend that this and the following chapter be used in a complementary fashion. Chapter 20 provides an overview of the organizational and administrative aspects of management of emergencies in the office environment. Chapter 21 gives the details of each procedure likely to be encountered in this setting. Thus, Chapter 20 should be read and frequently reviewed by everyone in the office setting, including office managers and nursing staff. It can be used to guide the establishment of emergency equipment boxes and of treatment and communications protocols, as well as for training of staff. Chapter 21, by contrast, may be used as a reference in the event of an actual emergency in the office.

highlights information that helps physicians prepare their offices for pediatric emergencies.

TRIAGE

Triage in the medical office can be thought of as the process by which staff members identify seriously ill patients. The most commonly encountered office emergencies are respiratory distress, seizures, and obstructed airways. Fortunately, patients in shock and cardiac arrest are not often seen in the office setting. Although status epilepticus is usually obvious to most observers, impending respiratory failure and partial airway obstruction are less readily recognized and require training in order for these conditions to be reliably identified.

Education of all staff members is the first step in providing urgent medical care. We recommend that *all* office staff members be trained in basic life support (BLS).* Courses are available through the American Academy of Pediatrics, the American Heart Association, the Red Cross, and, in many areas, EMS agencies. Physicians, nurses, and nurse practitioners should also be trained in pediatric advanced life support (PALS).

Staff members should be familiar with the patients in their practice who are at high risk for seizures or respiratory compromise, such as asthmatics with repeated hospital admissions and patients with known seizure disorders. The staff should also be aware of certain conditions that predispose patients to seizures, respiratory problems, or other serious illnesses, including hydrocephalus, ventriculoperitoneal shunts, severe prematurity, congenital heart disease, and immunocompromise, among many others. Patients with such problems require careful evaluation. Many common and otherwise minor childhood ailments can result in serious compromise for such patients.

Telephone triage is an expanding part of primary care and can be a difficult skill to master. Standardized telephone triage protocols help identify seriously ill patients and prompt the medical professional to make urgent referrals and/or to activate EMS when appropriate.

STABILIZATION

Priorities for stabilization of a sick patient in the office are the same as in the emergency department or in the field. "ABC" is the mnemonic used to reinforce the order of the primary survey: evaluate the (1) **a**irway, (2) **b**reathing, and (3) **c**irculation. Only after these areas are evaluated and stabilized does one proceed to the remainder of the physical examination. Continual reassessment of the patient and complete vital signs (including blood pressure) are fundamental to

*The principles of pediatric resuscitations are covered in detail in BLS and PALS courses and are beyond the scope of this chapter. The procedures used in resuscitation are described in Chapter 21 of this text.

BOX 20-1 SUGGESTED EMERGENCY EQUIPMENT FOR THE PEDIATRIC OFFICE

Need to Have

Oxygen supply
100% nonrebreather masks
Bag-valve-mask ventilator with reservoir
Infant, child, and adult masks
Suction (portable)
Broselow tape
Infant, child, and adult blood pressure cuffs
Latex-free gloves

Nice to Have

Oximeter
Laryngoscope with Miller blades
Endotracheal tubes
Intravenous catheters and tubing
Intraosseous needles
Backboard

all well-run resuscitations. Careful attention to these areas can prevent a full-blown cardiorespiratory arrest from developing.

In every resuscitation, it is imperative to clearly identify all participants' roles. Tasks that need to be assigned include airway management, chest compressions, administration of medications, intravenous line placement, and recording. One person must clearly lead the resuscitation effort.

Written protocols that highlight staff members' roles in emergencies should be readily available and reviewed by all staff on a regular basis. These guidelines should specifically indicate who is responsible for activating EMS.

Mock resuscitations are a useful means of preparing for emergencies. In addition to reviewing the skills learned in BLS and PALS, role-playing in a mock emergency forces staff to retrieve seldom-used equipment and to review dosages of unfamiliar medications. This practice can be very instructive. Mock codes help identify strengths and weaknesses in the emergency response team, in addition to maintaining skills.

Pediatricians' offices need not be equipped as if they were emergency departments because purchasing and maintaining seldom-used equipment and supplies can be costly. Basic equipment and drugs required to stabilize seriously ill patients should be available (Boxes 20-1 and 20-2). When preparing an office for pediatric emergencies, the first priority (after staff education) should be to acquire the tools necessary to stabilize airways and ventilate patients. Consequently, oxygen and a bag-valve-mask should be available in all medical offices. A set of masks sized to fit infants, children, and adults should be included.

Oxygen saturation has been described as the fifth pediatric vital sign. Therefore pulse oximeters are often helpful in resuscitations. Oximeters are also useful when caring for less severely ill patients, such as those with pneumonia, bronchiolitis,

BOX 20-2 SUGGESTED EMERGENCY MEDICATIONS FOR THE PEDIATRIC OFFICE

Need to Have

Oxygen (portable)
Albuterol
Dextrose
Epinephrine

Nice to Have

Lorazepam
Normal saline
Broad-spectrum antibiotic such as Ceftriaxone
Diphenhydramine
Methlyprednisolone
Glucagon

and asthma. Although oximeters can be expensive, primary care physicians might consider adding this valuable tool to their office equipment.

Color-coded, length-based tapes such as the Broselow tape are designed to help deliver emergency care to infants and small children. First, the tape is used to estimate the patient's height (measured from heel to crown). Then predetermined medication doses and sizes of emergency equipment are easily found on the tape. Alternatively, precalculated resuscitation worksheets can be used to ensure appropriate medication doses during an emergency.

Emergency equipment and medications should be organized and labeled so that they are readily available. A staff member should be assigned to maintain all emergency supplies and to periodically check them for completeness.

MEDICOLEGAL ISSUES RELATING TO COBRA/EMTALA

Because stabilization and transport of acutely ill children in the office raises legal as well as medical issues, we include here a discussion of some of the relevant U.S. statutes. In 1986, Congress added to its annual Consolidated Omnibus Budget Reconciliation Act (COBRA) amendments that were designed to prevent the practice of "patient dumping." There was some concern that private hospitals were transferring indigent patients to less-capable public hospitals for financial reasons. Conversely, private hospitals were refusing the transfer of indigent patients from smaller hospitals.

COBRA 86 defined a detailed statutory duty for hospitals and physicians. Since then, several additions and refinements have been made. The statute is now referred to as the Emergency Medical Transport and Active Labor Act (EMTALA), and it creates three duties for the hospital and the physician. Each patient must be screened, stabilized, and (if necessary) provided with an appropriate transfer. This mandate covers patients who are sent to the hospital by their private physician to receive medications in the emergency department.

EMTALA *appropriate transfer* has the following five basic requirements:

1. Transferring hospitals must provide medical treatment within their capacity to minimize risks to the patient's health and, if a woman is in labor, the health of the unborn child.
2. Transferring hospitals must contact receiving hospitals, which must agree to accept the patient in transfer and to provide appropriate medical treatment, including having available space and qualified personnel for treatment.
3. Transferring hospitals must effect patient transfer through qualified personnel and transportation equipment, including necessary life support measures.
4. Transferring hospitals must send the receiving hospitals all medical records related to the emergency medical condition available at the time of transfer and list the name and address of any on-call physician who refused or failed to appear within a reasonable time to provide necessary stabilizing treatment.
5. Transferring physicians must sign a certification that the benefits reasonably expected outweigh the risks of not receiving appropriate medical treatment at another facility.

TRANSPORT

Office-based pediatricians should know what EMS are available in the area where their offices are located. Pediatricians should be familiar with the emergency medical transport system (i.e., ground transport, air transport), the nearby emergency departments, and the nearest pediatric tertiary care center. The referring physician is responsible for arranging appropriate transportation and continued medical care for the sick child until the patient reaches the destined facility.

Transportation by family automobile, physician's automobile, or taxi is not appropriate for anyone with a serious medical condition and may have adverse medicolegal consequences, in addition to the obvious adverse medical outcomes. One study showed that physicians used family automobiles for transport to the emergency departments not because of lack of service or cost issues, but simply because they were not aware of the EMS personnel's pediatric training.

At the national level, there are four levels of prehospital care providers:

1. *First Responders (FR):* Provide basic first aid to callers until definitive treatment and transport arrive. May include the use of an automated external defibrillator.
2. *Basic Emergency Medical Technician (EMT-B):* Provides BLS care and transportation. The Basic EMT class includes 100 to 200 hours of training.
3. *Intermediate Emergency Medical Technician (EMT-I):* Provides BLS care and selected ALS care. Can give intravenous fluids, glucose, naloxone, and albuterol. Intermediates must complete the Basic class and an additional 100 to 200 hours of training.

4. *Paramedic (EMT-P):* Provides the highest level of prehospital care. Includes BLS and ALS treatment. Paramedics must complete the Basic class and an additional 500 to 1000 hours of training.

If 911 services are not available, specific numbers for ambulance services should be posted near all office phones and included in the emergency protocol book.

COMMUNICATION

Written and/or verbal contact between the office physician and the emergency physician is essential to ensure accurate transfer of information. Pediatricians should provide detailed but succinct medical histories for all seriously ill patients. A thorough review of the precipitating events and any treatment given in the office will be helpful to the receiving medical team. As always, lists of allergies and medications should be included. When transferring patients with chronic illnesses or special needs, additional information such as advance directives and "do not resuscitate" (DNR) status is essential.

Debriefing sessions for office staff are critically important after providing emergency medical care. Reviewing the management of a seriously ill patient allows staff to express their emotions and may help them refine the skills necessary to treat the next emergency patient.

DOCUMENTATION

Documentation is an essential aspect of medical practice. In the face of any possible litigation, recollection of the events surrounding the evaluation is limited and, therefore, the medical record becomes more important. The following are some important points to include in the documentation for all patients requiring emergency management and care:

- The initial presentation, assessment, and any interventions should be documented in order and as detailed as possible.
- Parental consent is not needed in an emergency situation; if children present without a legal guardian, care should not be delayed because of consent issues. As time permits, efforts to obtain parental consent over the telephone should be made and documented.
- If parents refuse medical treatment for their children and no immediate danger or potential for a serious impairment is posed, then competent parents can sign a form stating that they took this course against medical advice. It should be documented, however, that parents had a normal mental status, understood the potential risks, and had the opportunity to ask questions but refused the offered treatment.
- All contacts made and information given and sent with patients should be documented.

- Finally, it is always helpful to document the frequent reassessment after each intervention and the final status on disposition.

CONCLUSION

All children with urgent medical needs who present to their physicians' offices should expect to receive appropriate medical care followed by safe, competent transportation to an emergency department.

SUGGESTED READINGS

Alteri M, Bellet J, Scott H: Preparedness for pediatric emergencies encountered in the practitioner's office, *Pediatrics* 85:710, 1990.

American Academy of Pediatrics: Policy statement—The emergency physician and the office-based pediatrician: an EMSC team (RE9742), *Pediatrics* 101:936, 1998.

Baker D, Ludwig S: Pediatric emergency transport and the private practitioner, *Pediatrics* 88:691, 1991.

Brown JL: *Pediatric telephone medicine: principles, triage, and advice,* ed 2, Philadelphia, 1994, JB Lippincott.

Davis C, Rodewald L: Use of EMS for seriously ill children from the office, *Prehosp Emerg Care* 3:102, 1999.

Fuchs S, Jaffe D, Christoffel K: Pediatric emergencies in office practices: prevalence and office preparedness, *Pediatrics* 83:931, 1989.

Katz HP: *Telephone medicine, triage and training: a handbook for primary health care professionals,* Philadelphia, 1990, FA Davis.

Mower WR et al: Pulse oximetry as a fifth pediatric vital sign, *Pediatrics* 99:681, 1997.

Schmitt BA: *Pediatric telephone advice,* ed 2, Philadelphia, 1999, Lippincott-Raven.

Sullivan DJ: Minors and emergency medicine, *Emerg Med Clin North Am* 11:841, 1993.

Tsai AK et al: Evaluation and treatment of minors: reference on consent, *Am Emerg Med* 22:1211, 1993.

Zumpft CW: The correction of interhospital "dumping" by legislation, *J Emerg Med* 6:443, 1998.

CHAPTER 21

Emergency Procedures

Robert J. Freishtat
Gretchen R. Volk
Frank A. Maffei

The sudden and unexpected need to perform an emergency procedure on a child evokes anxiety among even the most experienced practitioners. Minimizing anxiety and maximizing proficiency are best done through thoughtful preparation. Although cognitive skills can be maintained with periodic review of emergency techniques, motor skills can deteriorate rapidly without practice. Therefore emergency procedures should be rehearsed on a regular basis. For practitioners who regularly encounter infants and children, this task is best accomplished by maintaining current certification in the American Heart Association/American Academy of Pediatrics (AHA/AAP)–sponsored courses in neonatal and pediatric advanced life support. This chapter summarizes the following emergency procedures:

- Emergency childbirth
- Neonatal resuscitation
- Pediatric resuscitation
- Foreign body/choking management
- Advanced airway management
- Cardiac arrhythmia management

EMERGENCY CHILDBIRTH

Background and Introduction

Most deliveries occur in the controlled setting of a labor and delivery ward; however, on rare occasions, an unexpected delivery may occur. Preterm labor may progress so quickly that safe transfer to an obstetrical unit is not possible. Multiparous women in active labor can deliver after a very brief labor. In addition, adolescents may come to the physician's office for evaluation of abdominal pain and, despite months of amenorrhea and weight gain, be in denial that they are pregnant and in labor. A calm and systematic approach to performing a vaginal delivery is essential to minimize both infant and maternal morbidity.

Indications

- Imminent birth with strong, frequent contractions (less than 2 minutes apart) and a bulging perineum

Contraindications

- Delivery that is not imminent and conditions that allow safe transport
- False labor or Braxton-Hicks contractions (irregular contractions of unchanging intensity without dilation of the cervix)

High-Risk Situations

- Prolapsed cord (The infant needs to be delivered immediately, usually by Cesarean section. Until delivery occurs, the baby's presenting part needs to be lifted off the cord to relieve the compression.)
- Placenta previa/abruptio
- Chorioamnionitis
- Meconium-stained amniotic fluid
- Suspected cephalopelvic disproportion
- Breech presentation
- Fetal distress (Listen to the fetal heart rate after a contraction, and suspect this complication if it is less than 120 or more than 160 beats per minute. In these cases, provide mothers with oxygen and intravenous [IV] fluids, and have them lie on their left side to improve blood flow to the uterus.)

Supplies and Equipment

Need to have

- Blankets for the baby
- Bulb syringe
- Double-grip cord clamp
- Kelly clamps, 2 medium
- Large basin for the placenta
- Scissors

Nice to have

- Doppler ultrasound to assess the fetal heart rate
- Heated isolette

- Infant resuscitation equipment
- Intravenous fluid for mother
- Sterile gauze 4 × 4s
- Sterile gloves
- Sterile towels

Procedure

1. Activate emergency medical services (EMS).
2. Place the patient in the dorsal lithotomy position.
3. If available, use sterile gloves and drape the perineal area with sterile towels.
4. Perform a vaginal examination to determine the baby's presenting part (occiput in more than 95% of term deliveries) and examine for a prolapsed cord.
5. Encourage the mother to pant and not push during contractions to allow for a slow delivery.
6. When the baby's head begins to crown, apply gentle pressure to the occiput with your palm to prevent rapid expulsion.
7. With a sterile towel in your second hand, apply gentle upward pressure against the fetal chin through the perineum (modified Ritgen maneuver). This may offer added control when delivering the head.
8. Support the baby's head as it passes through the vaginal opening and allow it to rotate naturally to one side.
9. If the membranes are still intact, snip them at the base of the baby's neck and pull them away from the face.
10. Slide your finger around the baby's neck to determine if the umbilical cord is there. If it is loosely wrapped around the neck, slip it over the head and shoulder. If it is tightly wrapped, clamp it in two places and cut it.
11. Clear the baby's mouth and nose of secretions with a bulb syringe.
12. Gently guide the head down to deliver the anterior shoulder.*
13. Gently guide the head upward to deliver the posterior shoulder. The body of the baby should deliver easily at this point. If not, apply moderate traction on the baby's head in the longitudinal axis.
14. Suction the baby's mouth and nose again.
15. If you haven't already cut the cord, apply two clamps and cut between them.
16. Apply the umbilical clamp 2 to 3 inches away from the infant's body.
17. Dry the infant and keep the mother and baby warm.
18. Expect delivery of the placenta in about 20 minutes. The uterus will become firm and begin contracting. The umbilical cord will lengthen, and there may be a sudden gush of blood. Apply gentle pressure to the uterus through the

*Shoulder dystocia: In the event of difficulty delivering the anterior shoulder, two simple maneuvers may allow easier passage. First, flex and abduct the maternal hips onto the abdomen (McRobert's maneuver). If this fails, have an assistant apply suprapubic downward pressure to help dislodge the impacted anterior shoulder. More invasive maneuvers (posterior shoulder and arm delivery, Wood's corkscrew maneuver, and intentional clavicular fracture) are rarely successful unless performed by experienced practitioners.

mother's abdomen to help the delivery. Do not put traction on the umbilical cord because this could lead to uterine inversion.

Possible Complications

- Shoulder dystocia
- Maternal hemorrhage
- Neonatal asphyxia
- Uterine inversion

Aftercare Instructions

- Keep the infant warm and dry.
- Observe the mother for signs of excessive bleeding and shock.
- Feel for a boggy or atonic uterus. Prevent relaxation of the uterus by frequent massage.
- Examine the mother for lacerations.
- If necessary, arrange for transport of mother and infant to a hospital.

Modifications for Situations of Limited Resources

- Clean towels, clean scissors, and strong string may be substituted for sterile supplies.
- A stethoscope may be used to assess the fetal heart rate instead of a Doppler ultrasound.

NEONATAL RESUSCITATION

Background and Introduction

Approximately 5% to 10% of newborns require some form of resuscitation at birth. Therefore all practitioners must understand the systematic approach to the assessment and management of critically ill newborns.

Assessment

The Apgar score was developed to quickly assess a neonate at various stages of transition to extrauterine life. It represents the status of several vital parameters in a newborn during the first minutes of life (Table 21-1). Scoring occurs at 1 and 5 minutes.

Indications

- Respiratory insufficiency
- Bradycardia (usually secondary to hypoxia)
- Central cyanosis unresponsive to 100% blow-by oxygen

TABLE 21-1
Apgar scoring system

	2 points	1 point	0 points
Heart Rate	>100 bpm	<100 bpm	None
Respirations	Good	Hypopnea	Apnea
Color	Pink	Acrocyanosis	Central cyanosis
Tone	Good	Hypotonic	Atonic
Reflex Irritability	Strong	Poor response	Unresponsive

High-Risk Situations

- Prematurity
- Difficult delivery
- Congenital anomalies
- Hydrops fetalis

Contraindications

- Extreme prematurity, *typically less than or equal to 22 weeks based on physical assessment*

Supplies and Equipment

Need to have

- Bulb syringe
- Butterfly needles: 23- and 25-gauge
- Curved iris forceps
- DeLee suction trap
- Dextrose 10% solution
- Endotracheal tubes: 2.5 mm (10-Fr), 3.0 mm (12-Fr), 3.5 mm (14-Fr), 4.0 mm (16-Fr)
- Epinephrine 1:10,000 (0.1 mg/ml)
- Feeding tubes, 5- and 8-Fr
- Glucose test strips
- Hemostats
- Infant ventilation bag (750 ml) with appropriate masks
- Laryngoscope with straight (Miller) blades, sizes 0 and 1
- Meconium aspirator
- Naloxone (0.02 mg/ml)
- Normal (0.9%) saline
- Oxygen
- Peripheral intravenous catheters: 24-gauge
- Scalpel
- Scissors

- Sodium bicarbonate 4.2% (0.5 mEq/ml)
- Spare bulbs and batteries
- Sterile gauze
- Sterile towels
- Stethoscope
- Suction catheters: 6-, 8-, and 10-Fr
- Stylets
- Syringes: 1, 3, 5, and 10 ml
- Timer
- Umbilical tape
- Umbilical venous catheters: 3.5- and 5.0-Fr
- Wall suction (80 mmHg)
- Warm towels

Nice to have
- Albumin 5% solution
- Anesthesia bag and manometer for controlling inspiratory pressures
- Atropine (0.1 mg/ml)
- Blood gas analysis
- Calcium chloride (100 mg/ml)
- Calcium gluconate (100 mg/ml)
- Defibrillator
- Glucagon
- Heart-rate monitor and pulse oximeter
- Intraosseous needle
- Oral airways
- Radiant warmer with light
- Sterile plastic bags for exposed organs (e.g., gastroschisis, neural tube defects)
- Three-way stopcocks
- Tincture of benzoin

Procedure

The resuscitation team should, at minimum, consist of a leader responsible for airway management and direction of the resuscitation as well as an assistant to assess the heart rate and perform other tasks as needed. Ideally, a third team member should be present to administer medications and prepare supplies.

In order to have the appropriate supplies on hand, the anticipated neonatal weight should be estimated from the gestational age (Table 21-2).

Warm, dry, stimulate
1. Receive, dry, and stimulate the baby vigorously under a radiant warmer with warm towels.
2. Suction secretions from the oropharynx and then the nose.
3. Have the leader promptly assess respiratory effort and color while the assistant listens for the heart rate. An infant with a heart rate greater than 100 beats per

TABLE 21-2
Estimated neonatal weight

Gestational age (weeks)	Birth weight (grams)
24	700
26	900
28	1100
30	1350
32	1650
34	2100
36	2600
38	3000

minute (bpm) and good respiratory effort can be observed with blow-by oxygen as needed.

Airway and ventilatory management

1. If an infant's respiratory effort is inadequate, begin bag-mask ventilation (BMV) with 100% oxygen.
   - Note that BMV is contraindicated in neonates with gastroschisis or a diaphragmatic hernia who require ventilatory support. These infants should be promptly intubated because of the increased risk of bowel ischemia with gaseous distension from BMV.
   - Infants with small mandibles, as in the Pierre-Robin sequence, may benefit from an oral airway in conjunction with BMV.
2. Ventilate the infant at a rate of 40 breaths per minute.
   - Keep inspiratory pressures less than 40 cm H_2O.
   - Tidal volumes should approach 6 ml/kg.
3. Confirm bilateral equal breath sounds and chest wall rise. The absence of these signs suggests a poor mask seal, low inspiratory pressure or tidal volume, airway obstruction, or pulmonary volume limitation (e.g., tension pneumothorax, gastric distension). Be sure the face is dried and mouth cleared of secretions to achieve a good seal.
4. Proceed with endotracheal intubation if BMV is ineffective or prolonged.
   - Before performing intubation in an infant who may be drug-depressed, an intramuscular injection of naloxone can be attempted.
   - Prolonged BMV requires the placement of a nasogastric or orogastic tube.
   - In addition to aiding ventilation, endotracheal intubation also provides a route for some cardiac resuscitation medications in case they become necessary.
   - Intubation instructions can be found in the section on Advanced Airway Management.

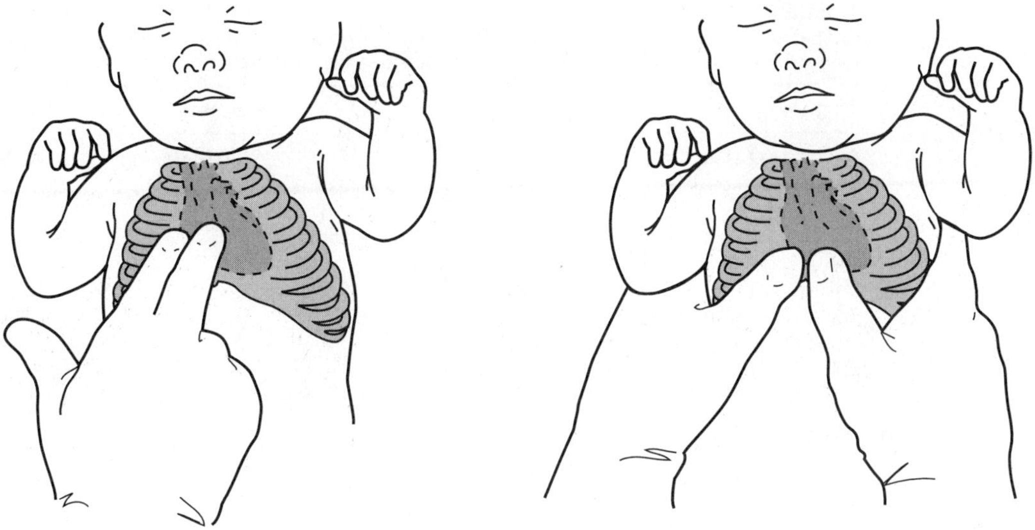

FIG. 21-1. Begin chest compressions, between 60 to 80, at a rate of 120 bpm with two fingertips or thumbs on sternum along intramammary line.

Circulatory management

Note: Optimizing oxygenation is the primary treatment for bradycardia in the newborn.

1. While initial stabilization is progressing, have the assistant continuously report the heart rate to the leader by tapping out each beat with a finger.
2. If after 30 seconds of BMV, the heart rate is:
   - Greater than 100 bpm, the infant can be reassessed without ventilatory support.
   - Greater than 60 bpm and rising, the infant should be reassessed with continued ventilatory support.
   - Between 60 and 80 and not increasing, begin chest compressions at a rate of 120 bpm with two fingertips or thumbs on the sternum along the intramammary line (Fig. 21-1).
   - Less than 60 bpm, begin chest compressions as described previously.
3. Continue compressions until the heart rate is greater than 80 bpm. If the heart rate remains below 80 bpm after 30 seconds of chest compressions, continue compressions and administer resuscitation medications.

Resuscitation Medications (Table 21-3)

- Low-dose epinephrine 1:10,000 (0.1 mg/ml) is indicated for bradycardia that is not responsive to oxygen and hypotension. It is the first drug to be administered for a heart rate less than 80 bpm after 30 seconds of chest compressions.

TABLE 21-3
Neonatal resuscitation medications. Routes of medication administration include via an endotracheal tube, umbilical venous catheter, peripheral intravenous line, or intraosseous line.

Drug	Indications	Dose	Route
Atropine (0.4, 0.8, 1 mg/ml)	Bradycardia	0.01-0.03 mg/kg	IM/IV/IO/ETT
Calcium chloride 10% (100 mg/ml)	Hypocalcemia, hyperkalemia	20 mg/kg	IV
Calcium gluconate 10% (100 mg/ml)	Hypocalcemia, hyperkalemia	100 mg/kg	IV
Dextrose 10%	Hypoglycemia	2-4 ml/kg	IV
Epinephrine (high-dose) 1:1,000 (1 mg/ml)	Asystole, bradycardia, hypotension	0.1-0.3 ml/kg	ETT
Epinephrine (low-dose) 1:10,000 (0.1 mg/ml)	Asystole, bradycardia, hypotension	0.1-0.3 ml/kg	IV/IO
Naloxone (0.4 mg/ml)	Narcotic depression	0.1-0.2 mg/kg	IM/IV/IO/ETT
Normal (0.9%) saline	Hypotension	10 ml/kg	IV/IO
Sodium bicarbonate 4.2% (0.5 mEq/mL)	Metabolic acidosis	1-2 mEq/kg	IV/IO

- Sodium bicarbonate is indicated to correct metabolic acidosis.
- Normal (0.9%) saline (10 ml/kg aliqouts) is indicated for hypotension.

Complications

- Bradycardia
- Hypoxia
- Pneumothorax

Modifications for Situations of Limited Resources

Ventilation can take place as mouth-to-mouth-and-nose or mouth-to-mask. Cardiopulmonary resuscitation (CPR) can be performed as usual until medications become available.

PEDIATRIC RESUSCITATION

Background and Introduction

Despite recent advances in resuscitation medicine and more widespread training in pediatric CPR, the outcome of pediatric cardiac arrest remains dismal. Intact neurological survival approaches only 10% under the best circumstances. In contrast, when early interventions preclude further deterioration to cardiac arrest, primary respiratory arrest has a more favorable outcome (up to 80% intact survival). If at all possible, recognition and intervention absolutely must occur before circulatory collapse.

Preparation

Successful resuscitations require careful preparation, which is best done in two phases. *Long-term preparation* consists of multiple ongoing educational and physical tasks that include the following:

- Clinician certification in the AAP/AHA-sponsored pediatric advanced life support (PALS) course
- Resuscitation room preparation, including easy access to all equipment and easy visualization of resuscitation algorithms and medication charts
- Resuscitation cart fully supplied (Box 21-1)
- Maintenance and scheduled testing of all equipment (e.g., bag-mask apparatus, cardiac monitor and defibrillator, glucometer)
- Resuscitation practice via "mock codes"

In the event of being forewarned by EMS of an incoming arrest, *immediate preparation* should commence and include the following steps:

- Identification of a resuscitation team leader
- Assignment of roles to team members that include (personnel permitting):
  — Airway management
  — Airway vascular access (up to two individuals)
  — Airway cardiac compressions
  — Airway medication preparation
  — Airway circulator
  — Airway recordkeeper
  — Airway family support/information provider
- All individuals prepare the equipment needed for their specific roles. If EMS provides an accurate age and body habitus, equipment size and medications can be estimated. Once the child arrives, more accurate selection of drugs and equipment can be facilitated using a Broselow tape.

Indications

- Respiratory insufficiency
- Shock
- Cardiopulmonary arrest

High-Risk Situations

- No response to bystander and EMS CPR
- Upper airway obstruction, difficult airway
- Underlying chronic disease, immunocompromise
- Chronic medication use (i.e., beta-blockers, steroids)

BOX 21-1 OFFICE CODE CART CONTENTS

Airway

Endotracheal tubes: uncuffed sizes 2.5 to 7.5, cuffed sizes 5.0 to 8.0
Stylets, 6-F and 14-F
Laryngoscope handles (extra batteries and bulbs)
Laryngoscope blades: Miller sizes 0 to 3
Suction catheters sizes 6-, 8-, 10-, 12-, and 14-Fr
Yankauer suction tip, regular and fine tip
Oral airways in infant, small child, child, small adult, and medium adult sizes
Nasopharyngeal airways sizes 12-, 16-, 20-, 24-, and 28-Fr
Magill forceps in child and adult sizes
End-tidal CO_2 detectors, disposable
Pulse oximeter probes
Bulb syringes
Tracheostomy tubes

Breathing

Bag-mask-valve devices in infant, child, and adult sizes
Oxygen masks in infant, child, and adult sizes
Nebulizer face masks
Oxygen extension tubing
Respiratory saline
Tracheostomy mist collar
Oxygen, tank

Circulation

IV catheters 24-, 22-, 20-, 18-, and 16-gauge
Butterfly needles
Blood pressure cuffs in sizes newborn, infant, child, and adult
Intraosseous catheters
Tourniquets: large, small, and rubber bands
Bags of normal saline
Syringes in sizes 1, 5, 10, 20, and 50 cc
Three-way stopcocks
Extension tubing
Arm boards, short and long

Emergency Medication

Epinephrine, 1:10,000 and 1:1000 concentrations
Atropine, 0.1 mg/ml prefilled syringes
Dextrose 50% (D_{50}) prefilled syringes
Naloxone 0.4 mg/ml
Lorazepam 2 mg/ml
Syrup of ipecac
Activated charcoal
Albuferol for inhalation
Methylprednisolone: oral liquid and tablets

Miscellaneous

Broselow tape
Harriet Lane handbook
Critical care flowsheets
Foley catheters in sizes 5-, 8-, 10-, and 12-Fr
Urine bags
Nasogastric tubes in sizes 5-, 8-, 10-, 12-, 14-, and 18-Fr
Replogle tube, 10-Fr
Glucometer and BG chemstrips
Labels for medications and drips
Masks and safety goggles
Gloves and sterile gloves, including latex-free
Alcohol and iodophor pads
Benzoin
Xylocaine jelly
Surgilube
Christmas tree oxygen adaptor
Razor blades
Tape
Lumbar puncture tray, infant and adult
Spinal needles 18-, 20-, and 22-gauge and 1½- and 3½-inch
Flashlight with replacement batteries
2 x 2 gauze
Backboard (can be strapped to the back of the cart)
Sterile towels and fenestrated drapes
Hard cervical collar, small and medium sizes

Supplies and Equipment

See Box 21-1 for code cart supplies.

Procedure

Adhering to the ABCs of advanced life support remains the cornerstone of all resuscitative efforts. The following procedure provides a systematic approach to all critically ill children using an expanded ABC approach. Please refer to subsections of the text for specific procedures.

Airway

1. Assess for air movement and patency of the airway.
2. If there is history of trauma, stabilize the cervical spine before performing any airway maneuver.
3. Begin with simple airway maneuvers, such as the head tilt–chin lift (contraindicated in suspected cervical spine injury) or jaw thrust, to improve air movement.

Breathing

1. Look for chest wall rise and auscultate for breath sounds.
2. Check color, respiratory rate, work of breathing, and, if available, pulse oximetry.
3. If respiratory failure or insufficiency is noted, begin BMV with 100% oxygen.
4. If the child has some spontaneous respirations, attempt to coordinate BMV with the child's breaths.
5. In the apneic child, ventilate at approximately 24 to 28 breaths per minute (bpm) for infants, 16 to 20 bpm for children, and 12 to 16 bpm for adolescents.
6. If BMV is prolonged and/or difficult or the patient is apneic, secure the airway by intubating the trachea.

Circulation

1. Assess circulatory status by checking pulse rate and quality (comparing distal to central), color, temperature, capillary refill, and blood pressure.
2. Note mental status and urine output as measures of end organ perfusion.
3. Quickly check cardiac rhythm in two leads because pulseless ventricular tachycardia and fibrillation require immediate defibrillation (three shocks at 2 J/kg, 4 J/kg, 4 J/kg; maximum shocks 200 J, 360 J, 360 J)

Pulselessness

1. Begin compressions and coordinate them with ventilation (five compressions: one breath). In an infant, use both the index and middle fingers on your dominant hand or encircle the chest and use both thumbs to compress the sternum. Compressions should occur one finger's breadth below the nipple line.
2. Compress the chest of an infant at a depth of 1 inch and at a rate of at least 100 times per minute. Pause every fifth compression to administer a positive pressure breath.
3. In a child, compress the lower half of the sternum using the heel of one hand at a depth of 1.5 inches and a rate of 100 times per minute. Pause every fifth compression to administer a positive pressure breath.
4. As compressions are underway, have other team members attempt intravascular or intraosseous access (see following).
5. Administer resuscitation medicines (e.g., epinephrine, atropine, lidocaine, and naloxone) via the endotracheal tube pending vascular or intraosseous

access. Epinephrine is indicated in asystolic arrests, pulseless ventricular tachycardia, ventricular fibrillation (after defibrillation attempts), and in symptomatic bradycardia.

- Epinephrine, first dose:
  - IV/IO 0.01 mg/kg (1:10,000, 0.1 ml/kg)
  - Endotracheal tube (ETT) 0.1 mg/kg (1:1000, 0.1 ml/kg)
- Epinephrine, second and subsequent doses:
  - IV/IO/ETT 0.1 mg/kg (1:1000, 0.1 ml/kg) every 3 to 5 minutes

Bradycardia

Adequate oxygenation and perfusion correct most bradyarrhythmias seen in arrest situations. Rarely, epinephrine and atropine may be necessary.

- Epinephrine:
  - IV/IO 0.01 mg/kg (1:10,000, 0.1 ml/kg)
  - ETT 0.1 mg/kg (1:1000, 0.1 ml/kg)
- Atropine:
  - IV/IO 0.02 mg/kg (minimum 0.1 mg, maximum 1 mg)
  - ETT 0.04 mg/kg

Hemodynamic instability

Peripheral IV access needs to be obtained. This is often the most difficult hurdle to overcome in resuscitation. Short, large-bored catheters are preferred. In an arrest situation, if IV access cannot be obtained in the first 90 seconds, attempts at an intraosseous line should be made.

Once access is obtained, administer resuscitation medicines as indicated and begin rapid volume expansion.

- Crystalloid: Normal saline or lactated Ringer's 20 ml/kg

If signs of circulatory compromise are present, additional volume should be administered as rapidly as possible and repeated until an adequate clinical response is achieved (i.e., improved distal perfusion and blood pressure, reduction in heart rate, improved mental status and urine output). Children in shock may require up to 100 ml/kg in the first hour to maintain perfusion.

Acidosis seen in arrest situations is most often caused by respiratory insufficiency and hypoperfusion. Therefore mild to moderate acidosis is ideally corrected by restoring ventilation and perfusion. Severe acidosis can be treated with sodium bicarbonate.

- HCO_3: 1 mEq/kg (8.4%, 1 mEq/ml)

Infants, usually under 2 months of age, may present in shock because of a congenital heart lesion that depended on a patent ductus arteriosus for systemic blood flow (i.e., coarctation of the aorta, hypoplastic left heart syndrome). Once the ductus closes, profound shock may ensue. The practitioner must have a high index of suspicion in such cases because the administration of prostaglandin E_1 (PGE_1) may be life-saving. Because of potentially serious and common side effects of apnea, hypotension, and hypoglycemia, administration of PGE_1 is best done in conjunction with a pediatric cardiologist or pediatric intensivist.

- PGE_1: 0.05 to 0.1 μg/kg/min

3Ds: disability, dextrose, and drugs

Disability

A rapid neurologic assessment is necessary in any critically ill or injured child. Using the "AVPU" method, determine if the child is **A**lert, responsive to **V**erbal stimuli, responsive to **P**ainful stimuli, or entirely **U**nresponsive. Check for signs of raised intracranial pressure and/or herniation that include hypertension, bradycardia, irregular respiration, bulging fontanel in an infant, and pupillary inequality and/or unresponsiveness. If raised intracranial pressure is suspected, 0.5 to 1 gm/kg of mannitol should be administered. Reserve hyperventilation for impending herniation. Optimal cerebral perfusion is best maintained by careful attention to oxygenation and mean arterial pressure.

Dextrose

Without exception, every critically ill child should have a rapid glucose determination performed within minutes of arrival. Hypoglycemia may accompany many processes that cause critical pediatric illness (e.g., sepsis, trauma, and ingestion). Treat hypoglycemia with 0.5 to 1 gm/kg of dextrose (2 to 4 ml/kg D_{25} or 1 to 2 ml/kg D_{50}).

Drugs

Inquire about both therapeutic medications and possible accidental ingestions. Also, consider the need for specific medications in an ongoing resuscitation (e.g., intubation medications, antidotes for poisonings, inotropes, and/or pressors).

Euthermia/Equipment

1. Treat hypothermia by rewarming. Remove wet clothing and place children under warm blankets.
2. Administer warmed IV fluids and humidified oxygen.
3. Treat fever with 15 mg/kg of acetaminophen administered orally or rectally.
4. Check equipment for proper functioning. During resuscitative efforts, an acute decompensation, such as hypoxia, may not be physiological but rather caused by equipment failure (i.e., disconnected oxygen source).

Foley catheter

Insert a bladder catheter to better assess urine output during volume expansion.

Gastric tube

When the airway is secured, insert a gastric tube and decompress the stomach. This is especially important if prolonged BMV occurred before intubation. A nasogastric tube is contraindicated with head and facial trauma.

Hydrocortisone and hemoglobin

Consider the need for steroids. Stress dosing is required for children on long-term steroid treatment (e.g., severe asthma, nephrotic syndrome, malignancy, collagen vascular disease) and those on physiological replacement (e.g., hypopituitarism, Addison's disease, congenital adrenal hyperplasia). An initial dose of at least 2 mg/kg of hydrocortisone should be administered in such cases.

Consider the need for packed red blood cell (PRBC) transfusion when concomitant anemia is present in a child with poor oxygenation or circulatory instability. An initial transfusion of 10 ml/kg of PRBCs may be necessary.

As any resuscitation progresses, the practitioner in charge must identify the need for additional help and take appropriate steps to mobilize further resources. Early communication with a pediatric tertiary center is essential. Involvement of subspecialty services, such as pediatric emergency medicine, anesthesia, critical care, and surgery, may prove life-saving.

Complications

- Hypoxia
- Hemorrhage
- Myocardial injury
- Pneumothorax
- Pulmonary contusion
- Chest wall injury

Aftercare Instruction

Postresuscitation care continues with optimizing ventilation, oxygenation, and perfusion and preventing secondary organ injury. Arrangements for transport to a pediatric intensive care unit (intrahospital or interhospital) should be made directly with the receiving physician.

FOREIGN BODY/CHOKING MANAGEMENT

Background and Introduction

Foreign body (FB) aspiration is a common cause of accidental death in children under 1 year of age. Because 85% of foreign bodies are cleared before EMS arrives, knowledge of airway FB management by potential first responders is a necessity. This section describes the maneuvers available to practitioners managing an obstructed airway.

Indications

- Complete airway obstruction: Unable to speak, poor air movement
- Cyanosis

Contraindications

- Effective coughing
- Abdominal thrusts should be replaced with chest thrusts for infants and pregnant women.

Supplies and Equipment

Need to have
- Practitioner

Nice to have
- Laryngoscope with appropriate blade
- Magill forceps

Procedure

Children and adolescents
Conscious and upright (Fig. 21-2)
1. From behind, place your arms around the patient's waist.
2. Make a fist with one hand, wrapping your other hand around it.
3. Just above the patient's navel, thrust forcefully inward and upward, bracing the patient's body against yours.
4. Repeat the thrusts until the airway is clear or the child falls unconscious.

Unconscious and supine (Fig. 21-3)
1. If loss of consciousness is witnessed during an FB obstruction, open the airway using a tongue-jaw lift maneuver (grasp both the tongue and lower jaw between your thumb and finger and lift) and, if visualized, remove the object with a finger sweep.
2. Attempt rescue breathing, repositioning the head if initial attempts are unsuccessful. If ventilation remains unsuccessful, proceed with steps 3 to 6.
3. Kneel beside the patient and place the heel of one hand just above the navel.
4. With the second hand overlying the first, give five forceful upward abdominal thrusts.
5. Check the oropharynx for the presence of the FB.
   - If the FB is seen, remove it, but do not attempt a blind finger sweep.
   - Direct laryngoscopy and removal of the FB with Magill forceps can be attempted (Fig. 21-4).
6. Repeat steps 2 to 5 until ventilation is successful or the FB is removed, and activate EMS if necessary.

Infant
1. While sitting, grasp the infant face down, firmly holding the jaw with your hand and resting the torso along your forearm. Rest your arm along your thigh for added support. Be sure the head is held lower than the torso.

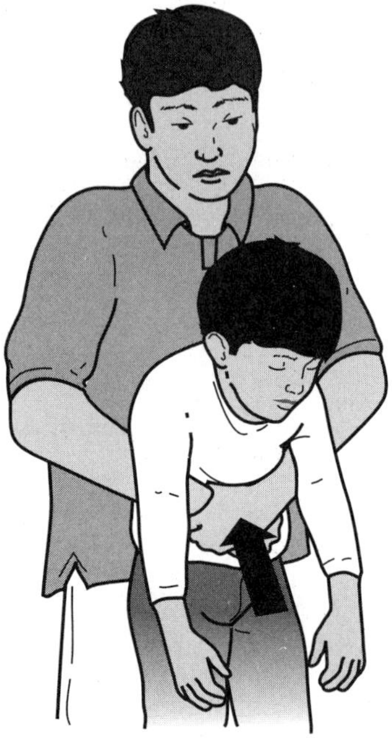

FIG. 21-2. Relief of foreign body obstruction in conscious children (Heimlich maneuver).

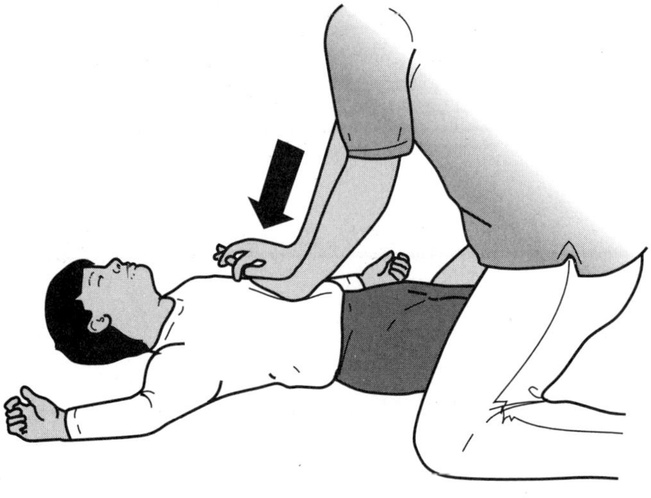

FIG. 21-3. Heimlich maneuver for unconscious child, lying supine.

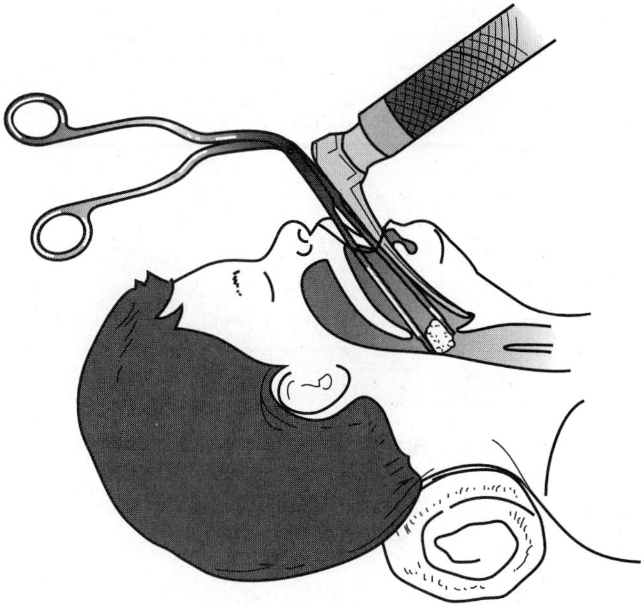

FIG. 21-4. Using Magill forceps to remove foreign body.

2. Give five firm back blows with the heel of your hand between the infant's scapulae (Fig. 21-5, *A*).
3. Turn the infant over. One hand should stabilize the infant's head and neck against your thigh while the other is used for chest thrusts.
4. Placing two fingers one finger's breadth below the nipple line, deliver five quick downward thrusts (Fig. 21-5, *B*).
5. Repeat this cycle until the FB is expelled or the infant loses consciousness. If the infant becomes unconscious, open the airway using a tongue-jaw lift and, if visualized, remove the object with a finger sweep.
6. Attempt rescue breathing with repositioning the head if initial attempts are unsuccessful.
7. If ventilation remains unsuccessful, repeat steps 1 to 6 and activate EMS.

Complications

- Abdominal organ injury
- Hemorrhage
- Vomiting

A 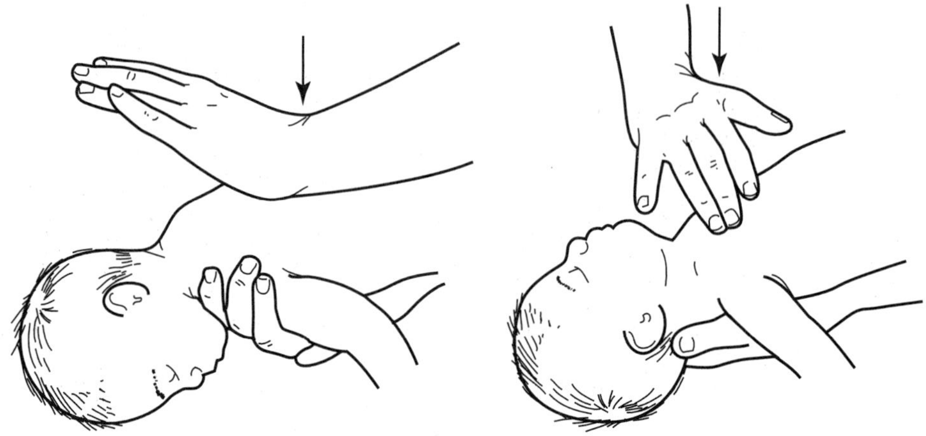 B

FIG. 21-5. Relief of foreign body obstruction in infants. **A,** Backblows. **B,** Chest thrusts.

Aftercare Instructions

All patients, including those who have stable airways, should be taken to a medical facility for confirmation of airway clearance and further care.

Modifications for Situations of Limited Resources

Management of FB airway obstruction can proceed without any equipment. The only limitation is regarding visualization and removal of the FB.

ADVANCED AIRWAY MANAGEMENT

Background and Introduction

When BMV is prolonged or cannot provide adequate ventilatory support, several airway management options exist. Those discussed in this section are orotracheal intubation, the laryngeal mask airway, and percutaneous translaryngeal ventilation. Additionally, it would be inappropriate to outline the use of these airway management techniques without addressing the use of proper sedation. These artificial airways are noxious to conscious patients, so indications and medications for sedation and paralysis are described.

Relevant Anatomy

For each of these procedures, it is essential to understand normal airway anatomy (Figs. 21-6, 21-7, 21-8).

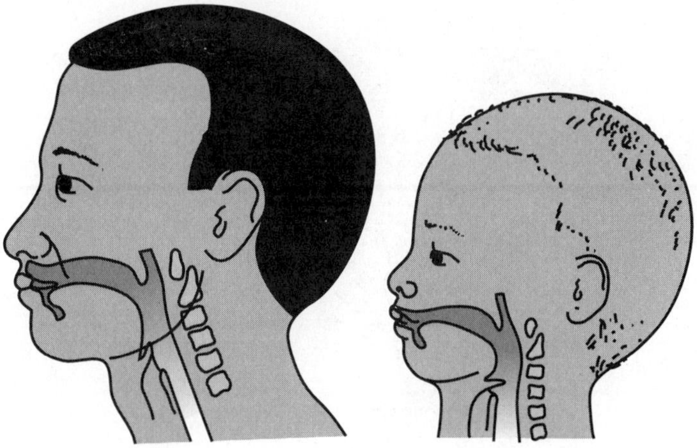

FIG. 21-6. Comparative anatomy of adult and infant airways.

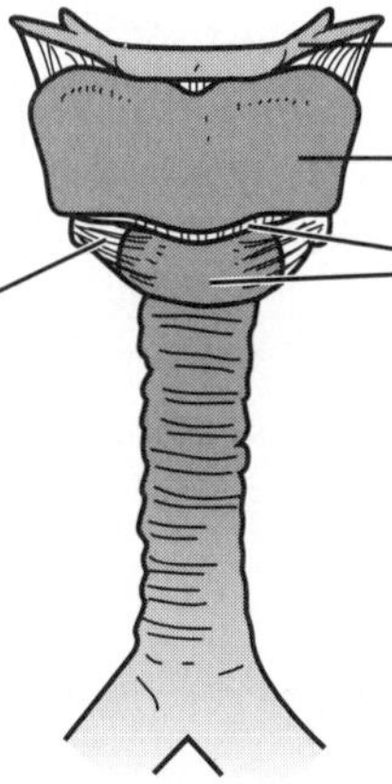

FIG. 21-7. Normal anatomy of infant larynx. Note position of thyroid cartilage lying under hyoid bone. Cricothyroid membrane attaches from superior border of cricoid to thyroid cartilage.

Contraindications

Never attempt to intubate children with upper airway obstructions who are maintaining a functional airway by body position. These children require immediate in-hospital management. If intubation is necessary in children with upper airway obstruction or in children with a difficult airway, a paralytic is absolutely contraindicated. It is best to maintain some respiratory drive in these situations in the event of an unsuccessful intubation.

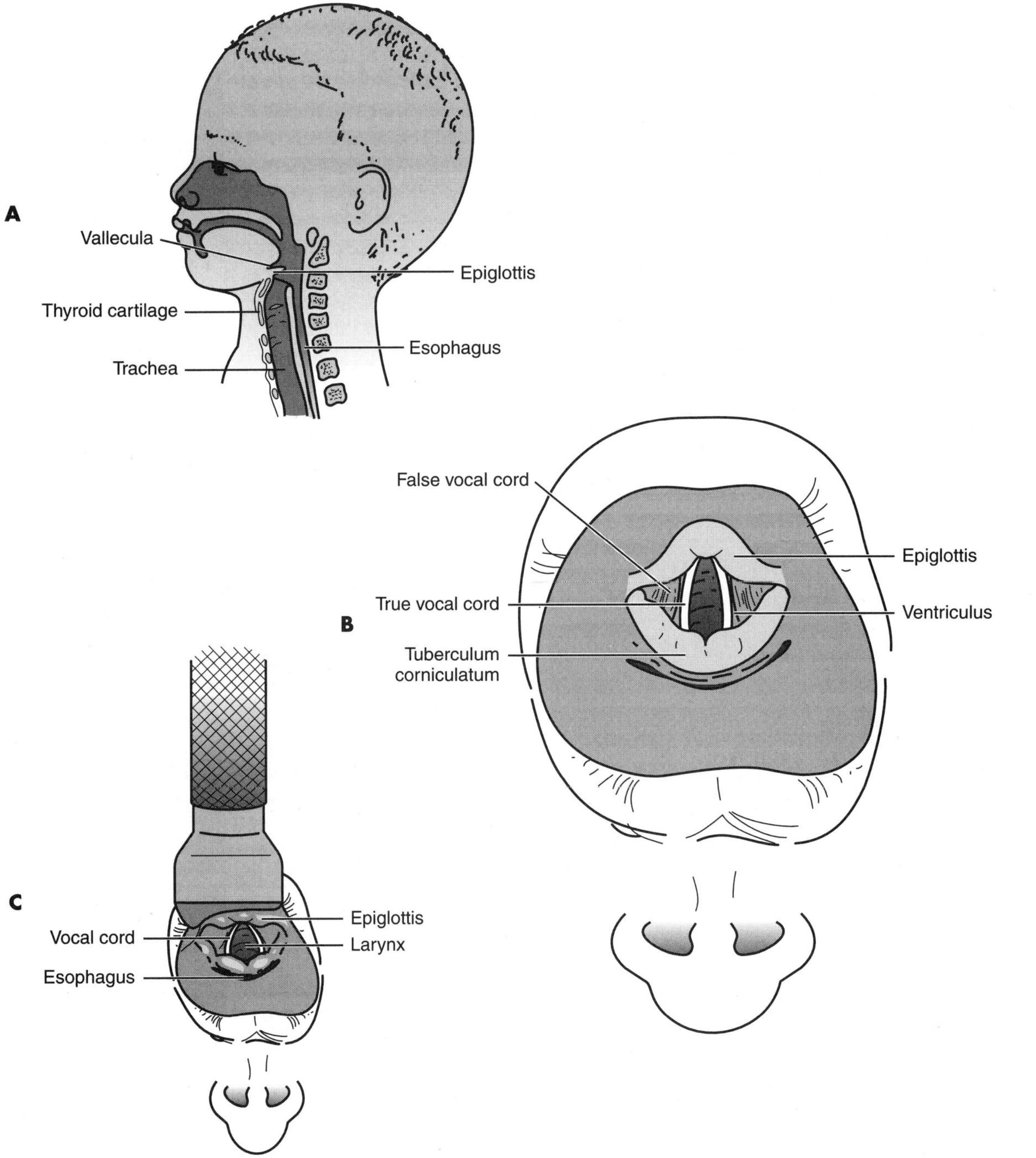

FIG. 21-8. Relationship of vallecula, epiglottis, and base of tongue; note cephalad position of larynx in infant. **A,** An older child's larynx is positioned more caudally. **B,** Laryngeal structures as viewed from above. **C,** Small size and relative position of vocal cords, epiglottis, and larynx as viewed through laryngoscope.

Orotracheal Intubation

Indications

- Ineffective or prolonged BMV
- Upper airway obstruction
- Airway protection

Supplies and equipment

Need to have

- Bag-mask apparatus connected to 100% oxygen
- Endotracheal tubes (Use the formula $\frac{16 + \text{age in years}}{4}$ to estimate tube size.)
- Laryngoscope
- Malleable stylets
- Spare bulbs and batteries
- Straight (Miller) and curved (Macintosh) blades
- Suction apparatus
- Syringe (10-ml) for cuff inflation

Nice to have

- Carbon dioxide detector
- Cardiopulmonary monitor with oximeter

Procedure

1. Prepare equipment and personnel. Using the mnemonic memory device "SOAP," prepare **S**uction tubing and catheters, **O**xygen delivery systems (bag-mask apparatus), **A**irways (endotracheal tubes of size predicted and one size smaller), and **P**harmaceuticals, if necessary.
2. Hyperoxygenate with 100% oxygen if the situation allows in a spontaneously breathing patient.
3. Position the patient's head in the sniffing position. In a child older than 2 years, this may be accomplished by placing a folded towel beneath the head and neck (Fig. 21-9).
4. Have an assistant apply cricoid pressure (Sellick maneuver) to prevent aspiration.
5. Open the patient's jaw by pushing the teeth apart with your right thumb and index finger.
6. Carefully insert the laryngoscope blade along the right edge of the tongue.
   - Sweeping the tongue to the left, advance the blade toward the epiglottis (Fig. 21-10).
   - If using a straight blade, slide the tip beneath the epiglottis and lift straight upward, exposing the vocal cords (Fig. 21-11, *A*).
   - With a curved blade, place the tip in the vallecula and lift. The epiglottis will rise out of the way (Fig. 21-11, *B*).
7. Pass the ETT along the right side of the mouth, between the vocal cords, and into the trachea (Fig. 21-11, *C*).

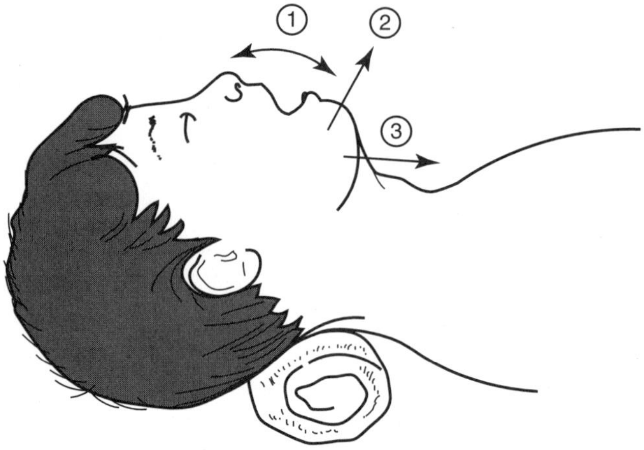

FIG. 21-9. Triple jaw maneuver. *1,* Mouth open. *2,* Mandible displaced anteriorly and *3,* downward. Note: in a child older than 2 years, place folded towel beneath head and neck to achieve this action.

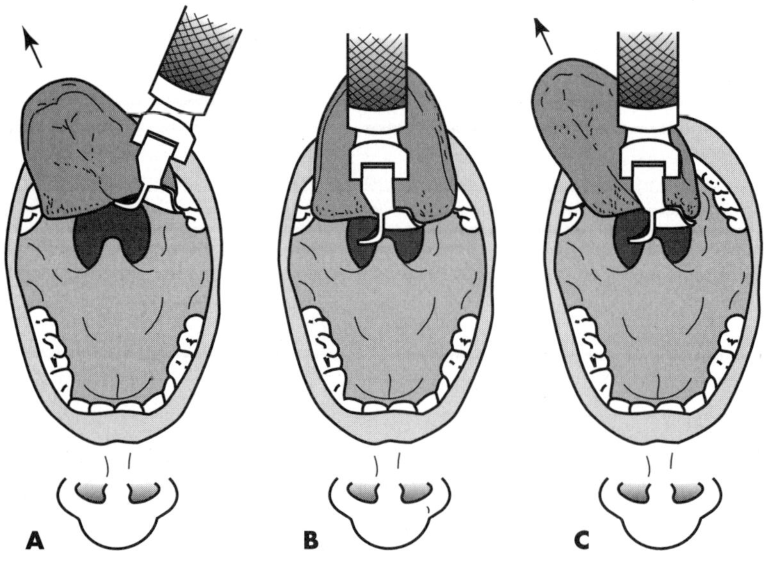

FIG. 21-10. Laryngoscope is inserted into right side of mouth. Tongue is swept from right to left. **A,** Incorrect: Laryngoscope has not returned to the middle. **B,** Incorrect: Tongue hangs over right side of blade. **C,** Correct: final position.

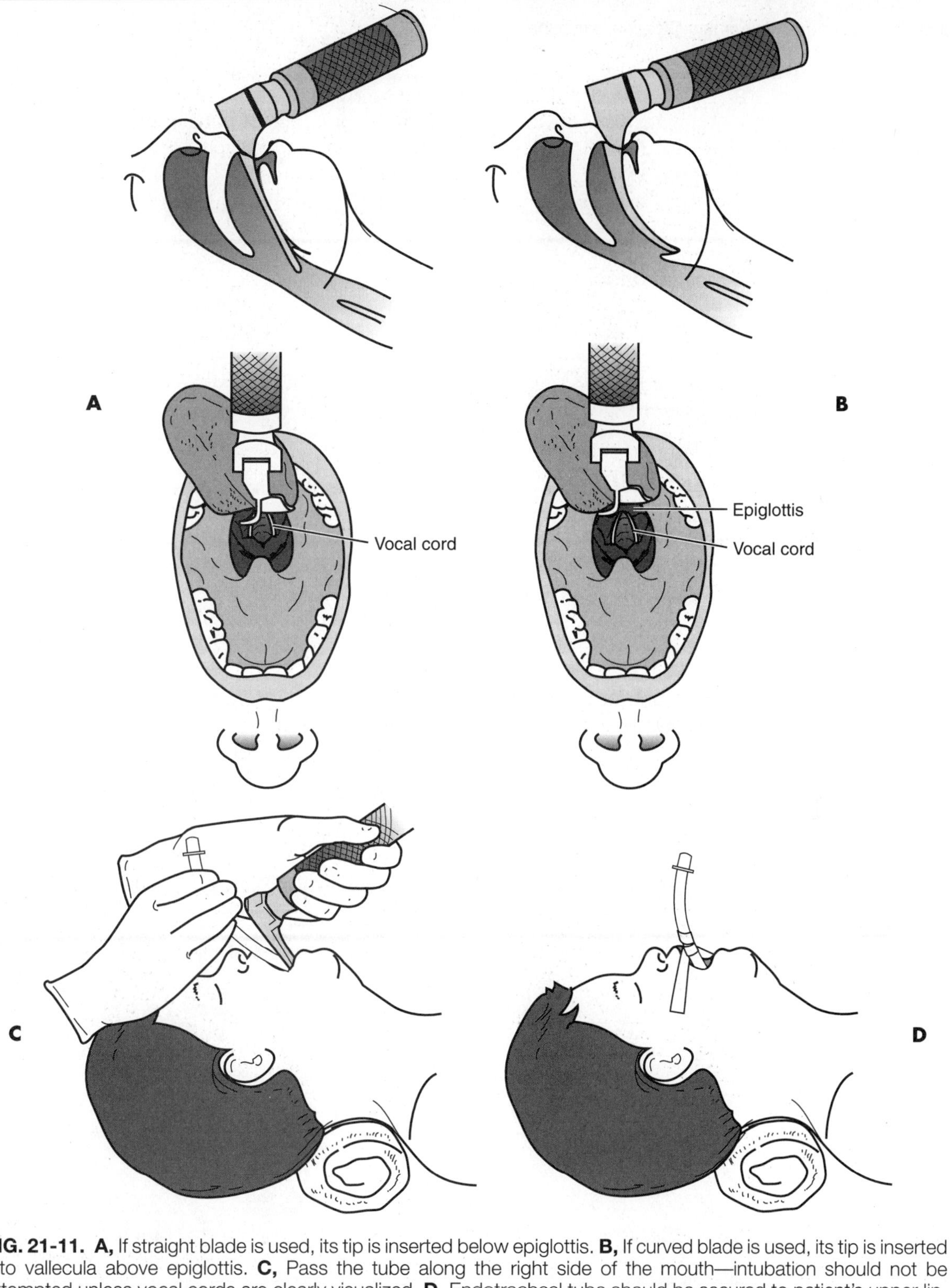

FIG. 21-11. A, If straight blade is used, its tip is inserted below epiglottis. **B,** If curved blade is used, its tip is inserted into vallecula above epiglottis. **C,** Pass the tube along the right side of the mouth—intubation should not be attempted unless vocal cords are clearly visualized. **D,** Endotracheal tube should be secured to patient's upper lip. If tape is used, ensure that tape is waterproof. Place two loops of tape around tube to reduce chances of accidental extubation.

8. If using a stylet, carefully remove it now.
9. Ventilate via the ETT and confirm the presence of equal breath sounds.
10. Adjust the tube depth for optimal breath sounds. The formula depth (cm) = 3 × ETT size (mm) can be used as a guide.
11. Secure the tube in place and confirm its position with a chest radiograph (Fig. 21-11, *D*).

Complications

- Esophageal intubation
- Tracheal or esophageal perforation
- Aspiration
- Vocal cord injury
- Bradycardia

Managing the Difficult Airway

The laryngeal mask airway

Indications

The laryngeal mask airway (LMA) is recommended by the American Society of Anesthesiologists for managing the difficult airway when intubation and ventilation are not possible, but before the use of percutaneous translaryngeal ventilation.

Supplies and equipment

- Bag-mask apparatus connected to 100% oxygen
- Laryngeal mask airways (Six LMA sizes are available; the appropriate size is chosen based on the patient's weight.) (Table 21-4)
- Syringe (15-ml) for cuff inflation

Procedure

1. With the left hand, position and maintain the patient's head in the sniffing position as for endotracheal intubation.
2. Pull open the mouth by lowering the mandible.

TABLE 21-4
Laryngeal mask airway size for patient weight

Weight (kg)	LMA Size
Less than 6.5	1
Up to 20	2
Up to 30	2.5
Up to 60	3
Up to 80	4
Greater than 80	5

3. With the right hand, insert the LMA into the mouth and hold it against the palate with the index finger.
4. Carefully slide the LMA into the posterior oropharynx and insert it caudally until it meets resistance with the upper esophagus.
5. Inflate the cuff. The black line on an appropriately sized LMA should move in line with the upper lip or incisors.
6. Ventilate with a bag-mask apparatus and place a bite block to prevent damage to the LMA from patient chewing.

Complications

- Aspiration
- Posterior pharyngeal bruising
- Later dysarthria

Percutaneous translaryngeal ventilation

Indications

- Facial trauma
- Inability to ventilate by bag-mask apparatus, endotracheal tube, and LMA

Percutaneous translaryngeal ventilation (PTLV) is a temporizing measure intended to establish airways in and oxygenate patients who have failed repeated attempts at endotracheal intubation and LMA placement, if available. Once translarygeal ventilation is established, these patients must be taken immediately to a facility where cricothyrotomy or tracheostomy can be performed.

Supplies and equipment

Need to have

- High-pressure 100% oxygen source (50 psi)
- Large-bore angiocatheters: 12- and 14-gauge
- Oxygen tubing
- Three-way stopcock

Nice to have

- Suction catheters: 18- and 20-F

Procedure

1. Puncture the inferior aspect of the cricothyroid membrane (Fig. 21-12, *A*) with a large-bore IV catheter, angling slightly toward the lungs (Fig. 21-12, *B*).
2. While advancing the catheter, remove the needle.
3. Attach the stopcock to the catheter (Fig. 21-12, *C*).
4. Connect oxygen tubing to the stopcock or interpose a suction catheter (Fig. 21-12, *D*). Run oxygen at 25 psi (7.5 L/min), advancing to 50 psi (15 L/min) as chest rise and breath sounds confirm the catheter position.
5. If using a stopcock alone, open the flow to the patient for 1 second and then to the outlet for 2 to 4 seconds. Switch the stopcock back and forth in this manner to allow for inspiration and expiration.
6. If using a suction catheter, open the stopcock to the patient. Using the same

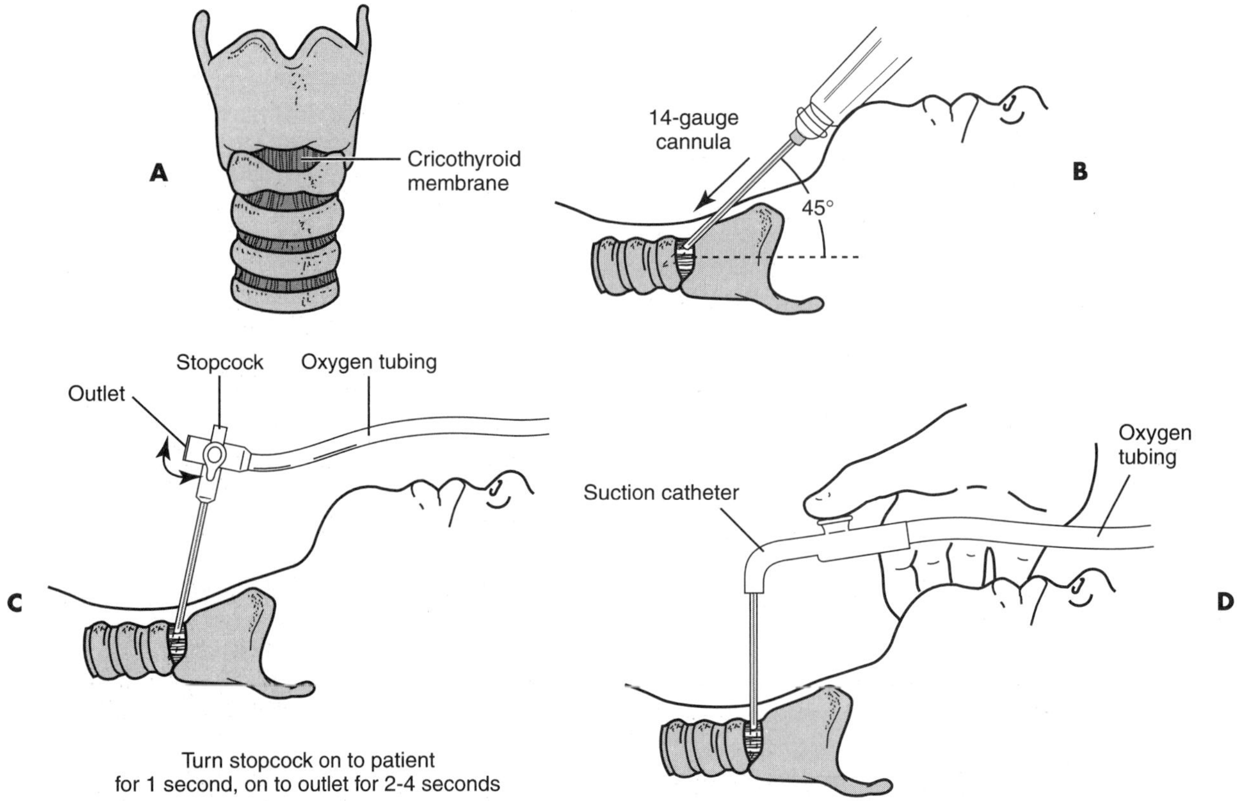

FIG. 21-12. Cricothyrotomy. **A,** Anatomical view. **B,** Insertion of 14-gauge IV cannula. **C,** Three-way stopcock to control inspiration and expiration. **D,** Suction catheter to control inspiration and expiration.

tempo as in the previous step, close and open the suction opening with a finger to provide inspiration and expiration. A 3.0 endotracheal tube adapter may be placed directly into the catheter hub, allowing bagged ventilation (Fig. 21-13).

7. Secure the catheter in place and transport the patient for further care.

Alternative connection apparatus for PTLV

An alternative apparatus for connecting the oxygen source and the intratracheal catheter has been recently reported. This apparatus uses a standard nasal cannula device as follows.

Procedure

1. Cut a side hole in a standard nasal cannula tubing before it bifurcates.
2. Adjacent to the nasal prongs, cut through the tubing and fit the free end into the hub of the catheter.

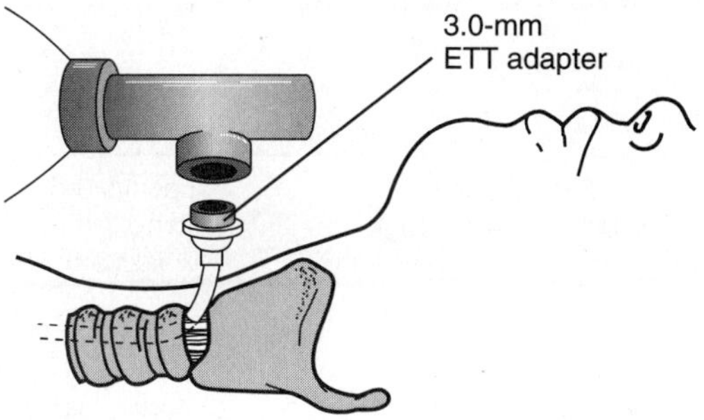

FIG. 21-13. Bag attached to 3.0 endotracheal tube adapter connected to IV cannula.

3. Tightly tie off the other limb of tubing that attaches to the nasal prongs.
4. Connect the apparatus to the oxygen source as usual for a nasal cannula.
5. Operate as outlined previously, occluding the side hole with a finger for inspiration.

Possible complications

- Hemorrhage
- Airway occlusion
- Subcutaneous emphysema
- Pneumothorax, pneumomediastinum
- Air embolism
- Esophageal rupture

Aftercare Instructions

Subsequent to intubation, LMA placement, or PTLV, a physician trained in advanced airway and ventilator management must care for the patient.

Modifications for Situations of Limited Resources

Without appropriate equipment, a difficult airway can still be managed by modifying PTLV. By incising a small hole in the cricothyroid membrane and inserting a large-bore catheter or tube, mouth-to-catheter ventilation can take place.

Rapid-Sequence Techniques for Intubation

Rapid-sequence intubation (RSI) is indicated for airway management in conscious patients with a full stomach. It involves administering a series of medications aimed toward increasing the chance of a successful intubation while decreasing noxious stimulation and the risk of gastric aspiration.

TABLE 21-5
Rapid-sequence intubation medications

Patient	Premedication	Sedative	Paralytic
General	Atropine 0.02 mg/kg IV (min 0.1 mg, max 1 mg) Midazolam 0.1-0.2 mg/kg IV	Thiopental 3-5 mg/kg IV or Fentanyl 3-5 μg/kg IV and Midazolam 0.1-0.2 mg/kg IV or Propofol 1-3 mg/kg IV or Ketamine 1-2 mg/kg IV	Rocuronium 0.6-1 mg/kg IV or Vecuronium 0.2-0.3 mg/kg IV or Succinylcholine 1-2 mg/kg (max 150 mg) IV or Cisatricurium 0.2 mg/kg IV
Hypotension	Atropine 0.02 mg/kg IV (min 0.1 mg, max 1 mg)	Etomidate 0.2-0.4 mg/kg IV or Ketamine 1-2 mg/kg IV	Rocuronium 0.6-1 mg/kg IV or Vecuronium 0.1-0.2 mg/kg IV or Cisatricurium 0.2 mg/kg IV
Head injury	Lidocaine 1 mg/kg IV	Thiopental 3-5 mg/kg IV or Etomidate 0.2-0.4 mg/kg IV or Propofol 1-3 mg/kg IV	
Head injury with hypotension	Lidocaine 1 mg/kg IV	Etomidate 0.2-0.4 mg/kg IV or Thiopental (low-dose) 1-3 mg/kg	
Seizures	Midazolam 0.1 mg/kg IV	Thiopental 3-5 mg/kg IV or Propofol 1-3 mg/kg IV	
Asthma	Atropine 0.02 mg/kg IV (min 0.1 mg, max 1 mg)	Ketamine 1-2 mg/kg IV or Propofol 1-3 mg/kg IV	Rocuronium 0.6-1 mg/kg IV or Cisatricurium 0.2 mg/kg IV

RSI, by definition, does not include BMV; however, in reality, many patients receive BMV before intubation. The medication pathway does not have to be altered for this circumstance, but the practitioner must be wary of, and take steps to counter, the increased risk of aspiration in patients with gastric distension from BMV.

Typically, RSI involves pretreatment with a sedative followed by a muscle relaxant. This general pathway remains largely the same for most patients, although the choice of sedating and paralyzing agents as well as any additional medications depends on the specific clinical scenario (Table 21-5).

TREATMENT OF CARDIAC ARRHYTHMIAS, VAGAL MANEUVERS, CARDIOVERSION, AND DEFIBRILLATION

Background and Introduction

Arrhythmias can be categorized as primary or secondary. Primary arrhythmias arise from inherent cardiac pathology, such as an aberrant pathway or an ectopic focus. Arrhythmias can also be secondary to systemic pathology, such as hypoxia or drug toxicity. Regardless of the origin of the arrhythmia, the basic ABCs of resuscitation must be addressed during stabilization of the cardiac rhythm. The following section describes treatment of supraventricular tachycardia (SVT), ventricular tachycardia (VT), and ventricular fibrillation (VF). Please see the section on Pediatric Resuscitation for treatment of asystole and bradycardia.

Supraventricular Tachycardia

Background and introduction

SVT is the most common primary arrhythmia in children. It is usually caused by reentry of the electrical impulse to the atrioventricular (AV) node via an accessory AV connection (AV reentry tachycardia) or an accessory pathway within the AV node (AV-nodal reentry tachycardia). AV reentry tachycardia is the most common form of SVT, especially in children under 12 years. AV-nodal reentry tachycardia does not become clinically significant until adolescence. A narrow-complex QRS characterizes SVT 90% of the time. When aberrant conduction coincides with SVT, the QRS complex can be wide, making it look similar to VT. Treat this rhythm as VT until proven otherwise.

Differentiating SVT from sinus tachycardia can be difficult. Distinguishing points include the following:

- The rate in sinus tachycardia is usually less than 200, whereas in SVT, it is generally greater than 200.
- P-waves are always present in sinus tachycardia. In SVT, the P-waves may be absent, abnormally shaped, or inverted in leads II, III, and a VF.
- In sinus tachycardia, beat-to-beat variation in the heart rate is commonly seen, whereas in SVT the heart rate is extremely regular.
- On a rhythm strip, the onset or termination of the tachycardia is gradual in sinus tachycardia and abrupt in SVT.

Vagal maneuvers/adenosine

Increasing vagal tone slows conduction through the AV node and may convert SVT to a sinus rhythm. Several maneuvers are known to increase vagal tone: abdominal pressure (valsalva maneuver), rectal stimulation, eliciting gagging with a tongue depressor, carotid massage, and applying ice to the face. Application of an ice-water bag to the face has been most effective and is described below.

Adenosine blocks antegrade conduction through the AV node block, thereby interrupting reentrant tachycardias. Although adenosine cannot terminate non-reentrant tachycardias (i.e., atrial flutter, atrial fibrillation), it may slow conduction through the AV node long enough to better elucidate the underlying arrhythmia. Adenosine is rapidly metabolized (half-life = 10 seconds); therefore it must be given as a rapid bolus close to the central circulation. Central access is preferred, but for practical purposes, an antecubital IV will suffice.

Indications

- Hemodynamically stable patients with narrow-complex tachycardia

Contraindications

- Hemodynamically unstable patients with narrow-complex tachycardia (Go directly to cardioversion.)

Supplies and equipment

Need to have

- Adenosine 0.1 mg/kg, not to exceed 6 mg for a first dose and 0.2 mg/kg up to 12 mg for a repeat dose
- Bag-valve-mask
- Cardiac monitor
- Defibrillator/cardioversion machine with pediatric paddles and electrode gel
- Ice bag large enough to cover the child's face and wrap around to the ears, filled two-thirds with ice water
- EKG machine
- IV access (IV catheter, alcohol swab, normal saline)
- Normal saline flush, 5 ml
- Resuscitation medications (epinephrine, atropine, lidocaine)
- Suction equipment

Procedure

If children are unstable, go directly to cardioversion.

1. Place children on the cardiac monitor.
2. Obtain a continuous oximetry reading.
3. Obtain IV access, preferably in the antecubital vein.
4. Immobilize young children. Explain procedure to older children and ask them to hold their breath.
5. Apply the ice bag to children's face until conversion to sinus rhythm or for a maximum of 15 seconds. Be sure to cover the mouth and nose. This may be repeated twice if children remain stable.
6. If the arrhythmia persists and children are still hemodynamically stable, proceed to adenosine.
7. Rapidly inject adenosine and follow immediately by a normal saline flush. This is best accomplished by inserting the needles of the adenosine syringe and flush syringe in the injection port nearest to the hub of the needle. Clamp the IV line just above the port to prevent backflow. Rapidly inject the adenosine and follow instantaneously with a rapid injection of the flush. If the rhythm does not change, double the adenosine dose (maximum single dose 12 mg or 0.3 mg/kg) and repeat the process.

Complications

- Asystole is usually brief and followed by sinus rhythm. It can be seen after vagal maneuvers alone.
- Bronchospasm and vasodilation can be induced by adenosine.

Synchronized cardioversion

Cardioversion provides a depolarization to the myocardium that is timed with patients' own intrinsic electrical activity. An electrical impulse is provided to patients immediately after their own QRS complex is generated. This minimizes the risk of precipitating VF.

Indications

- Unstable SVT, VT with a pulse, atrial fibrillation, and atrial flutter (See section on Defibrillation for pulseless VT.)
- Stable SVT that is unresponsive to vagal maneuvers and pharmacotherapy

Contraindications

- Absent pulse

High-risk situations

- *Digitalis toxicity:* There is a higher incidence of VT and VF after cardioversion. In this instance, prepare patients for cardioversion with lidocaine (1 mg/kg) and Digibind. Use lower energy than you would ordinarily in this circumstance.
- *Chronic atrial fibrillation:* Clots that have formed over time may become dislodged with cardioversion and lead to cerebral emboli. Stable patients should be anticoagulated before undergoing cardioversion.

Supplies and equipment

Need to have

- Advanced cardiac life support (ACLS) equipment: oxygen, airway and intubation equipment, suction, IVs, emergency drugs
- Commercial gel for the paddles (Saline-soaked gauze pads may be used instead, but care must be taken not to allow the saline from one pad to contact that of the other, leading to a short circuit.)
- Defibrillator/cardioversion unit
- ECG monitor
- Paddle electrodes (infant paddles if less than 1 year old or less than 10 kg; adult paddles for all others)

Nice to have

- Lidocaine
- Sedation (midazolam 0.1 mg/kg and fentanyl 2 to 4 μg/kg)

Procedure

1. Place the patient on a flat, dry surface and provide continuous monitoring.
2. If the patient is unstable, proceed immediately with cardioversion.
3. If the patient is stable, secure IV access and give oxygen and sedation.
4. Apply electrode gel to the paddles.
5. Turn on the cardioversion machine.
6. Select the lead that displays the tallest R-wave.
7. Make sure the synchronize function is *on.*
8. Select the starting energy dose of 0.5 J/kg and wait for the signal that the machine is charged.
9. Place one paddle on the upper right chest below the clavicle. Place the other paddle to the left of the left nipple.
10. Confirm the cardiac rhythm with the "Quick Look" function.

11. Make sure everyone (including yourself!) is cleared from the table. If providing artificial ventilation, stop at this point.
12. Press firmly on the electrode paddles and depress the discharge buttons.
13. Hold the paddles in place for several moments, until discharge occurs.
14. If the rhythm persists, repeat steps 1 through 13 using an energy level of 1 J/kg. This may be repeated one additional time, providing three total shocks of 0.5 J/kg, 1 J/kg, and 1 J/kg.

With extreme tachycardia, the machine may be unable to deliver a synchronized shock. Keep the paddles on the chest with the discharge buttons depressed for a full 10 seconds. If the patient's condition is deteriorating, you may need to deliver the shock in the asynchronous mode.

Complications

- Atrial and ventricular ectopy is common, especially in the first 15 to 30 minutes.
- Skin burns from the paddles
- Electrical shock for anyone in contact with the patient or the bed
- Recurrence of the original arrhythmia
- Asystole
- Ventricular fibrillation (If this occurs, immediately recharge the machine in asynchronous mode and prepare for defibrillation.)
- Myocardial damage
- Emboli

Aftercare instructions

- Start a lidocaine bolus (1 mg/kg) and drip (20 to 50 μg/kg/minute) after successfully cardioverting VT.
- Correct any underlying cause that may have led to the arrhythmia.

Ventricular Tachycardia

This rhythm, which is defined as three or more repetitive beats originating from an ectopic ventricular focus, is unusual in children. Various possible etiologies include underlying heart disease, cardiac tumors, myocarditis, hypoxia, acidosis, hypokalemia or hyperkalemia, sympathomimetic drugs, and prolonged QT because of either congenital syndromes or secondary to medications such as tricyclic antidepressants. EKG findings suggestive of VT include the following:

- Regular rate, greater than 120
- Wide QRS complex (exceeding 0.08 seconds in infants and 0.09 seconds in children)
- Unusual QRS morphology, often a right bundle branch block in infants and a left bundle branch block in children
- AV dissociation (P-waves and QRS complexes are independent of each other)
- T-waves and QRS complexes point in the opposite directions
- Fusion beats occur when a sinus impulse fuses with an ectopic ventricular impulse. The morphology of the complex is intermediate between the two.

The therapy for VT depends on the hemodynamic status of the patient. A stable patient with a pulse and VT is treated initially with lidocaine bolus of 1 mg/kg followed by a continuous infusion of 20 to 50 μg/kg/minute. A hemodynamically unstable patient (i.e., poor perfusion, hypotension) with a pulse and VT is treated with synchronized cardioversion (see previous section). Pulseless VT is treated like VF with immediate defibrillation (see following section).

Ventricular Fibrillation

This uncommon pulseless rhythm in children is caused by disorganized depolarization of the myocardium. The ECG will show a course or fine oscillating line. After confirming that this is not caused by lead artifact, the treatment is immediate defibrillation.

Defibrillation

Defibrillation provides a large electrical impulse to the myocardium. If a sufficient amount of the myocardium can be depolarized, it may be refractory to its own underlying chaotic rhythm, allowing the sinoatrial node to resume control.

Indications

- Pulseless ventricular tachycardia
- Ventricular fibrillation

Contraindications

- Asystole
- Ventricular tachycardia with a pulse

Supplies and equipment

- ACLS equipment: oxygen, airway and intubation equipment, suction, IVs, emergency drugs
- Commercial gel for the paddles (Saline-soaked gauze pads may be used instead, but care must be taken not to allow the saline from one pad to contact that of the other, leading to a short circuit.)
- Defibrillator/cardioversion unit
- ECG monitor
- Paddle electrodes (infant paddles if less than 1 year old or less than 10 kg; adult paddles for all others)

Procedure

1. Determine pulselessness and confirm VT or VF in more than one lead.
2. Begin or continue CPR.
3. Activate EMS.
4. Secure airway.
5. Attempt IV/intraosseous access but do not delay defibrillation.
6. Turn on the defibrillator.

7. Make sure the synchronize function is *off.*
8. Place one paddle on the upper right chest below the clavicle. Place the other paddle to the left of the left nipple.
9. Select a starting energy dose of 2 J/kg (maximum 200 J) and wait for the signal that the machine is charged.
10. Stop chest compressions and recheck the rhythm on the monitor.
11. Make sure everyone (including yourself!) is cleared from the table. If providing artificial ventilation, stop at this point.
12. Press firmly on the electrode paddles and depress the discharge buttons.
13. If the pulseless VT or VF persists, repeat steps 7 through 12 using an energy level of 4 J/kg (maximum 360 J). This may be repeated one additional time, providing three total shocks of 2 J/kg, 4 J/kg, and 4 J/kg.
14. After the initial series of three shocks, administer epinephrine if VT or VF persists.
    - Epinephrine, first dose:
      — IV/IO 0.01 mg/kg (1:10,000, 0.1 ml/kg)
      — ETT 0.1 mg/kg (1:1000, 0.1 ml/kg)
15. Defibrillate 4 J/kg 30 to 60 seconds after each medication.
16. Administer lidocaine
    - Lidocaine: IV/IO 1 mg/kg
17. Defibrillate 4 J/kg 30 to 60 seconds after each medication.
18. Administer second epinephrine dose.
    - Epinephrine, second and subsequent doses:
      — IV/IO/ETT 0.1mg/kg (1:1000, 0.1 ml/kg) every 3 to 5 minutes
      — Consider bretylium 5 mg/kg first-dose IV, 10 mg/kg second-dose IV

Complications

- Atrial and ventricular ectopy is common, especially in the first 15 to 30 minutes.
- Skin burns from the paddles

TABLE 21-6
Age-specific vital signs

Age	Weight (kg)	Systolic BP (mm Hg)	Heart rate (bpm)	Respiratory rate (breaths/min.)
6 months	7	70 to 105	110 to 170	30 to 50
1 year	10	80 to 105	90 to 150	25 to 35
3 years	15	80 to 105	70 to 140	20 to 30
6 years	20	80 to 110	65 to 130	20 to 30
8 years	25	80 to 110	60 to 130	15 to 30
10 years	30	90 to 115	60 to 130	10 to 20
12 years	40	90 to 120	60 to 120	10 to 20
Adolescent	50	110 to 135	60 to 100	10 to 20
Adult	70	110 to 140	60 to 100	10 to 20

- Electrical shock for anyone in contact with the patient or the bed
- Recurrence of the original arrhythmia
- Asystole
- Myocardial damage
- Emboli

Aftercare instructions

See aftercare instructions in Pediatric Resuscitation section.

Quick reference tables

Tables 21-6, 21-7, and 21-8 provide general information as well as sizes of equipment and doses of medications appropriate for specific ages and sizes of children.

TABLE 21-7
Orotracheal intubation specifications

	ETT		
Age	Size (mm)	Depth (cm)	Laryngoscope blade
6 months	3.5	11	1 straight
1 year	4.0	12	1, 2 straight
3 years	4.5	14	2 straight
6 years	5.5	16	2 straight
8 years	6.0	18	2 straight
10 years	6.5	20	2 straight, curved
12 years	7.0	21	2, 3 straight, curved
Adolescent	7.5	22	2, 3 straight, curved
Adult	7.5	24	3 straight, curved

TABLE 21-8
Nasogastric, chest tube, femoral central line, peripheral intravenous line specifications

			Femoral Central Line		
Age	NG tube Size (F)	Chest tube Size (F)	Size (F)	Depth (cm)	IV line (Gauge)
6 months	8	12	4	40	24
1 year	8	16	4	45	24
3 years	10	18	5	55	22
6 years	10	20	5	60	22
8 years	12	24	5	60	22
10 years	12	28	5	60	20
12 years	12	32	5	60	20
Adolescent	12	34	5	60	18
Adult	14	36	5	60	18

SUGGESTED READINGS

Emergency Childbirth

Cunningham FG et al, editors: Conduct of normal labor and delivery. In *Williams obstetrics,* ed 20, Stamford, CT, 1997, Appleton and Lange.

Gianopoulos JG: Emergency complications of labor and delivery, *Emerg Med Clin N Am* 12:201, 1994.

Higgins S: Emergency delivery, prehospital care, emergency department delivery, perimortem salavage, *Emerg Med Clin N Am* 5:3, 1987.

Schrader K, Budassi S: Emergency childbirth, *J Emerg Nursing* 5:2, 1979.

Williams C: Emergency childbirth, *Nursing* 16:3, 1986.

Neonatal Resuscitation

American Heart Association/American Academy of Pediatrics Neonatal Resuscitation Program Steering Committee: *Manual for neonatal resuscitation,* Dallas, 1995, American Heart Association.

Frand MN, Honig KL, Hageman JR: Neonatal cardiopulmonary resuscitation: the good news and the bad, *Pediatr Clin of North Am* 45:587, 1998.

Gomella TL, Cunningham MD, Eyal FG, editors: *Neonatology: management, procedures, on-call problems, diseases and drugs,* ed 3, Norwalk, CT, 1994, Appleton and Lange.

Kattwinkel J et al: ILCOR advisory statement: resuscitation of the newly born infant: an advisory statement from the pediatric working group of the international liaison committee on resuscitation, *Eur J Pediatr* 158:345, 1999.

Young TE, Mangum OB: *Neofax: a manual of drugs used in neonatal care,* ed 12, Raleigh, NC, 1999, Acorn Publishing.

Pediatric Resuscitation

Chameides L, Hazinski MF, editors: *Textbook of pediatric advanced life support,* Dallas, 1997, American Heart Association.

Goetting MG: Mastering cardiopulmonary resuscitation, *Pediatr Clin North Am* 41:6, 1994.

Young KD, Seidel JS: Pediatric cardiopulmonary resuscitation: a collective review, *Ann of Emerg Med* 33:2, 1999.

Foreign Body/Choking Management

Andazola JJ, Sapien RE: The choking child: what happens before the ambulance arrives? *Prehosp Emerg Care* 3:7, 1999.

Chameides L, Hazinski MF: *Textbook of pediatric advanced life support,* Dallas, 1997, American Heart Association.

Fitzpatrick PC et al: Pediatric airway foreign bodies, *J LA State Med Soc* 150:138, 1998.

Pfenninger JL, Fowler GC, editors: *Procedures for primary care physicians,* St Louis, 1994, Mosby.

Rubio QF et al: Magill forceps: a vital forceps, *Pediatr Emerg Care* 11:302, 1995.

Seidel J: Preparing for pediatric emergencies, *Pediatr Rev* 16:466, 1995.

Advanced Airway Management

Chameides L, Hazinski MF, editors: *Textbook of pediatric advanced life support,* Dallas, 1997, American Heart Association.

Gerardi MJ et al: Rapid-sequence intubation of the pediatric patient, *Ann Emerg Med* 28:55, 1996.

Peak DA, Roy S: Needle cricothyroidotomy revisited, *Pediatr Emerg Care* 15:224, 1999.

Tintinalli JE, Ruiz E, Krome RL, editors: *Emergency medicine: a comprehensive study guide,* ed 4, New York, 1996, McGraw-Hill.

Tobais JD: The laryngeal mask airway: a review for the emergency physician, *Pediatr Emerg Care* 12:370, 1996.

Tobias JD, editor: *Pediatric critical care: the essentials,* Armonk, NY, 1999, Futura Publishing.

Yamamoto LG, Yim GK, Britten AG: Rapid sequence anesthesia induction for emergency intubation, *Pediatr Emerg Care* 6:200, 1990.

Treatment of Cardiac Arrhythmias, Vagal Maneuvers, Cardioversion, and Defibrillation

American Heart Association and American Academy of Pediatrics, *Textbook of pediatric advanced life support,* Dallas, 1998, American Heart Association.

Erickson C: Acute treatment of tachyarrhythmias. In Dieckmann R, Fiser D, Selbst S, editors: *Pediatric emergency and critical care procedures,* St Louis, 1997, Mosby.

Fisher D et al: Rapid sinus tachycardia, differentiation from supraventricular tachycardia, *Am J Dis Child* 137:164, 1983.

Meldon S et al: Pediatric ventricular tachycardia: a review with three illustrative cases, *Pediatr Emerg Care* 10:294, 1994.

Robinson B et al: Is that fast heartbeat dangerous (and what should you do about it?) *Contemp Pediatr* 13:52, 1996.

Scarfone R: Cardioversion and defibrillation. In Henretig FM, King C, editors: *Textbook of pediatric emergency procedures,* Baltimore, 1997, Williams and Wilkins.

Zuber T, Pfenninger J: Cardioversion. In Pfenninger J, Fowler G, editors: *Procedures for primary care physicians,* St Louis, 1994, Mosby.

APPENDIX A

Unique Travel Issues for Children

Tamara Thomas

Traveling with children presents parents with many unique demands that require special preparation. Although traveling with healthy children is challenging, traveling with sick children is even more so, particularly if travel includes remote locations or developing countries where sanitation issues arise. Planning, planning, planning is the hallmark for an enjoyable and smoothly running trip. Not all circumstances can be prepared for; however, early travel planning, knowledge of necessary precautions and available medical care, and traveling with a medical kit may be helpful.

Despite the challenges, traveling with children provides opportunities for life-changing experiences, family adventures, and togetherness that are not experienced at home where parents and children are in their work and school routine. International travel affords many educational opportunities and allows the entire family to "stretch their horizons."

Infants and children may be more vulnerable to travel-related illness and injury than adults because of a less mature immune system and different physiologic protective mechanisms. Although children come in various shapes and sizes—from 3-kg infants to 70-kg adolescents—some issues unique to all children that should be considered when traveling to remote or foreign locations.

SIZE

Children are smaller than adults, with a larger surface-to-volume ratio. In addition, infants and younger children have a larger head relative to their body size. These factors predispose children to environmental exposure risks at both extremes of hot and cold.

TEMPERATURE

Thermoregulation is less efficient in children. Children traveling to warm subtropical and tropical climates acclimatize more slowly and are at risk for hyperthermia. Because of their increased surface-to-volume ratio, they gain heat more rapidly than adults, but their cooling mechanisms are less efficient.

Conduction, convection, and radiative heat losses are diminished when the ambient temperature exceeds skin temperature, leaving evaporation (sweating) as the only effective means of heat loss. In addition, travel to tropical climates with high humidity decreases the effectiveness of sweat evaporation as a means to cooling.

Similarly, children's increased surface-to-volume ratio causes children to cool more rapidly. On average, children have less subcutaneous fat to insulate them and a less efficient shivering mechanism. Getting warm requires adaptive behavior responses for which infants and young children must depend on their parents.

HYDRATION

Infants and small children can become dehydrated rapidly in warm, tropical climates. Parents should be advised to encourage children to drink plenty of fluids when traveling in warm climates. Also, parents should be educated on appropriate fluid replacement in ill children. The use of oral rehydration solution should be explained.

TRAVEL CONSIDERATIONS

General Travel

When planning for the trip, take into account the children's ages, location and purpose of trip, and duration of stay. Parents should be prepared for children to have some coping difficulties and restlessness during long trips. An activity pack with small toys, pencils, crayons, cards, games, sticker books, portable tape player with tapes, or small, handheld computer games may help. Open both familiar and new toys at various points of the trip to keep young children entertained. Be prepared to tell stories, play games, or read to the children.

Involve children in planning the trip in order to prepare for travel, arrival, and destination activities. Talk about things you will do after arriving at your destination. A few treats such as pretzel packages, gummy bears, and other nonmessy items will help keep children satisfied.

Remote Travel

Acute mountain sickness (AMS) in preverbal children may manifest itself by fussiness, poor appetite, vomiting, playfulness, and inability to sleep. Incidence of AMS in preverbal children has been reported similar to that of adults.

Foreign Travel

Barriers to foreign travel include food and water sanitation issues. Research food options and water availability, water purification needs, lodging possibilities, and transportation issues. Study the culture you will be visiting and help set the children's expectations for the trip by acquainting them with local customs, teaching them foreign phrases, and showing pictures of where you will be traveling. Prepare them for types of food to expect and sample "foreign dishes" at home before departure.

Air Travel

Bulkhead row seats have more floorspace for infants to play and may provide cots. Having the parent sit on the aisle allows some movement for the child during long flights.

Eustachian tube dysfunction

Ear pain is experienced by approximately 15% of children during altitude and pressurization changes and occurs from pressure difference between the eustachian tube and the atmosphere. Children may relieve ear pain by yawning, chewing gum, or swallowing, and infants may be helped by drinking from a bottle or breast when taking off or landing.

Warm towels to cover a hurting ear may temporize ear pain. The heat warms and expands the air in the middle ear and decreases the negative pressure that retracts the tympanic membrane. Predeparture treatment with pseudoephedrine has been shown to be effective in decreasing earaches in adults; however, a study in young children showed no improvement.

Motion sickness

Children undergoing air or water travel commonly experience motion sickness. Children ages 2 through 12 are more susceptible to motion sickness. Chemoprophylaxis should be considered for children who regularly suffer from it. Most therapeutic agents are muscarinic receptor antagonists or histamine H1-receptor antagonists and tend to make children drowsy. Dimenhydrinate (1 to 1.5 mg/kg/dose) 1 hour before and every 6 hours during nausea-provoking trips is commonly recommended. Caution should be used when administering these medicines to infants and young children.

Sedation of Young Children During Travel

Sedating children during travel is controversial because most sedative agents have side effects. In addition, ethical concerns are raised if the purpose of sedating children is the comfort of the adults traveling with them. Because of these side effects, as well as altitude considerations encountered with air travel, no routine recommendations are made for travel sedation in young children.

Sedatives, such as diphenhydramine (1 mg/kg/dose every 4 hours), have been suggested to help children sleep during extended flights but have no proven efficacy in altering the effects of jet lag or in improving overall travel comfort. Fischer et al. suggests a test dose before the trip to determine whether children

TABLE A-1
Age-specific expectations for wilderness travel

Age	Expectation	Safety issues
0-2 yr	Distance traveled depends on the adults; child carriers used	Provide "safe play area," e.g., tent floor, extra tarp laid out; bells on shoes; ipecac syrup
2-4 yr	Difficult age; stop every 10-15 min; hike ½ to 2 miles on own	Dress in bright colors; teach how to use whistle; ipecac syrup
5-7 yr	Hike 1-3 hr/day; cover 3-4 miles over easy terrain; rest every 30-45 min	Carry whistle: three blows = "I'm lost," 2 blows = "We are coming"; carry own pack with mini first aid kit and water
8-9 yr	Hike a full day with easy pace; cover 6-7 miles over variable terrain; if taller than 4 feet, can use framed pack	As for 5-7 yr, plus: reach map use and route finding; precondition by increasing maximum distances by ≤10%/week; watch for overuse injuries; keep weight of pack ≤20% of body weight
10-12 yr	Hike a full day at moderate pace; cover 8-10 miles over variable terrain	As for 8-9 yr
Teenagers	Hike 8-12 miles at adult pace; may see a decrease in pace or distance with growth spurt	As for 8-9 yr

From Kennedy BC, Gentile DA: *Children in the wilderness,* ed 3, St Louis, 1995, Mosby.

have a paradoxical reaction of excitability. Others believe that parents who are tempted to use sedatives for their traveling children should be discouraged from this practice because antihistamine effects can be unpredictable.

Age-Specific Considerations

Children of varying ages have different travel needs. Distance traveled, pace, and safety issues should be matched to the children's ages and abilities (Table A-1).

PRETRIP PLANNING/PREPARATION

Planning your trip in advance determines whether a trip is a successful, enjoyable vacation or a stressful example of what not to do. Many travel preparation resources are available that can assist in your planning (Box A-1).

Medical Care

Research available medical facilities with English-speaking physicians (if necessary). For those children with underlying illness, research what medical specialists are available in the country you are visiting.

BOX A-1 RESOURCES

Center for Disease Control
 Voice information Service 888/232-3228; Fax 888/232-3299 (24 hours per day)
 Travel health information: http://www.cdc.gov/travel/travel.html
 CDC Yellow book: http://www.cdc.gov/travel/ybint
 Malaria hotline for health care providers: 404/332-4555; Fax 404/332-4565
World Health Organization: http://www.who.ch
U.S. Department of State (travel warnings): http://travel.state.gov/travel_warnings
Travel reference links: http://www.saintafpr.com/travel
International Association for Medical Assistance to Travelers: http://www.sentex.net/~iamat/
Sources of Medical Travel Supplies
 Travel Med, Inc.
 351 Pleasant St. Suite 312
 Northampton, MA 01060
 800/TRAV-MED
 http://www.travmed.com
 Chinook Medical Gear
 2805 Wilderness Place
 Boulder, CO 80301
Additional travel supplies
 Magellan's International Travel Corporation (free 60-page catalogue)
 Essentials for the International Traveler
 Box 5485
 Santa Barbara, CA 93150-5485
 800/962-4943; Fax 805/568-5406
 http://www.magellans.com

Confirm your regular medical insurance coverage before departing. Your medical policy may not cover care received outside the country. Medical coverage and evacuation insurance plans can be easily and economically obtained. When purchasing evacuation insurance, check on any restrictions the policy may have as well as where you will be evacuated.

Location

Research climatic conditions where you will be visiting. Consider the need for raingear, comfortable walking shoes, and lightweight comfortable clothes that can be layered. Safety issues to be considered include health, injury prevention, and local political climate. Educate yourself on local sanitation, common local illnesses, and pertinent safety issues at your destination.

Activities

In addition to plane reservations to your destination country, investigate ground transportation options. Getting from point A to point B can be challenging, and in remote locations your options may be limited. Traveling with a guided tour may help novice travelers with these details.

Travel Documents

U.S. passports

To obtain a U.S. passport for the first time, apply in person at a passport agency or post office. Be prepared to show proof of U.S. citizenship, two identical 2x2-inch photographs, and proof of identity. Adults receive a 10-year passport, which can be renewed by mail. Children younger than 18 years receive a 5-year passport, which must be applied for again.

Stolen infants' passports are marketable in some countries. Make copies of your passport, visa, and trip itinerary and place them in your carry-on bag and each checked bag to facilitate resolving problems. It may also be helpful to leave one copy of documents at home with a friend or family member.

Lost passport—*What to do*

Go to the closest consulate with the following items:

- Police report documenting loss/theft
- Four passport-size photos
- $65 U.S.
- Photocopy of lost passport

Single parents may benefit from carrying custody papers when crossing international borders with children, particularly if their last names are different. Noncustodial parents should carry a notarized parental consent form for their minor children traveling with them.

Visa

Visa requirement information can be located at the Bureau of Consular Affairs Home page at http://travel.state.gov/.

TRAVEL ADVICE

Approximately 1.5 million children travel internationally each year.[1] Generally, children and young adults are more likely to become ill with travel-related illness. In addition, accidents are a common cause of morbidity and mortality for travelers abroad. Hargarten reports that a traveler's chance of dying in a motor vehicle accident while traveling is 4 to 18 times greater than it is in the United States. Although children are exposed to similar travel risks as adults, they are more vulnerable to these environmental hazards, and extra care should be taken for injury prevention. In addition, insufficient information exists on safety and efficacy of travel medications and vaccines for young children's use.

Primary care pediatricians are often called on to provide travel advice (Box A-2). Traveling children's health should focus on prevention of illness and injury. Risks faced by children traveling may be minimized by providing and applying advice about safety, comfort, routine and special immunizations, food/water hygiene, and medications.

BOX A-2 TRAVEL HEALTH PLANNING

Travel Recommendations
- Identify location
    - Weather/seasonal variations
    - Length of trip
    - Purpose
    - Identify safety issues

Health Considerations
- Determine access to and quality of local medical care
- Confirm medical insurance coverage
- Identify medical evacuation issues and need for insurance policy
- Refill regular prescription medications
- Immunization
    - Plan early for vaccination series
        - Update **routine, standard immunizations**
        - Give **routine travel vaccines** (Hepatitis A, typhoid)
        - Evaluate need for **geographic specific immunizations** (Japanese B, Yellow fever, Meningococcus, etc.)
        - Evaluate need for **chemoprophylaxis**
- Medical kit

Safety Issues

Ingestions

Because infants tend to put everything in their mouths, it is advisable to carry syrup of ipecac. Keep all medications, as well as malaria chemoprophylaxis, in childproof bottles because they are toxic when taken in large doses.

Shoes

Covered shoes should be worn to avoid infection with skin-penetrating parasites (Strongyloides stercoralis and hookworm).

Food

Research what types of food are available in the area you are traveling to. "Exotic" or unusual foods may not be welcome by infants, toddlers, or grade-school children. Offer children a similar food at home before traveling to help familiarize them with what they will be eating. Lightweight snacks may be appreciated.

Getting lost

Toddlers are often difficult to keep track of because they are small, fast, and energetic explorers. Dressing them in bright colors may help you see them in a crowd. Teaching 3- or 4-year-olds to use a whistle when they do not see you may be helpful. It has been suggested that older children with a whistle be taught a code to give messages such as two blows for "I am lost."

It is important to discuss with your children the possibility of getting lost and to formulate an emergency plan. Tell the children to stay in one place and wait for help when they realize they are lost. Have the children carry their name, citizenship, passport number, hotel address, and phone number, as well as the embassy phone number, pinned to their clothing.

Hotels have business cards at the desk with addresses and phone numbers in English on one side and in the local language on the other. Have older children carry a hotel card and taxi fare with them at all times, which they may show to a taxi driver if they are separated from parents and need to be returned to the hotel. In congested train stations, markets, or airports abroad, it may be helpful to use a chest harness on toddlers with a tether to an adult.

Avoiding injury

Traveling with infants in remote or underdeveloped countries can be challenging because they require constant attention as their activity increases. Inspect play areas and try to devise safe areas for them to play in. Electrical cords and outlets encountered by infants playing on the floor may not be up to North American standards. If possible, obtain car seats for children.

It is important for parents to have realistic expectations for children's activities. Walking for miles in a foreign country may not be realistic or enjoyable for young children. Estimate the distance they can comfortably walk at home. Schedule frequent breaks with snacks for young children.

Parent Education

Pretravel advice to parents should be practical. Safety issues, wound care, and rehydration principles, as well as any particular health needs of the children, are reasonable starting points. Risks of travel in young infants and children should be discussed with their parents. In addition, immunizations, vaccinations, and prophylactic medications should be discussed, or patients should be referred to a reputable travel clinic. Discuss with parents what reasonable, early interventions to take if their children become ill in a remote location.

Health Recommendations

Many resources are available for the physician offering travel advice to patients. World Wide Web sites from reputable sources can be helpful. Checking more than one source may also be beneficial because authoritative recommendations still contain some element of opinion, and even major sources such as the Centers for Disease Control (CDC) and the World Health Organization (WHO) can disagree on some areas. Reputable Internet resources are also useful because disease patterns change and electronic information updating may be more timely than in written sources.

Travel consultation

The first step in providing travel advice is to obtain a basic medical history as well as pretravel history. Initial travel consultation should take place 6 to 8 weeks before travel in order to plan immunizations. A systematic stepwise approach should include the following:

- Routine travel advice: Pretravel history should include travel itinerary (including stopovers), time of year, purpose and duration of visit, activities planned, and access to and quality of medical care the travelers will experience.
- Routine immunizations: Routine, standard childhood immunizations should be confirmed and updated as necessary. Infants can receive some routine immunizations on an accelerated time course if travel to endemic areas of the diseases is anticipated. (Check American Academy of Pediatric and Centers for Disease Control guidelines for accelerated immunization timetables.)
- Routine travel immunizations: Next, routine travel immunizations, such as typhoid and hepatitis A, should be considered when traveling to most countries, except Canada, Australia, New Zealand, Japan, or Western Europe. Children under 2 years of age cannot receive the hepatitis A vaccine and require immunoglobulin.
- Geographic-specific immunizations/chemoprophylaxis: Geographic area dictates the need for yellow fever, meningococcus, Japanese B encephalitis vaccines, and malaria chemoprophylaxis.
- Unique risks or circumstances: Prolonged stays in a foreign country may affect travel advice. Special circumstances may indicate hepatitis B, rabies, or cholera vaccines.

The CDC Website, Yellow Pages, or voice phone lines are valuable up-to-date resources that assist in immunization planning.

Prophylaxis

Malaria

Malaria is transmitted by the female anopheles mosquito, which feeds primarily between the hours of dusk until dawn. Therefore limiting outside exposures during these hours; wearing clothing that covers head, arms, body, and legs; applying insect repellent; sleeping under a mosquito net; and using permethrin-impregnated mosquito nets all decrease malaria transmission. Other mosquito-borne diseases that are also decreased by protecting children from bites include encephalitis, dengue, leishmaniasis, filariasis, trypansomiasis, and cutaneous myasis.

The most proven insect repellent for skin use is N, N diethyl-meta-toluamide (DEET). Adequate protection is provided with 30% to 35% DEET, and childhood use of DEET is usually limited to less than or equal to 30% to 35% DEET. Other sources recommend lower percentages of DEET in children and state that these less potent mixes are effective but need to be applied more often. "Skeddadle," an insect repellent designed for children, contains 6.5% DEET and a polymer that prevents drug absorption by 70%. High DEET concentrations are reported to cause rashes, and systemic exposure leads to seizures and encephalopathy. Spraying permethrin, an insect repellent and insecticide, on clothes, linens, tents, and mosquito nets offers further insect protection. Permethrin should not be used on skin because of potential toxicity.

Malaria chemoprophylaxis in children is similar to that of adults, except doxycycline use should be avoided in children less than 8 years old. Parents should be advised that no chemoprophylaxis is 100% effective. Check the CDC Website for information about the locations where travel is being planned.

Mefloquine is recommended in most areas of chloroquine-resistant *Plasmodium falciparum,* although several areas have developed mefloquine resistance. Some sources question giving mefloquine to children weighing less than 15 kg. Mefloquine has not been studied extensively in children, but it has been reported as acceptable preventive therapy in infants and children by the CDC with a routine dose of 5 mg/kg weekly and 4.6 mg/kg in children weighing less than 15 kg. There is no liquid form of this drug. Mefloquine is contraindicated in children with a history of seizure disorder, psychiatric disorder, or cardiac conduction abnormalities.

Chloroquine has been shown to be safe and effective in children at a dose of 5 mg/kg/dose weekly; however, because of resistance, chloroquine chemoprophylaxis is inadequate in many areas of the world. The malarial parasite in Central America, Mexico, and a few areas of the Middle East is reported to be chloroquine-sensitive. Chloroquine and mefloquine are available only as bitter-tasting pills in the United States. Both medications are initiated 1 week before arrival, weekly while traveling, and 4 weeks after leaving. Pills can be crushed and mixed with chocolate syrup to mask the bitter taste. At the Duke University Children's Primary Care International Travel Clinic for Children, the Duke pharmacy crushes, weighs, and repackages chloroquine in gelatin capsules according to the patient's weight and dosing guidelines. Parents are then instructed to open the capsules and mix chloroquine with chocolate syrup.

Proguanil (3 mg/kg/ dose daily) purchased abroad has been added for chloroquine-resistant areas because it is unavailable in the United States. Both mefloquine and doxycycline are reported to be more effective alternatives. Doxycycline (1.5 mg/kg daily) can be used in children older than 8 years. Advise those traveling to sunny, tropical areas of the photosensitivity risk.Advise parents that malaria can occur despite taking antimalarials and educate them to recognize signs of malaria (e.g., fever, chills, myalgias, headache) and to seek immediate medical care. Fansidar (sulfadoxine-pyrithmethamine one-half pill per kg body weight) is primarily used for emergency self-treatment of malaria in travelers who are unable to take malaria prophylaxis or who are observing prophylaxis but are unable to obtain medical care within 24 hours. Travelers experiencing signs of presumptive malaria should take Fansidar immediately, continue their weekly prophylaxis drug, and seek medical care as soon as possible. Check current resources for areas of resistance to Fansidar before prescribing.

Diarrhea

Risk for adults to develop travelers' diarrhea (TD) over a 2-week trip has been reported as high as 20% to 50%. TD in children has not been extensively studied; however, Pitzinger et al. reported that most severe diarrheal disease and the highest attack rates occur in the less than 3-year-old age group. Careful eating and clean water is the best way to prevent TD. The adage of "boil it, cook it, peel it, or forget it" is a reasonable starting point but has not been scientifically proven. Because handwashing is more difficult for children in the remote environment, carrying premoistened, individually wrapped antiseptic wipes is helpful. Emphasis should focus on prevention of dehydration.

Consider medications for both prophylaxis and presumptive treatment for TD. Preventive medications include bismuth subsalicylate and antibiotics, but these drugs are not routinely recommended for children. Bismuth subsalicylates have a protective, prophylactic effect in adults; however, caution should be used in children because of the large salicylate exposure and risks of toxicity or Reye's syndrome.

The cornerstone of TD treatment is adequate fluid resuscitation. Oral rehydration should focus on a carbohydrate-to-sodium ratio of approximately 1:1. Oral rehydration solutions can be purchased, or recipes to prepare them are available. Formula and breastfeeding should be continued during rehydration. Presumptive treatment with antibiotics is generally more accepted, and parents can be instructed to start antibiotics after diarrhea has started.

Trimethoprim/sulfamethoxizole is a reasonable presumptive treatment for children; however, resistance is increasing in some areas. If traveling to Mexico or a location where *Campylobacter* is common, add a macrolide (erythromycin or azithromycin) to preventive treatment. Azithromycin has also been shown to be effective against *Shigella*. Furazolidone can be used in children more than 1 month of age and is effective against enteric diarrhea and *Giardia*. Furazolidone is the suggested treatment for pediatric cholera, although some strains in Asia are resistant. Ciprofloxacin, the recommended treatment in adults, should be avoided for children less than 12 years old because of the risk of cartilage abnormalities and arthropathies proven in animal studies; however, a lack of human safety data exists.

Fluoroquinolone use in children is again being addressed in light of fluoroquinolone treatment for resistant pediatric pseudomonas infections. It is hoped that these studies will more effectively address the safety profile. For children traveling in a remote location with a life-threatening diarrheal illness, an isolated fluoroquinolone course may be the best available option.

Antimotility drug use in children is controversial. Some authorities generally do not recommend using antimotility agents in young children. Loperamide hydrochloride may be beneficial in treating diarrhea, but its use has not been extensively studied. Others believe loperamide to be safe for children more than 2 years of age unless they have bloody diarrhea and fever, which may indicate a more invasive organism that may theoretically prolong illness. Loperamide in children younger than 2 years of age was reported to cause drowsiness but showed a decrease in stool volume in the sickest children admitted to a hospital with dehydration requiring intravenous therapy.

TRAVEL MEDICAL KIT

Be practical when planning what to take in your medical kit, and keep things as lightweight as possible (Box A-3). Anticipate needs that are specific to the area where you are traveling.

BOX A-3 PERSONAL TRAVEL MEDICAL KIT

Supplies
- Insect repellent (DEET, permethrin)
- Mosquito net
- Sunscreen/sunglasses
- Female sanitary supplies
- Adhesive bandages, butterfly bandages
- Ace wrap
- Alcohol wipes
- Antibacterial soap
- Antiseptic wipes (premoistened)
- Safety pins
- Water purification device and/or tablets
- Oral rehydration solution packets
- Thermometer tape
- Mole skin
- Flashlight

Medications
- Nonprescription
  - Ipecac
  - Oral rehydration salt packets
  - Topical antibiotic
  - Antifungals
    - Topical
    - Desitin ointment
  - Pepto Bismol tablets
  - Pain/fever
    - Acetominophen (Tylenol)
    - Ibuprofen
  - Topical steroid cream
  - Cold preparations
    - Antihistamines
    - Decongestants
    - Throat lozenges
- Prescription
  - All routine, personal prescription medications should be carried in your carry-on bag. Include some backup prescription medications in a second bag.
  - Antimalarials
  - Antibiotics
    - Oral
  - Gastrointestinal
    - Antinausea
    - Antidiarrhea
  - Motion sickness

Supplies

Rather than trying to procure everything in your medicine cabinet, try to include items that will enhance comfort, protect from the elements, and that might be difficult to obtain at your destination country.

- Insect repellent—DEET, permethrin: Simple protection strategies should be considered as well as repellent. Mosquito nets and proper dress (i.e., long sleeves, long pants) should be used during the right times of the day.

- Sunscreen
- Raincoat
- Mole skin for possible blisters
- Water purification tablets or device (Include powdered drink mix to cover iodine taste and make fluids more palatable to children.)
- Oral rehydration salt solution packets
- Female sanitary supplies
- Adhesive bandages, butterfly bandages
- Alcohol wipes
- Ace wrap
- Antibacterial soap
- Antiseptic wipes (premoistened and individually wrapped are very convenient)
- Safety pins
- Tissues (Tissue sports/travel packs are helpful for respiratory needs as well as for remote restrooms without toilet paper.)
- Syringe (medication administration)
- Rice cereal

Medications

Nonprescription medications for minor injury and illness may enhance travel comfort. Decongestants, analgesics, antidiarrheals, and therapy for insect bites and sunburn may be helpful during travel in remote areas.

Prescription medications in adequate amounts with a reserve should be left in original labeled, childproof bottles with a certifying note from a physician. Similarly, diabetics traveling with syringes and insulin should travel with a physician's note certifying medical necessity for syringes to display at customs.

PHYSICIAN INTERNATIONAL TRAVEL KIT

Physicians have many opportunities for international travel, both short and long term. Often, groups traveling to a remote location want a physician as a group member. As a "traveling" physician, identifying your role assists you in setting appropriate group expectations and helps you bring appropriate equipment. Your role as a physician could be a potentially supportive one for a group, actual practice of medicine for a group, or as a practitioner for the local population. As a pediatrician, you may be asked to evaluate complaints that are less familiar to you, such as chest pain in elderly patients, on the trip.

Once your role is identified, consider what type of support is appropriate. Medical practice in the developing world should be practical and both technologically and culturally appropriate. Understand what medical resources are available. Does the local health care infrastructure support the type of medical care you are planning? Consider distance from and accessibility to existing health care facilities. Think about resuscitation issues. Packing endotracheal tubes for travel to a remote location where no ventilators are available may not be reasonable.

When you consider what supplies to take, define where to start and where to stop (Box A-4). Anticipation of supply needs depends entirely on the quality of information obtained about the travel destination. Resuscitation supplies can include airway equipment, cardiac monitors, IV supplies, and resuscitation drugs, some of which would be impossible to get to a remote location. Talk to other physicians who have served in similar roles. Ask them about the most common medical conditions they saw, what supplies they ran short of, and what they neglected to bring. When you're serving as physician for a tourist group, the most common things you see are the most common things you see at home. Infectious diarrhea and upper respiratory infections account for most travel-related morbidity.

Although shipping supplies ahead of a medical team's arrival may be helpful, remember that shipping and transport to developing countries may be unreliable. Hand-carried supplies have the best chance of arriving at the site when the medical team is there. Have other team members assist in carrying supplies. Be prepared to treat viral illness in fatigued travelers. Use practical solutions when possible. A formal letter from your sponsoring organization explaining the purpose of your expedition, team member names, purpose of medical supplies you are carrying, and names of contact people in the country you are visiting may facilitate getting through customs.

Medical Kit

Be practical and carry lightweight medications that can be used for more than one condition. For example, erythromycin may cover respiratory illness and skin infections. Carry lighter-weight tablets or powder forms rather than liquids, which tend to spill in luggage.

Supplies

A multipurpose tool that includes a knife, tweezers, and scissors is invaluable. Diagnostic tools such as a portable otoscope with AAA batteries and a stethoscope are helpful.

Other

Wound care supplies tend to be in demand in large groups. Marantha-type building project participants often sustain splinters, abrasions, lacerations, and significant sunburns. Evaluate your role as trip physician and local resources before including extensive resuscitation supplies.

Medications

- Analgesics/antipyretics: Acetaminophen as well as a nonsteriodal antiinflammatory (e.g., Ibuprofen) is helpful for injuries, musculoskeletal pain, or viral syndromes. Musculoskeletal injuries are commonly seen when you serve as a physician for international building projects.

BOX A-4 PHYSICIAN MEDICAL KIT

Principles to follow:
- Be practical.
- Keep everything as lightweight as possible.
- Choose medications that you can use for more than one condition.
- Identify the most common medical conditions encountered.

Supplies

- Diagnostic
  - Blood pressure cuff
  - Otoscope/ophthalmoscope
  - Stethoscope
  - Thermometer
  - Tongue depressors
  - Urine dipsticks
  - Glucosticks
  - Urine HCG
  - Peak flow meter
  - Multipurpose tool (Leatherman, Swiss army knife, etc.)
  - Fluoroscein strips
  - Guaiac cards with developer
  - Gloves
  - Flashlight, extra batteries
- Other
  - Syringes
  - Needles
  - Sterile normal saline in 5-ml bottles for mixing IV or oral solutions
  - Method for dispensing medications (such as small sealable bags)
  - ACE wrap
  - Ankle brace, aircast
  - Splints
  - Airway supplies*
    - Endotracheal tubes
    - Laryngoscope
  - Intravenous access*
    - IV catheters
    - Intraosseus
    - IV solution
      - Normal saline
    - IV tubing
  - Wound
    - Normal saline (in canister under pressure for contact lens) works nicely for irrigating wounds
    - Betadine swaps (keep in a sealable bag)
    - Adhesive bandages, butterfly bandages
    - Steristrips
    - Benzoin
    - Dermabond
    - Antiseptic wipes
    - Staples
    - Suture kit
    - Suture, assorted
    - 4 × 4-inch gauze
    - Tape
- Medications
  - Analgesics/antipyretics
    - Acetominophen (tabs, suspension)
    - Ibuprofen (tabs, suspension)
  - Antimicrobials
    - Ophthalmic
      - Natural tears
      - Opthaine/alcaine
      - Antimicrobial drops
    - Otic — Floxin
    - Oral
      - Amoxicillin
      - Augmentin
      - TMP/SMX
      - Atypicals
        - Erythromycin
        - or
        - Azithromycin
    - Parenteral
      - Rocephin (1-gram vials—powdered)
    - Antihelminths
    - Antifungals
      - Diflucan is a one-time treatment, and the tablets are easier to pack than ointment.
  - Allergy
    - Epi-pen†
    - Diphenhydramine
    - Phenergan
  - Dermatology
    - Topical
      - Antimicrobial
        - Polysporin/Neosporin
        - Mupirocin
      - Antifungal
      - Anesthesia
        - Lidocaine 1%†
      - Hydocortisone cream
  - Gastrointestinal
    - Antacids
    - H_2 blockers
    - Antinausea
      - Compazine tabs or suppositories
        - Antimotility
    - Antimotility
      - Loperamide (1 mg/5 ml or 1 mg tabs)
  - OB-GYN
    - Antifungal for yeast vaginitis (Diflucan, a single treatment tablet, is a good choice.)
  - Pulmonary
    - Albuterol inhaler
    - Prednisone
    - Decongestant
    - Antihistamine
  - Tropical
  - Antitoxin

*Include if necessary, after doing a complete needs assessment.
†Caution with extremes of temperature, better to include in carry-on bag.

- Antimicrobials
  - — Ophthalmic: Opthaine and fluoroscein strips are helpful on work sites of building projects where corneal abrasions can be plentiful. Remember to bring antimicrobial drops to keep conjunctivitis from spreading from children to the rest of the trip members.
  - — Oral: Be sure to cover respiratory illness and possible traveler's diarrhea as well as skin infections. Try to bring antibiotics that can be used for more than one purpose. Those traveling to tropical regions should research the types of diseases that may be seen. Antihelminths, antifungals, and antiparasitics should be included, if necessary. These drugs may be purchased more economically in the country to which you are traveling because many developing countries do not require prescriptions. Make sure your information sources are reliable, however, because you do not want to be caught short of necessary medications.
  - — Allergy: An Epi-pen is simple for both medical providers and lay persons to use. Allergy kits including injectable epinephrine and oral diphenhydramine are available. Epinephrine should not be subjected to extremes of temperature and should be placed in your carry-on bag.
  - — Dermatology: Many skin lesions and infections occur in warm and moist tropics. Topical medications should cover bacterial and fungal infections as well as atopic dermatitis.
  - — Gastrointestinal: Antacids should be included for those travelers who have digestion difficulties with new foods. H_2 blockers may also help with this condition. Pepto Bismol, antimotility agents, and antibiotics should be included for presumptive treatment of travelers' diarrhea.
  - — OB-GYN: Include an antifungal for yeast vaginitis, which occurs commonly in the tropics.
  - — Pulmonary: Medications for the routine treatment of asthma (e.g., Albuterol inhalers, tablets, prednisone, vanceril inhaler) should be included in any kit. Basic pulmonary medications for symptomatic treatment of congestion and cough are also often used.
  - — Antitoxin: Check before leaving to see if the area to which you are traveling puts travelers at risk for rabies exposure and if rabies immunoglobulin is available.

SUGGESTED READINGS

Blair DC: A week in the life of a travel clinic, *Clin Microbiol Rev* 10:650, 1997.

Buchanan BJ, Hoagland J, Fischer PR: Pseudoephedrine and air travel associated ear pain in children, *Arch Pediatr Adolesc Med* 153:466, 1999.

Cossar JH et al: A cumulative review of studies on travelers, their experience of illness and implications of these findings, *J Infect* 21:27, 1990.

Dexter W: Hypothermia, *Postgrad Med* 88:55, 1990.

Dick L: Travel medicine: helping patients prepare for trips abroad, *Am Fam Phys* 58:383, 1998.

Ericcson CD, Dupont HL: Travelers' diarrhea: approaches to prevention and treatment, *Clin Infect Dis* 16:616, 1993.

Fischer PR: Travel with infants and children, *Infect Dis Clin North Am* 12:355, 1998.

Foster JA, Watson B, Bell LM: Travel with infants and children, *Emerg Med Clin North Am* 15:71, 1997.

Freedman DO: Keeping current—travel medicine resources available on the internet, *Infect Dis Clin North Am* 12:543, 1998.

Group Diarrhea and Dehydrating Diseases: Loperamide in acute diarrhea in childhood: results of a double-blind placebo controlled multicenter clinical trial, *Br Med J* 298: 1263, 1984.

Hargarten SW: Epidemiology of travel related deaths. In Jong ED, Keystone JJ, McMullen R, editors: *Travel medicine advisor,* Atlanta, 1993, American Health Consultants.

Johnson PC, Dupont HL, Ericsson CD: Chemoprophylaxis and chemotherapy of travelers diarrhea in children, *Pediatr Infec Dis J* 4:620, 1985.

Jong EC, McMullen R: Medical approach to the traveling patient. In Jong EC, McMullen R, editors: *The travel and tropical medicine manual,* Philadelphia, 1995, WB Saunders.

Juckett G: Malaria prevention in travelers, *Am Fam Phys* 59:2523, 1999.

Kennedy BC, Gentile DA: Children in the wilderness. In Auerbach P, editor: *Wilderness medicine,* St Louis, 1995, Mosby.

Knirsch CA: Travel medicine and health issues for families traveling with children. In *Advances in pediatric infectious diseases,* St Louis, 1999, Mosby.

Leggat FA, Speare R, Kedarune U: Traveling with children, *J Travel Med* 5:142, 1998.

Montella KR, Jong EC: Travel advice for pregnant women, infants, and children. In Jong EC , McMullen R, editors: *The travel and tropical medicine manual,* Philadelphia, 1995, WB Saunders.

Motala C et al: Effect of Loperamide stool output and duration of acute infectious diarrhea in infants, *J Pediatr* 117:467, 1990.

Pitzinger B: Incidence and clinical features of travelers diarrhea in infants and children, *Pediatr Infect Dis J* 10:7190, 1991.

Reyes I, Shoff W: General medical advice for travelers, *Emerg Clin North Am* 15:1, 1997.

Rizvon MK, Qazi S, Ward LA: International travel and vaccinations, *West J Med* 170:97, 1999.

Rose SR: *International travel health guide,* ed 7, Northampton, MA, 1996, Travel Medicine.

Thanassi WT, Weiss EL: Immunizations and travel, *Emerg Med Clin North Am* 15:43, 1997.

Wagner JA et al: Heat tolerance and acclimatization to work in heat in relation to age, *J Appli Physiol* 33:616, 1972.

Walter EB, Clements DA: Travel consultation for children in a university-affiliated primary care setting, *Pediatr Infect Dis J* 17:841, 1998.

Yaron M et al: The diagnosis of acute mountain sickness in preverbal children, *Arch Pediatr Adolesc Med* 152:683, 1998.

APPENDIX B

Aftercare Instructions

VENOUS SAMPLING

General Instructions

Blood drawing and intravenous lines (IV)

- The site of the needle puncture may ooze blood for just a few minutes after the needle is removed.
- Often, no bandage at all is required, and the skin can be treated normally.
- If a bandage was placed, please leave it on for 24 hours, then gently remove it.
- It is quite common to have a small bruise for a day or two after blood drawing or IV placement. The bruise will fade away within a week.
- There should be very little pain at the site of the needle stick, though younger children often refer to their hurt for a day or two.
- Some IV sites may have had an "infiltrate," if some of the IV fluid went out of the vein and into the arm or leg. Your doctor or nurse will tell you if this has happened. If your child has an infiltrate, you may apply warm (not hot) compresses to the area a few times each day to allow the fluid to be absorbed. In most cases there are no further problems. If pain, redness, or other skin changes occur, please call your doctor immediately.
- Very young children sometimes experience fears and anxiety after a painful procedure. This is normal, and you can help them through this with calm reassurance; let them know that you know that they are frightened.
- If your child is likely to need frequent blood drawing or IV placement because of his or her condition, ask your doctor to prescribe EMLA, which is an anesthetic cream you can apply at home before coming in for the blood drawing or IV placement. When placed on the skin for more than an hour, EMLA can make the skin almost completely numb, so that the procedure is much less painful. This can help your child avoid being excessively anxious about visiting the doctor's office or the hospital.

URINE SAMPLING

General Instructions

Collecting urine from small children is a very common procedure with very few side effects. Here are a few tips about what to expect following the use of a catheter or the performance of a "bladder tap." Your nurse or doctor will tell you which procedure was performed.

☐ Catheter

A catheter (small, flexible tube) is often used to get urine directly from a child's bladder. This helps us to get urine that is clean and free of outside germs. The catheter was carefully placed into your child's bladder by the doctor or nurse and was removed when the urine sample had been taken out.

- Some children experience an urgent need to urinate for the first few times they urinate after a catheter has been used. If this urgency continues longer than that, please get in touch with your nurse or doctor.
- Occasionally children will complain of some pain or a burning feeling the first few times they urinate after a catheter has been used. Again, if this lasts longer, please get in touch with your doctor or nurse.
- Any visible bleeding after a catheter has been used is not normal, and if you see bleeding or blood in the urine, please get in touch with your nurse or doctor right away.

☐ "Bladder Tap"

A "bladder tap" is used to get urine directly from the bladder in very small infants. In this procedure, a small needle was placed through your baby's skin into the bladder, and urine was withdrawn for testing. Although this might sound very serious, babies do not suffer any bad effects.

- Your baby will have a bandage on his or her belly at the place where the needle was used. This can be removed in 24 hours.
- Babies usually do not have any pain or discomfort after the procedure is finished. If your baby seems too fussy or cries during urination, please let your doctor or nurse know.
- Any visible bleeding after a "bladder tap" is not normal, and if you see bleeding or blood in the urine, please get in touch with your nurse or doctor right away.

LUMBAR PUNCTURE

General Instructions

Your child has had a lumbar puncture ("spinal tap") done to test for infection and for pressure within the brain. While many parents are naturally very frightened by this procedure, it is actually quite safe. Newborn infants and very young babies usually do not have any effects afterwards. Some older children and teenagers may complain about a headache for a few hours after the test is completed. This may be avoided by having the child remain in a lying-down position for a few hours.

Care of the puncture site

Your nurse or doctor will have covered the needle puncture site with a bandage or gauze pad. You should leave this in place for one day, and then remove it. No further dressing or special care is required.

When to call the doctor or nurse back

A small drop of blood is normal at the puncture site. If you see persistent oozing of blood or clear fluid from the area, though, please call your nurse or doctor right away. If your older child or teenager develops a severe headache or vomiting that doesn't stop, please call right away. And if you notice redness, swelling, or tenderness at the needle puncture site, also call immediately.

CEREBROSPINAL SHUNT TAP (VP SHUNT TAP)

General Instructions

Your child's shunt was tapped today to measure the pressure in the shunt system and to take out some fluid for testing. There are very few major complications of this procedure. Children rarely report pain at the site of the needle puncture over the shunt. You should watch your child carefully for any of the following signs, and if any occur, please call your doctor or nurse immediately.

- Redness, swelling, or discharge from the site of the needle puncture
- Fever—if fever develops, please be sure to check with your nurse or doctor before you give any medicines such as Tylenol or ibuprofen
- Fussiness or irritability
- Unusual sleepiness or lethargy
- Vomiting more than once or twice
- Complaint of a severe headache, blurry vision, or difficulty walking

Remember—it is unlikely that the shunt tap would cause any of these events, but any of them might be signs that the original problem is getting worse. If any occur, you call your doctor or nurse right away.

ARTERIAL SAMPLING

General Instructions

Your child has had blood taken from an artery so that your nurse or doctor could do some specialized tests. Taking blood from an artery is not much different from taking blood from a vein, but there are a few important differences.

- Taking blood from an artery hurts a little more, so your child may complain of pain after the blood is taken.
- Arteries may bleed for much longer after the needle is taken out. Your doctor or nurse will have held pressure over the artery for about 5 minutes, and will have put a tight bandage over the site. Do not remove the bandage for 24 hours.
- It is normal to notice some bruising at the site of the needle stick, but if you see swelling or persistent bleeding, please call your nurse or doctor right away.
- If your child complains of pain, numbness, or tingling in the hand or foot where the blood was drawn, or if that area looks extremely pale, call right away.

SEDATION

The medicines your child has received can sometimes cause excessive sleepiness, shallow breathing, confusion, or clumsiness. For the next 24 hours, it is important that you keep an extra close eye on your child at all times.

Discharge Instructions

The ride home

Do not leave your child unattended at any time in a car seat. If the child falls asleep in the car seat, be sure to watch the child continuously to make sure that he or she does not have any problems breathing.

Eating and drinking

In order to reduce the chance of vomiting, we recommend not eating for at least 2 hours following the sedation. Once your child is completely awake and alert and has no nausea, you may begin offering something to drink. Begin with clear fluids and advance to solids as tolerated. If your child is an infant, half a normal feeding may be given 1 hour after discharge as long as he or she is awake and alert.

Sleeping

If your child is sleepy, he or she should not be left alone. Your child should be awakened from sleep every hour for the next 4 hours. If your child's breathing does not appear normal or if you are unable to wake up your child, call 911 or return to the hospital immediately.

Playing

For the next 24 hours, your child should not engage in any play that requires coordination because it may result in injury. This includes activities such as biking, skating, climbing, or playing on a swing set.

Swimming

Your child should not swim or use machines that might potentially result in injury for the next 24 hours without adult supervision.

Bathing

An adult should supervise all playing or bathing for the next 8 hours.

Things to watch and return for

Return immediately to the emergency department for repetitive vomiting, any problems breathing, strange or unusual behavior that does not seem normal for your child, or any other worrisome symptoms.

If you have any questions, please do not hesitate to ask the person giving you these instructions now, or feel free to call us at any time after you leave.

WOUND CARE

General Instructions

- Keep the wound as clean and dry as possible.
- If the wound gets wet, you may pat it with a towel and let it air dry, but avoid rubbing.
- See your doctor in 2 days for a wound check.
- Watch for signs of infection (redness, pus, swelling, warmth, red streaks, fever, increasing severe or persistent pain).
- Apply any of the over-the-counter antibiotic ointments to the wound 3 to 4 times a day (Bacitracin, Polymixin, Neosporin).
- The wound may be covered or left open, depending on activities (the goal being to keep it clean and dry).
- No swimming until the wound is healed and/or the sutures have been removed.

☐ Wounds That Are Sutured or Stapled

- Follow the general instructions listed above.
- Have the sutures removed as directed. In general, sutures on the face should be removed in 3 to 5 days, those on the scalp and body in 7 days, and those that are deeper or on a moving extremity in 7 to 10 days.

☐ Wounds That Have Been Glued

- Follow the general instructions listed above, however DO NOT USE ANY OINTMENTS on the wound—it will dissolve the glue prematurely.
- You may bathe, but pat dry afterward and try to keep the area as dry as possible.
- During the first several hours after the wound is glued do not put any bandage on the wound because it may stick to the glue.
- The glue will gradually break up and fall off over the next 5 to 7 days, depending on thickness of application.

☐ Wounds That Have Been Steri-Stripped

- Follow the general instructions listed above, however DO NOT USE ANY OINTMENT as long as the steri-strips are in place because it will weaken their ability to hold. You may begin using ointment after the steri-strips have fallen off.
- The steri-strips should be left to fall off naturally. This will usually occur in 1 to 3 days.

☐ Wounds That Have Been Packed

- Follow the general instructions listed above, however DO NOT USE ANY OINTMENT.
- In general, the packing should be removed in 1 day, or, if directed by your physician, it may need to be changed and repacked daily at home.

BURN CARE

General Instructions

- Keep the burn as clean and dry as possible.
- If the burn or dressing gets wet, you may pat it with a towel and let it air dry, but avoid rubbing.
- See your doctor in 2 days for a burn check.
- Watch for any signs of infection (redness, pus, swelling, warmth, red streaks, fever, increasing severe or persistent pain).
- No swimming until the burn is healed.
- Sunlight should be avoided for a full year after a burn because it may cause uneven coloration of the skin. Avoid direct sunlight, keep the area covered, and/or use a sunscreen.

Burns Involving the Body

- Silvadene is the most common type of dressing used for burns involving the body.
- Silvadene is applied in a thin layer approximately 1/16 of an inch deep and a sterile gauze dressing is applied over the top. The dressing is changed twice a day.
- When changing the dressing the old layer of silvadene should be removed by gentle washing with mild hand soap. After the old layer is removed, the area is patted dry, and a new layer of silvadene and dressing are applied.
- Dressings are usually continued for approximately 3 to 5 days or as long as the burn appears red.

Burns Involving the Face

- Burns of the face are treated with Bacitracin ointment, NOT Silvadene.
- The face requires reapplication of the ointment at least 4 times a day. The old layer should be gently removed by washing with a mild hand soap, the area should be patted dry, and then a new layer of ointment is applied.
- Dressings are generally not necessary on the face. If there is one particularly deep or open area, it may be covered as needed.

ORTHOPEDIC CARE

General Instructions

- Apply ice for the first 24 hours. Ice should never be placed directly in contact with the skin; there should always be a protective layer between the skin and the bag of ice—for example, a wash cloth or towel to prevent burning the skin.
- Keep elevated above the level of the heart to minimize swelling.
- Watch for signs of increased swelling that may interfere with the blood supply or motor function of the affected limb.
- Check for numbness, tingling, or pain by touching the area above and below the injury. If areas of numbness, tingling, or increasing pain develop, you should notify your doctor.
- Check capillary refill as a measure of circulation. Depress the fingernail or toenail such that the nailbed turns white and then release. It should return to its previous pink color rapidly (in less than 2 seconds). If it does not, you should notify your doctor.

☐ Ace Wraps

- The wrap should not be stretched to the point that one can see through it, and the wrap should be applied from the distal to the proximal part of the extremity.
- The wrap should be tight enough to provide support, but not so tight as to be painful or restrict circulation. As swelling progresses following an injury occasionally the ace wrap will become too tight. In such cases the dressing should be loosened, or removed and then reapplied.

☐ Plaster or Fiberglass Splints and Casts

- Fiberglass dries very rapidly, but plaster casts take 2 days to dry completely.
- Keep the cast supported on a pillow while it is drying to prevent dents from forming.
- Keep the cast dry. Cover it with a plastic bag if there is any chance of it getting wet.
- If itching occurs DO NOT stick anything into the cast or put powder in the cast. Instead, to help relieve itching use a hair dryer set on a cool setting.
- Heat and perspiration can make wearing the cast uncomfortable, therefore avoid exertional activities.
- Do not alter or trim your cast in any way.
- Casts are strong, but damage may occur. Be careful to avoid any additional trauma or damage to the area.
- Follow the general instructions listed above—keep the affected limb elevated and watch for signs of increased swelling that might affect circulation or motor function.

☐ Crutches

- Use the crutches as directed to aid in walking and to avoid pressure on the cast and affected limb.
- Avoid putting pressure on your underarms because it may cause nerve damage. Instead, use your forearms and wrists to support your weight.

EYE CARE

General Instructions

- If an anesthetic drop was used, the eye may become more painful as the medicine wears off. Patients may complain of photophobia (pain with bright lights) and excessive tearing.
- Oral pain medications may be prescribed for short-term relief of painful eye injuries or infections. In general, with appropriate treatment, most of the pain will subside within 24 hours as the underlying problem is treated.
- Topical antibiotics in the form of either drops or ointment (Sulfacetamide drops or ointment, Polytrim drops, Polysporin ointment) may be used to improve healing and reduce the chance of infection.
- Ointments are placed into the eye by pulling down on the lower lid and squeezing a ribbon of ointment onto the inside of the lower eyelid.
- Drops may be placed either directly into the eye, or, in small children, they may be placed indirectly. It is often difficult to hold a small screaming child's eye open to place a drop. Instead, you may place the drop into the inner corner of the eye near the nose while keeping the baby on his or her back. When the baby next opens the eye the antibiotic drop will automatically flow into the eye.
- Patching may be used in cases of trauma or for patient comfort. If a patch is placed, it should be left in place for approximately 24 hours. It should not be left in place for more than 24 hours unless it is rechecked.
- Adolescents that may be driving should be informed that they cannot drive or do other tasks requiring depth perception while one of the eyes is impaired or while a patch is in place.
- Call your physician for increasing severe or persistent pain, discharge from the eye, swelling of the eye, or new visual complaints.

EAR, NOSE, AND THROAT PROCEDURES

Your child has had one of the following procedures performed today. Your nurse or doctor will tell you which procedure was performed. Please be sure to follow the instructions carefully.

☐ Removal of an Object or of Wax from the Ear

- This is a common occurrence in children and is not dangerous.
- Your doctor or nurse used either some running water or a small instrument to pull the object (or the wax) from the ear. Small children are often frightened by this procedure, so you should pay special attention to comforting and reassuring your child.
- Because the skin of the ear canal is delicate, very often a small amount of bleeding follows removal of an object. This is normal, and is not dangerous to the ear or the eardrum.
- If bleeding continues for more than 24 hours, however, please bring your child back to be seen again.
- If you notice a discharge of pus or other material, please call your doctor or nurse.
- If your child complains of dizziness, ear pain, or of hearing a ringing sound in the ear for more than a few minutes, please call the office or come back in.
- Your doctor or nurse may have prescribed some ear drops to reduce inflammation after the object was removed. Please use these drops exactly as prescribed.
- Sometimes the object cannot be removed in the office. If that was the case, your nurse or doctor will refer you to see a specialist, who will remove the object within a few days. It is safe to wait that long. Please carefully follow instructions about that appointment.

☐ Nasal Packing for a Nose Bleed

- Most nose bleeds stop on their own, but your child's was severe enough to require a special packing. This packing is really just like a bandage inside the nose, which applies pressure to stop the bleeding.
- Do not remove the packing yourself, because this could make the bleeding start again.
- Please be sure to keep your follow-up appointment to have the packing removed. If the packing stays in longer, it could become a site of infection.
- If the packing becomes soaked with blood, starts to smell bad, or if your child complains that the packing feels like it has moved, please call or come back in immediately.
- Your nurse or doctor may have prescribed antibiotics to take while the packing is in place. Please be sure you give these to your child just as they are prescribed.

☐ Removal of an Object from the Nose

- This is a common occurrence in children, and is not dangerous.
- There is no special care to give your child after an object has been removed.
- For comfort, you may wish to run a cool mist humidifier in the room for a day or two.

☐ Tongue Lacerations (Cuts)

- Your child has had a laceration (cut) sewn closed in the tongue. This is just a cut like anywhere else on the body, but your child may complain of feeling the stitches for a day or two.
- Give your child a soft, bland diet for several days (mashed potatoes, ice cream, pureed vegetables, milk shakes, etc.)
- Rinse the child's mouth daily with a solution of 2 ounces of hydrogen peroxide and two ounces of water (older, cooperative children only).
- Continued pain, swelling, discharge, or foul odor should not occur. If they do, please call your doctor or nurse right away.

☐ Jaw Dislocation

- Your child had a dislocated jaw (also called a "TMJ dislocation"). There may be some pain and discomfort for a day or two because the muscles and joints may be swollen.
- Have your child be careful to avoid widely opening the mouth for 2 days to avoid having it happen again.
- Use a soft diet for a few days, such as mashed potatoes, noodles, ice cream, and milk shakes (avoid anything that might be hard to chew).
- You may give ibuprofen at the dose prescribed by your doctor or nurse. Please be sure to give it every 8 hours for at least 2 days to reduce the swelling.
- Follow up with a specialist as instructed by your doctor or nurse.
- If pain gets worse or your child has trouble chewing, please call us or return.

DENTAL PROCEDURES

Your child has had one of the following procedures performed. Please follow these instructions carefully, along with any that the dentist gave you.

☐ Replacement of a Tooth

- Teeth that have been knocked out may have a good chance of being restored if they are replaced soon enough, but sometimes they need to be taken out later.
- Your doctor or nurse worked with a dentist to replace and then splint the tooth to give it the best chance possible.
- Follow a soft diet for a few days (mashed potatoes, noodles, ice cream, milk shakes) and avoid foods that are hard to chew.

☐ Repair of a Laceration (Cut) in the Mouth

- Mouth cuts are common in children, and they usually heal very well.
- If your child is old enough to cooperate, have her or him rinse the mouth once a day with a solution of 2 ounces of hydrogen peroxide and 2 ounces of water, to cleanse the mouth.
- If your doctor, nurse, or dentist gave you antibiotics, please be sure to give them to your child exactly as prescribed.
- Some small amount of bleeding from a cut in the mouth is normal for up to 24 hours.
- If your child complains of increasing pain, any discharge or pus is seen, or a fever develops, please call or return right away.

DERMATOLOGY PROCEDURES

General Information

Your child has had one of the following procedures performed. Your doctor or nurse will tell you which procedure was performed. Please read the information carefully, and be sure to follow all instructions. Call your doctor or nurse if you have any questions or concerns.

☐ Punch or Shave Biopsy

- This procedure was done to help identify the cause of your child's sore or other skin condition.
- Clean the wound twice daily with 3% hydrogen peroxide or with soap and water, then apply antibacterial ointment (such as neosporin or triple antibiotic ointment) and cover with a bandage.
- The crust over the site will fall off in 8 to 10 days.
- If a stitch was placed, it should be removed in ________ days.
- No restriction of activity is needed.
- If the wound becomes red, painful, or drains pus, or if your child develops a fever, please call your nurse or doctor.

☐ Cryosurgery

- Your doctor or nurse has performed a minor procedure called "cryosurgery" to remove a skin lesion or sore. It uses extremely cold liquid nitrogen to freeze the skin and the sore area.
- The area may be painful for a day or two following the procedure. Use acetaminophen (Tylenol) or ibuprofen as directed.
- Because some of the surrounding tissue is always damaged, a small scar is likely to occur just at the site of the procedure.
- Some temporary paleness of the skin may occur as well.
- If pain becomes severe or persistent, or if the area becomes extremely red, tender, or hot, please call your doctor or nurse.

☐ Patch Testing

- Your child has had a patch test placed to help know whether he or she has allergies to certain materials.
- The patches are taped to the skin and must remain in place for 48 hours. Keep the patches dry.
- Your doctor or nurse will read the test at 48 and 72 hours following the placement of the patch.
- Your nurse or doctor will interpret the test results. Even if you think there is no reaction, please be sure to keep the follow-up appointment to get a definite reading.

- Very rare reactions to this test include developing blisters at the site of the patch. If this should occur, please call your doctor or nurse right away.

☐ TB Testing (Mantoux Test—PPD)

- Your doctor or nurse has placed a skin test for tuberculosis (TB) on your child's arm. The area should not be painful after the injection is finished.
- In some cases, a second injection, called an "anergy test," is placed on the opposite arm. This may be necessary in interpreting test results.
- Your nurse or doctor will read the test in 48 to 72 hours.
- Even if you think there is no reaction, please be sure to keep your follow-up appointment to get a definite reading.

CARDIOPULMONARY PROCEDURES

General Instructions

Your child has had one or more of the following procedures done today. Your doctor or nurse will tell you which procedure was performed. Please read the information carefully, and be sure to follow all instructions.

☐ Electrocardiography

- Your child has had an electrocardiogram (ECG or EKG) done today. This is a test of the pattern of natural electrical activity in the heart.
- It is important that you understand that our office will have the ECG read later by a pediatric cardiologist (heart specialist), who may have more information to add to what your doctor or nurse told you today. In the meanwhile, your child may engage in normal activities.
- Please be sure to note any further symptoms that your child might have, and call the office if you have any concerns.

☐ Cardioversion

- Your child had an abnormally fast heart beat today, and your physician and nurses corrected it with either a "vagal maneuver" or with a medication called adenosine. In either case, your practitioner now feels that it is safe for your child to return home, but it is important that you follow these instructions carefully.
- There are no long-term side effects from the maneuver or the medication.
- Children who develop fast heart rates once may have it happen again at a later time.
- Observe your child closely for evidence of a problem, such as complaining of a funny feeling in the chest, or of a fast heart rate.
- Your doctor or nurse will teach older children how to perform the "vagal maneuver" themselves.
- Some children become very pale and lethargic. If any of these things happens, you should use "911" to call an ambulance and come to your closest hospital emergency room. Do NOT try to perform a "vagal maneuver" in that case.
- Your doctor may prescribe medication, or may recommend a special kind of surgery to correct the problem within the heart.
- Please be certain to keep all follow-up appointments.

☐ Thoracentesis or Chest Tube

- During your child's stay in the hospital, she or he had a procedure called thoracentesis, or had a chest tube placed. Both procedures are done to drain out blood, pus, air, or fluid from the chest. Now that your child is ready to go home, it is important for you to know what to expect.
- The tube and other instruments have been removed from your child's chest, and a small scar may be left. If a chest tube was placed, there may be one or two

stitches that have to be removed. Your nurse or doctor will tell you if this is the case.

- Your regular doctor should see the child before returning to any athletic activities.
- Pain can be managed with regular doses of acetaminophen (Tylenol).
- Carefully observe your child for any shortness of breath, severe cough, chest pain, being pale or blue, or fever. Come to the emergency department immediately if any of these things occur.

☐ Peak Flow Measurements

Your child has been given a device to measure "peak flow." This is a very useful tool in helping you and your child keep track of how well she or he is doing in managing the asthma. Please use the peak flow meter exactly as instructed. A few reminders:

- Use the peak flow meter twice each day: once as soon as the child is awake in the morning, before any medicine is taken, and again between noon and 2 P.M.
- Write down the number on the chart that your doctor or nurse gave you for this purpose. Without recording the measurements, the peak flow meter is useless.
- Always measure peak flow with the child standing up, and instruct the child to blow as hard as possible.
- You should determine the child's "personal best" peak flow over the course of several weeks when the asthma is not acting up. Measure it twice daily, record the numbers, and use these as the personal best standard.
- If your child's peak flow drops into the yellow range (50 to 80 percent of personal best), give a dose of inhaler or nebulizer medicine (usually Albuterol, Salbutamol, or Ipratropium). If the peak flow is in the red range (less than 50 percent of personal best), then give the medicine and call your doctor or come to the emergency department right away.
- Keep the peak flow meter clean and in a place where it is easy to find, and make it a daily habit to use it—just like brushing teeth!

GASTROINTESTINAL PROCEDURES

General Instructions

Your child has had one of the following procedures done. Your doctor or nurse will tell you which procedure was performed. Please read the information carefully, and be sure to follow all instructions.

☐ Nasogastric (or Orogastric) Tube Placement

- A tube was placed into your child's stomach through the nose (or mouth). This is done to remove material from the stomach, to find out a source of bleeding, or to provide certain kinds of liquids or medications. The tube has now been removed.
- Your child may complain of some pain in the nose, mouth, or throat for a day or two. This is normal, and can be treated with standard doses of acetaminophen (Tylenol) or ibuprofen.
- If your child develops a severe cough or trouble swallowing, please call your doctor or nurse right away.

☐ Gastrostomy Tube Replacement

- Your child's gastrostomy tube (G-tube) was replaced today. This is a simple procedure, and can even be done at home by parents. Normally there are no complications of replacing a G-tube.
- A small amount of blood is normally seen right at the insertion site.
- If your child develops severe abdominal pain, is uncomfortable or cries during the next feeding through the tube, or develops fever, please call your nurse or doctor right away.
- You may be given an extra tube to keep with you, in case the tube accidentally gets removed or damaged. Be sure you understand how to replace the tube yourself (your doctor or nurse will demonstrate how to do it).

☐ Oral Rehydration Therapy (ORT)

- Your child has received fluids by mouth to treat dehydration from diarrhea and/or vomiting. This is a very effective treatment, and helps to avoid painful and unnecessary intravenous fluids. Now that your child is rehydrated, it is time to take her or him home.
- It is important for you to continue to provide ORT at home, along with normal feedings.
- For an infant, continue breast or bottle feeding as you normally do. Offer the infant one extra feeding using an oral rehydration solution between each regular breast or bottle feeding. Oral rehydration solutions such as Pedialyte, Infalyte, Rehydralyte, or the World Health Organization's packets are best.
- DO NOT give your infant or young child full-strength fruit juices, soda pop, or other high-sugar drinks such as Kool-Ade.

- Older children may do better with half-strength fruit juices and a supply of saltine crackers.
- All children should continue their normal healthy diet—do not stop feeding your child during the diarrhea.
- Some vomiting is normal, and children generally can drink more than they vomit, preventing dehydration.
- Remember that diarrhea usually lasts for 3 to 5 days, so don't be discouraged if it isn't all better within the next day or two.
- Call your doctor or return to be seen if your child develops a dry mouth, deeply sunken eyes, very little or very strong urine, or seems unusually sleepy or irritable.

☐ Hernia Reduction

- Your child has a hernia, which was reduced (pushed back in) today by your doctor. It is safe for you to take your child home now, but a follow-up visit with a surgeon will be needed within one week to arrange to have the hernia repaired.
- In the meanwhile, you should expect that the hernia may reappear, especially after your child coughs or strains. If you see the hernia come out again, you can usually push it back in yourself, with steady gentle pressure. You may feel a little "gurgle" as the hernia goes in.
- Reasons to return to the emergency department or to call your doctor are if you cannot push the hernia back in include if the child develops persistent vomiting, fever, or discoloration of the skin over the hernia, or if the child appears to be having abdominal pain.

☐ Rectal Prolapse

- Your child had an episode of rectal prolapse, in which some of the large intestine passes out through the anus. This is a sight that is usually very disturbing to parents, although it is not usually very uncomfortable for the child. Your doctor was able to return the rectum to its normal position.
- Rectal prolapse can happen more than once, however. Some things you can do to reduce the likelihood are to use a stool softener or increase the amount of fiber in your child's diet.
- Your doctor may order some additional tests to try to find out the cause of the prolapse. Be sure to keep any appointments you are given.
- Most children who have a prolapse simply outgrow it by the time they are 3 years old.
- If it happens again, please call your doctor or nurse right away.

GENITOURINARY PROCEDURES

General Instructions

Your child had one of the following procedures done. Your doctor or nurse will tell you which procedure was performed. Please read the information carefully, and be sure to follow all instructions.

☐ Vaginal Foreign Body

- Removal of an object from a child's vagina is usually very uncomfortable for the child. Your child may have been given some sedative medication to help her tolerate the procedure better, and she may need a few hours to recover completely from that medicine.
- After the removal of the object from the vagina, she may complain of pain in the area, especially when urinating. You can give her acetaminophen (Tylenol) or ibuprofen, and you may find that she is more comfortable urinating while sitting in a tub of warm water.
- The discomfort should go away within one or two days. If it does not, or if your child complains of worsening pain, has a vaginal discharge, or an unusual odor, please call your doctor or nurse right away.
- Be sure to give any medications that were prescribed, and to keep any follow-up appointments you were given.

☐ Repair of Vaginal Lacerations

- Your child had an injury to her vagina that required repair using stitches.
- After one day, you can begin having her take a lukewarm water bath once a day.
- If urinating is painful, some children find that they can urinate more comfortably while sitting in a warm bath.
- Either the stitches should be removed in ________ days.

  OR
- The stitches are the kind that will be absorbed and do not need to be removed.
- Any discomfort should go away within one or two days. If it does not, or if your child complains of worsening pain, has a vaginal discharge, or an unusual odor, please call your doctor or nurse right away.
- Be sure to give any medications that were prescribed, and to keep any follow-up appointments you were given.

TOXICOLOGICAL EMERGENCIES

General Instructions

Your child has had one of the following procedures done. Your doctor or nurse will tell you which procedure was performed. Please read the information carefully, and be sure to follow all instructions.

☐ Ocular Decontamination

- Your child has had an eye irrigated (rinsed out) to get rid of a substance that might have been harmful to the eye.
- Following this procedure, many children complain of mild eye pain or irritation.
- Children may have slight redness of the eye for up to a day.
- Your doctor or nurse may have applied eye drops or ointment as part of the treatment. If they prescribed more drops or ointment, be sure to use them as prescribed.
- If the eye becomes more red, swollen, begins to drain any material, or becomes more painful, please call immediately.

☐ Gastric Lavage

- Your child has had gastric lavage (stomach pumping) done to remove dangerous materials from the stomach.
- Many people have a sore throat and some minor pain with swallowing for a day after this procedure.
- Some spitting up of blood is normal for just a few hours.
- If vomiting occurs more than once or twice, or if vomiting blood persists, call your nurse or doctor.

☐ Activated Charcoal

- Your child was given activated charcoal to trap dangerous materials and prevent them from being absorbed into the bloodstream. Charcoal is a safe material, and is often given along with a cathartic (a powerful laxative) to encourage a bowel movement.
- Your child will make black stools for a day or two, and may have gas and diarrhea.
- If the child vomits within an hour or two after being given the charcoal, expect the vomit to be black.
- If your child develops severe abdominal pain or persistent vomiting, please call right away.

☐ Whole-Bowel Irrigation

- Your child was given a liquid to wash out the bowel and help eliminate dangerous materials. This liquid causes very watery bowel movements, which may last up to a day after the treatment was given.
- If severe abdominal pain develops or if the child vomits more than once or twice, please call right away.

Index

Page numbers followed by "t" indicate tables and boxes, *italic* page numbers indicate figures, and page numbers followed by "n" indicate footnote text.

B

C

V

W

X